Health Outcome Measures in Primary and Out-Patient Care

Health Outcome Measures in Primary and Out-Patient Care

edited by

Allen Hutchinson

Department of Public Health Medicine, University of Hull, UK

Elaine McColl

*Centre for Health Services Research,
University of Newcastle upon Tyne, UK*

Margaret Christie

Department of Psychology, University of York, UK

and

Carol Riccalton

*Centre for Health Services Research,
University of Newcastle upon Tyne, UK*

harwood academic publishers

Australia • Canada • China • France • Germany • India • Japan
Luxembourg • Malaysia • The Netherlands • Russia • Singapore • Switzerland
Thailand • United Kingdom

Emmaplein 5
1075 AW Amsterdam
The Netherlands

British Library Cataloguing in Publication Data

Health outcome measures in primary and out-patient care
   1. Medical care   2. Primary care (Medicine)   3. Medical care —
   Evaluation   4. Primary care (Medicine) — Evaluation   5. Outcome
   assessment (Medical care)
   I. Hutchinson, Allen
   362.1

   ISBN 3-7186-5899-2 (Hardcover)
   ISBN 3-7186-5900-X (Softcover)

CONTENTS

Contents

ACKNOWLEDGMENTS

The impetus for this book came from two workshops organised under the auspices of the Applied Psychology Research Group; we extend our thanks to the members of that group and to the participants in the workshops. Thanks also to the funders of the workshops, Glaxo and the medical division of Allen and Hanburys.

The efficient collation of material from a large number of authors, scattered through many countries, was facilitated by Christine Hutchinson, whose secretarial support in producing the chapters was invaluable. Technical assistance was also patiently provided by Barbara Ingman.

Finally our thanks must go to the team at Harwood, who have assisted and supported us on the long path to publication.

LIST OF CONTRIBUTORS

Martin Bardsley
North Thames Regional Health Authority,
London,
United Kingdom

Senga Bond
Centre for Health Services Research,
University of Newcastle upon Tyne,
United Kingdom

John Brazier
Sheffield Centre for Health
and Related Research,
University of Sheffield,
United Kingdom

John Cairns
Health Economics Research Unit,
University of Aberdeen,
United Kingdom

Margaret Christie
Department of Psychology,
University of York,
United Kingdom

Jos A G Dessens
Department of Methodology
and Statistics,
University of Utrecht,
The Netherlands

Martin Eccles
Centre for Health Services Research,
University of Newcastle upon Tyne,
United Kingdom

Duncan Fatz
Central Middlesex and Willesden Chest
Clinic, London,
United Kingdom

Pedro L Ferreira
Faculty of Economics,
University of Coimbra,
Portugal

Penny Fitzharris
Department of Medicine,
Wellington School of Medicine,
New Zealand

Alison Frater
Hertfordshire Health Agency,
Welwyn Garden City,
United Kingdom

Davina French
Department of Psychology,
University of Western Australia,
Australia

Andrew M Garratt
Department of Health Sciences,
University of York,
United Kingdom

Berit Rokne Hanestad
Department of Public Health and Primary
Health Care,
University of Bergen,
Norway

Jenny Hewison
Department of Psychology,
University of Leeds,
United Kingdom

Jan Heyrman
Department of General Practice, Catholic
University of Leuven, Belgium

Katelijne van Hoeck
Department of General Practice,
Catholic University of Leuven,
Belgium

Allen Hutchinson
Department of Public Health Medicine,
University of Hull,
United Kingdom

Max Jacobs
Department of General Practice,
University of Utrecht,
The Netherlands

Duncan Keeley
The Health Centre, Thame,
United Kingdom

Azim Lakhani
United Kingdom Department of Health,
London,
United Kingdom

Elaine McColl
Centre for Health Services Research,
University of Newcastle upon Tyne,
United Kingdom

Keith Meadows
Department of Public Health Medicine,
University of Hull,
United Kingdom

Fiona Moss
North Thames Regional Health Authority
and Central Middlesex Hospital, London,
United Kingdom

Carol Riccalton
Centre for Health Services Research,
University of Newcastle upon Tyne,
United Kingdom

Danny A Ruta
Tayside Health Board,
Dundee,
United Kingdom

Nick Steen
Centre for Health Services Research,
University of Newcastle upon Tyne,
United Kingdom

Fransje Touw-Otten
Department of General Practice,
University of Utrecht,
The Netherlands

Chapter 1 _____

HEALTH OUTCOMES FOR PRIMARY AND OUT-PATIENT CARE: AN EDITORIAL OVERVIEW

ALLEN HUTCHINSON, ELAINE McCOLL, MARGARET CHRISTIE AND CAROL RICCALTON

INTRODUCTION

Assessment of health outcome - the measurement of the impact of health care (or a lack thereof) on the well-being and quality of life of patients, and the utilisation of the information provided by such measurements - is becoming a recognised component of the evaluation and monitoring of care in many developed countries. There are a number of factors contributing to this development. Those who commission or purchase health care, such as national and regional governments, third party payers, managed-care programmes and, in some places, primary care physicians, are increasingly asking for evidence of the effectiveness of health care interventions and packages of care before placing contracts. Clinical audit is receiving increasing prominence as a means of ensuring high quality health care, by identifying and remedying deficiencies in health care provision. To this end, clinicians, who previously tended to rely on measuring the process of care, are also moving towards evaluation of health outcomes. Subjective, patient-oriented health outcomes, as opposed to objective clinical indicators, are being incorporated into assessments of new health technologies, including clinical trials of new drug therapies. Changing demographic structures, in particular increased life expectancy, and the emergence of effective treatments and preventive strategies for many acute conditions, has led to a shift in the work of health care professionals towards the treatment of chronic diseases, such as asthma, diabetes, arthritis, epilepsy and hypertension. For the majority of patients with chronic disease, a total cure is not a realistic option; rather, the aim of health care is to maintain the best possible quality of life or slow the natural deterioration. To this end, monitoring of the patient's progress on an on-going basis is an essential part of the process of care. Self-monitoring is also essential if patients are to be involved in the management of their own care, an avowed aim of many guidelines for the care of patients with chronic disease, such as the St Vincent Declaration on the care and quality of life of patients with diabetes (WHO / IDF, 1990) and the British Thoracic Society guidelines on the management of asthma (British Thoracic Society, 1994). The emphasis on consumer sovereignty also means that increasing attention is being paid to patients' views; patients' organisations and advocacy groups representing people with specific clinical problems are naturally interested in the outcome of health care, since representatives often have personal experience of the impact of clinical problems on day to day life.

Yet, as clinical and health services researchers have begun to address the practice as well as the theory of outcome assessment, it has become clear that there is still a considerable way to go before the evolving methods of assessment can be integrated into routine health care management and clinical practice. Many of the methods are relatively experimental and depend on new technologies which are unfamiliar to most clinicians and to many managers. Methods of measuring health status are increasingly available (e.g. McDowell and Newell, 1987; Bowling, 1991; Wilkin et al., 1992; Bowling, 1994). However, there are substantial scientific and practical differences between health status measurement and health outcome assessment. In particular, the application and utility of the information provided by health status measures and health outcome measures in routine practice is only now becoming clear. There is much to do, therefore, both on a theoretical and on a practical basis, before outcome assessment is likely to become part of everyday care.

Because of this complexity, there is a need to clarify issues at the interface between theory and practice. It is from researchers and practitioners with a perspective on turning outcome assessment into a practical tool for routine clinical practice, decision-making and policy formulation that the contributors of this book have come. The germs of the idea for a collection of papers on the state of the art on outcome assessment were laid at two workshops in late 1991. Both took place under the auspices of the Applied Psychology Research Group, a group with an established track record in facilitating communication across disciplinary and speciality boundaries and in encouraging multidisciplinary research and collaboration. The first workshop, entitled "Health Economics and Health Psychology: Converging Perspectives for Collaborative Research" and funded by an educational grant from Glaxo, focused on measuring benefits from clinical interventions and the barriers to achieving optimal benefits from treatment of care. The second workshop, organised together with the Centre for Health Services Research, University of Newcastle and supported by an educational grant from the

Medical Division of Allen and Hanburys, focused on "Outcome Measurement in Ambulatory Care". It brought together a number of research teams, clinicians and users of outcome measures, to review some of the technical problems of measuring health status and health outcome and the practical issues surrounding the application of such measures in commissioning health care, in clinical trials and in health services research.

At about the same time, other research groups with similar interests were coming together to form the European Research Group on Health Outcomes (called ERGHO in true European fashion). Despite its youth, ERGHO went on to win a substantial research grant from the European Commission, under its BIOMED initiative; this enabled the bringing together of eleven teams, from seven different countries, with a focus on ambulatory care outcomes research to compare and contrast experiences in health outcome assessment across a number of cultures and in a variety of settings.

AIMS OF THIS BOOK

In parallel with the development of the broad range of research programmes outlined above, there have been a number of useful scientific reviews of health status measurement (e.g. McDowell and Newell, 1987; Bowling, 1991; Wilkin *et al.*, 1992; Bowling, 1994; Jenkinson, 1994). Some useful and relevant experience has also been gained from similar work being carried out especially in North America (e.g. Feinstein, 1987; Lohr, 1989; Patrick and Deyo, 1989; Steinwachs, 1989; Tarlov *et al.*, 1989; Greenfield and Nelson, 1992; Davies *et al.*, 1994).

The purpose of this book is to build on this work by demonstrating the wide range of issues to be considered in health outcome assessment, with a particular emphasis on the chronic diseases which have such an impact on the health and well-being of communities and individuals, and which account for an increasing proportion of the resources allocated to health care provision.

There can be few more multidisciplinary approaches in health care than outcome assessment. Health and illness are complex concepts and their measurement, in anything other than the most straightforward biomedical terms, requires a mix of theoretical, scientific and practical approaches. We have therefore brought together authors from a variety of fields to demonstrate the state of the art. They are drawn, for the most part, from participants in the two workshops described above and from ERGHO; the inclusion of contributions from a number of western European countries is intended to show how differences in the organisation and delivery of care can provide contrasts through which a broader understanding of the salient issues may be gained. We have also sought expert input from a nursing perspective on outcome measurement and on the impact of outcome measurement on assessing health needs and planning for and monitoring health services provision at a national level.

The differing perspectives are intended to draw a broad readership from policy makers, researchers, clinicians and patients' representatives. Because many of the topics are in the field of ambulatory health care, clinicians from both hospital and primary care settings should find this book of interest. Indeed, health outcome assessment for patients cared for across the interface between primary and secondary care may be one of the most important quality improvement developments of the next decade. Whether in cancer care, with early detection and palliative care in the community and intensive therapies in hospitals, or in chronic diseases where there is a wide spectrum of severity of illness and treatment is a long-term affair, and the setting may vary over time, the assessment of outcomes of care and of effectiveness and cost-effectiveness will be a priority for health services.

GENERAL THEMES

Although the individual chapter authors come from a variety of disciplines and from different perspectives there are themes which are common to all or many of the chapters. Most obvious is that almost all health services in developed countries are in a state of change, with effectiveness and cost-effectiveness at the top of the agenda for most agencies who pay for health care. Outcome assessment has a proper role to play in these circumstances, but it is important to ensure that the methodologies are sound before decisions are taken on the results, since those subsequent actions may be far-reaching, with serious implications for patient care, if decisions are based on inappropriate information.

Within this changing environment, outcome assessment is of value in a number of contexts. Evaluation of the effectiveness of health technologies, both in the context of health services research and in clinical trials, is clearly an area where the methods are applicable. However, this is a relatively small market compared with the use of outcomes assessment in routine practice. Performance review and clinical audit require methods of assessing the impact of health care in quantitative terms. But here too there is a shift from process measures and biomedical indicators to a more patient-oriented approach. In particular, there is a need for multidimensional measures of health to take account of the broad impact of ill health. This is a recurrent theme throughout the whole book. In particular, the chapters by Jacobs and Dessens, by Steen and McColl, and by Hutchinson and colleagues illustrate some means of taking these factors into account.

Establishing the effectiveness of broader programmes of care, which may be commissioned by regional or national health services, requires different approaches. The contributions by Brazier and Cairns and by Lakhani show how the special perspective of the health economist and population level data can be applied in this regard. Bardsley uses the opportunity of changes in the British National Health Service to show how outcome measurement can be used to commission health care provision that is more closely directed to patient needs.

Contrasts between patient-centred approaches and population methods are also at the forefront of differences in the conceptualisation of health outcome. The conceptualisation of health is notoriously problematic but the direction taken by Garratt and Ruta, with their Patient Generated Index, by Hanestad, and by Heyrman and van Hoeck, demonstrate some of the innovative methods which are being adopted to bring together the conceptualisation of health and the measurement of health outcome.

In a number of the chapters, the scientific aspects of outcome assessment are dealt with in some detail; if measures are to form the basis of clinical decision-making it is important to ensure sound results. The essential attributes of validity, reliability and responsiveness to change are referred to in a number of chapters, both in terms of the underlying theory (Jacobs and Dessens) and the practical implications in the context of developing clinically useful instruments (for instance Steen and McColl, French and Christie, Garratt and Ruta). A different approach to these attributes is necessarily taken in Brazier and Cairns' discussion of the health economists' perspective on health outcome measurement.

Although a number of existing publications deal with the subject of selecting health status and health outcome measures (e.g. McDowell and Newell, 1987; Bowling, 1991; Fitzpatrick et al., 1992; Wilkin et al., 1992; Bowling, 1994), it is important in a book on the practice of outcome assessment to give consideration to methods of choosing appropriate measures. Jacobs and Dessens draw on the considerable experience of clinical researchers in the Netherlands and elsewhere as they outline the methods of measure selection which might be used at the beginning of an outcome assessment project.

It is in the field of application to specific service or clinical situations that this book has particular relevance. Despite becoming increasingly specialised, the nursing professions are numerically by far the greatest of the clinical disciplines and they are often the closest to patients, both in primary and in secondary care settings. Bond analyses the impact of outcome measurement on the nursing professions. In the field of obstetric care, an area which is increasingly viewed as being "over-medicalised", the concept of outcome assessment in pregnancy deserves attention. Pregnancy should be viewed as a natural condition, not a disease. Hence Ferreira's investigation of obstetric outcomes from a well-being perspective, rather than an illness viewpoint, is particularly interesting.

The two chapters which relate specifically to outcomes assessment in asthma provide a different sort of contrast. On the one hand, Moss and her colleagues take a pragmatic view of the process in an adult out-patient population, believing that there is a need to take a stepwise approach to using outcome data in patient monitoring and management, but recognising that multiple outcomes can prove complex to interpret. French and Christie rise to a different challenge in attempting to explore the ability of children to record their response to asthma at different stages in their development. This in turn contrasts with the multiple health problem approach which Heyrman and van Hoeck found necessary in assessing the outcome of care for older people.

A deliberate attempt has been made to bring together perspectives from different cultures to learn from differences in approaches. Close comparison between the experience of researchers and practitioners in different countries and settings is increasingly important, however. To this end, the work of Touw-Otten and Meadows is designed to show both the complexities and the opportunities of cross-cultural comparison, something which will become increasingly common between European countries and within multicultural societies

Our intention is both to demonstrate current progress on outcome assessment and to identify many of the methodological challenges which must be faced in bringing outcome assessment into routine practice. Running through many of the chapters is the recurring theme that the methodology of measurement is increasingly robust and available. It is in dealing with the challenge of assisting clinicians to understand the value and use of outcome assessment, an area in which developments in information technology could and should play a significant role, that the next concerted effort must lie.

REFERENCES

Bowling, A. (1991) *Measuring health: a review of quality of life measurement scales.* Buckingham: Open University Press.

Bowling, A. (1994) *Measuring disease: a review of disease specific quality of life measurement scales.* Buckingham: Open University Press.

British Thoracic Society (1993) Guidelines on the management of asthma. *Thorax*, **48**, S1 -S24.

Davies, A.R., Doyle, M.A., Lansky, D., Rutt, W., Orsolits Stevic, M. and Doyle, J.B. (1994) Outcomes assessment in clinical settings: a consensus statement on principles and best practices in project management. *Joint Commission Journal on Quality Improvement*, **20(1)**, 6-16.

Feinstein, A.R. (1987) *Clinimetrics.* New Haven: Yale University Press.

Fitzpatrick, R., Fletcher, A., Gore, S., Jones, D., Spiegelhalter, D. and Cox, D. (1992) Quality of life measures in health care. I: Applications and issues in assessment. *British Medical Journal*, **305**, 1074-1077.

Greenfield, S. and Nelson, E.C. (1992) Recent developments and future issues in the use of health status measures in clinical settings. *Medical Care*, **30**, MS23-MS41.

Jenkinson, C. (Ed.) (1994) *Measuring health and medical outcomes.* London: UCL Press.

Lohr, K. (1989) Advances in health status assessment. *Medical Care*, **27**, S1-S11.

McDowell, I. and Newell, C. (1987) *Measuring health: a guide to rating scales and questionnaires*. Oxford: Oxford University Press.

Patrick, D.L. and Deyo, R.A. (1989) Generic and disease-specific measures in assessing health status and quality of life. *Medical Care*, **27**, S217-S232.

Steinwachs, D.M. (1989) Application of health status measurement in policy research. *Medical Care*, **27**, S12-S26.

Stewart, A.L., Greenfield, S., Hays, R.D., Wells, K.B., Rogers, W.H., Berry, S.D., McGlynn, E.N. and Ware, J.E. (1989) Functional status and well-being of patients with chronic conditions: results from the Medical Outcomes Study. *Journal of the Americal Medical Association*, **262**, 907-913.

Tarlov, A.R., Ware, J.E, Jr., Greenfield, S., Nelson, E.C., Perrin, E. and Zubkoff, M. (1989) The Medical Outcomes Study: an application of methods for monitoring the results of medical care. *Journal of the American Medical Association*, **262**, 925-930.

Wilkin, D., Hallam, L. and Doggett, M.A. (1992) *Measures of need and outcome for primary health care*. Oxford: Oxford University Press.

World Health Organisation (Europe) and International Diabetes Federation (Europe) (1990) Diabetes care and research in Europe: the St Vincent Declaration. *Diabetic Medicine*, **7**, 360.

Chapter 2 _____

ASSESSING HEALTH OUTCOMES IN CHRONIC DISEASE

ALLEN HUTCHINSON, JENNY HEWISON AND MARTIN ECCLES

INTRODUCTION

As the requirements of policy makers and clinicians have focused on the measurement of health and health outcome as an important means of evaluating quality of care it has become clear that there is a substantial gap between theory and service practice. Experience from clinical audit and from commissioning health care in the United Kingdom (UK) so far suggests that very few measures of outcome are used, other than such crude indicators as mortality rates (Department of Health 1993). This theory-practice gap is partly a product of a lack of available outcome assessment techniques and partly the result of the relative complexity of making use of the results of outcome assessment, especially within the framework of routine clinical practice.

The purpose of this chapter is to review the principal practical issues for consideration in the assessment and implementation of health outcome measurement, in the context of chronic diseases. Such diseases have a significant impact on the lives of people with those illnesses, and on their carers. Although there is relatively sparse experience to draw on from clinical practice in the UK, enough evidence has been accrued from such studies as the Outcome Measures for Ambulatory Care project (McColl *et al.*, 1995) to provide practical guidance in this complex area.

When Davies and her fellow directors of outcome assessment initiatives in the United States (US) recently reviewed best North American practice in the field

(Davies *et al.*, 1994) they identified three main reasons for establishing an outcomes initiative, namely:
1) to describe, in quantitative terms, the impact of care on patients' lives
2) to establish a reliable basis for clinical decision-making by clinicians and patients
3) to evaluate effectiveness of care and to identify opportunities for improvement.

These three objectives fit well with the drive towards evidence-based health care and effective clinical practice which has led to initiatives such as the Cochrane Collaboration and the move by Oxman and colleagues (1993) to establish critical appraisal as a core clinical skill. But the fact that there is the need for such a movement at all suggests that it has been unusual for clinicians to take such a structured approach to the care of the populations of patients whom they serve. Although many British clinicians would probably subscribe to these aims and would consider that they are an implicit part of everyday care, it is actually unusual to address such aims explicitly.

However, there are now a number of initiatives in the UK National Health Service (NHS) which increasingly require a more proactive approach to establishing whether care is appropriate and effective. This movement is led both by the Royal Colleges, who act as the professional standard-setting bodies, and by policy makers who are interested in value for money and effective care for the population. This movement is mirrored in other countries where the clinical guidelines programme of the Dutch College of General Practitioners (Grol, 199?), is a good example of this professionally led approach.

In view of our current position in the UK it is therefore necessary to understand how such a process of outcome assessment might be managed in order to move from policy to practice. Shanks and Frater (1993) have attempted to clarify the concepts which are concerned with a move towards an outcomes-led health service. Their article defines a hierarchy of four key terms in outcome assessment:
1) *outcome* - a result
2) *health outcome* - an effect manifest as a change in health status
3) *health care outcome* - a result which is attributable and responsive to health care
4) *health outcome of health care* - a result evident in terms of health status which is attributable and responsive to health care.

Although there is by no means a consensus regarding these definitions, the Shanks and Frater taxonomy is helpful in exploring the complexity of the terms and concepts and in highlighting the many variables which impinge on the outcome of care for an individual. There may be a great many influences on a person's health, only some of which are related to the care received (or which should have been received) by that individual. For instance, a person may indulge in risk-taking behaviour despite appropriate provision of information regarding that risk. A person may be unemployed, a known health risk factor, and the state of that person's health may be poorer than the average as a result, even if their carer has taken action to treat the medical conditions from which the individual suffers.

Furthermore, there are conditions of unknown aetiology such as multiple sclerosis or Alzheimer's disease, where variation in clinical practice may be appropriate because there is no single agreed course of action. In circumstances such as these, when the links between treatment effect and patient health are more tenuous, it is more difficult to establish health care outcomes. Nevertheless, there are many situations where the assessment of health outcome could prove a valuable asset to clinical practice.

OUTCOME INDICATORS AND OUTCOME MEASURES

There are two principal ways in which outcome assessment can be used. In the first, an outcome *indicator*, a measure of health is used quantitatively to describe the health of a group of people in a particular setting (such as a general practice or an out-patient clinic), at a particular time point. Until recently most clinicians have depended on biomedical measures of health, such as forced expiratory volume in asthma or glycosolated haemoglobin in diabetes, in any attempt to describe the health of groups of patients. More recently it has become clear that the use of standardised health status measures can provide valuable additional information on populations of patients (see for instance, Fitzpatrick *et al.*, 1992), from which more informative contrasts may be made with future data collection exercises on the same population or with past or concurrent measurements on other populations.

In order to provide this information an outcome indicator requires the scientific attributes of validity and reliability but because indicators are essentially undertaking a descriptive task they do not need to be responsive to change over time, although they do need to be sensitive to cross-sectional differences. Steen and McColl deal with these attributes in more detail in Chapter 3. For many health status measures, both generic and condition-specific, there is published evidence of reliability and validity, meaning that such measures can be used as outcome indicators to provide standardised information, allowing improved decision-making by both clinicians and patients. The challenge here is to develop practical means of achieving this in a manner which does not intrude into the lives of patients or the work of clinicians.

Outcome *measures*, on the other hand, will be used over time to attribute observed changes to a particular intervention, in other words to infer causality. They are therefore valuable instruments for all three of the principal uses of outcome assessment (Davies *et al.*, 1994): describing the impact of care; providing information for reliable decision-making; and evaluating the effectiveness of care under defined circumstances. Outcome measures might be used to assess the impact of an intervention through the measurement of health status before and after that intervention. Taking the example of diabetes and asthma again, possible interventions may include a change of treatment from oral hypoglycaemic agents to insulin or the prescription of inhaled steroids for the first time.

In the case of outcome measures the scientific problem is rather greater than for indicators, while the practical problems remain the same. Not only must outcome measures be reliable and valid, but they must be responsive to changes over time. In the care of people with chronic disease some of these changes may be small and occur over quite extensive periods of time. People with osteoarthritis may be severely disabled but the deterioration may occur over years and the effect of a new therapy may be limited, though important. Few condition-specific or generic health status measures have proven evidence of responsiveness to change over time. So, although there is a tendency to see multidimensional health status measures as the principal method of measuring health outcome in chronic disease, it is important to recognise that few health status measures currently meet the scientific criteria and there is a need to begin to explore the development of these valuable clinical tools.

In addition to identifying the aims of an outcome assessment initiative Davies and her colleagues (1994) usefully highlight outcomes management as an important element of the assessment process and one which often seems to be missing in a peer review programme. It is outcomes management which takes the information provided as a result of measuring and monitoring outcomes and applies it to improving the care provided to patients with the aim of making beneficial changes. The process of measuring and monitoring becomes a sterile exercise unless it is accompanied by an approach which turns results into action. Hence a key element of outcomes management is to provide feedback of information to the clinicians who can then translate results into action.

TAKING THE DECISION TO ASSESS OUTCOME

Although the structure of health care services is very different in the US and the UK, it is interesting to note that there are substantial areas of agreement concerning many of the issues raised by Davies (1994) and those which arose during a major programme of outcome measure development and testing recently undertaken in British clinical practice (McColl et al., 1995). Furthermore, experience by the research team in the European Research Group on Health Outcomes, a multi-disciplinary health services research team evaluating ambulatory care outcomes assessment, has demonstrated that experience in North America is replicated in a number of Western European countries. Since much of our current information on assessment comes from experience in North America, it is important to consider other emerging work, and in this chapter we refer to the development of health outcome indicators and measures for asthma and diabetes in order to illustrate the opportunities and the pitfalls of outcome assessment in the ambulatory care field in a European context.

When considering the value of outcome assessment, it is important to acknowledge that outcome measurement is not the only method of evaluating the quality of health care or the impact of specific interventions. Under some conditions process measurement can provide a more useful approach or act as a proxy for outcome measurement. For instance, it is now clear that the prescription of a regular small dose of aspirin to people who have survived a myocardial infarction will, in many circumstances, improve their outcome by decreasing their risk of a subsequent vascular event. Considerable effort would be required to monitor the outcome of such a group of patients on a routine basis; a more effective and appropriate method of monitoring the care being provided for these patients may be to monitor process - for instance the prescription of aspirin.

Unfortunately, relatively few studies have shown anything more than a tentative link between process and outcome, with the result that process or activity monitoring alone is not able to provide the evidence that interventions improve the health of patients. For this reason, the recent shift in emphasis in the health systems of developed countries, from the mere provision of an enormous range of activity towards care which is effective and efficient, requires a critical approach in which the assessment of outcome must play a part. Furthermore there is an increasing recognition that a quality-improvement-led health service must provide both patients and health professionals with more sophisticated information about the health of people using the service, so that users and providers can make more informed judgements about levels and direction of care. Unfortunately it has proved surprisingly difficult to establish an outcomes-led service in practice, although some Health Maintenance Organisations in the US appear to be moving in that direction.

In view of the effort and difficulties involved, the decision to assess outcome is one that should not be made lightly. It should be taken in the knowledge of substantial potential gains for patients and professionals when the correct choice of subject and situation is made.

A PRACTICAL APPROACH TO OUTCOMES ASSESSMENT

The first step in an assessment is to recognise and take into account the main influential factors in any particular setting. Davies and her colleagues (1994) use their experience to list concisely the main factors which must be taken into account in undertaking an outcome assessment initiative. We have prioritised these based on our experience in the UK:
1) potential controversy surrounding the subject
2) objectives to be achieved

3) availability of measurement tools
4) organisational complexity
5) types of patients
6) number of patients
7) logistic complexity.

Many of these factors are easily recognisable to those clinicians involved in any form of performance review such as clinical audit, a subject on which substantial human and financial resources are currently spent in the UK NHS. Perhaps the Davies' team's (1994) most important point is "all outcomes assessment projects are difficult". They advise the prospective candidate to "start with the comparatively easy ones, then move to the harder ones after accruing some experience". This "start simple" approach suggests that an outcomes initiative will be more successful if, as a matter of policy, relatively non-controversial, straightforward subjects are tackled in the first instance.

Although clinicians are used to considerations of failed treatments and mortality as indicators of effectiveness (or its lack) in individual cases, the use of outcome information to manage change in clinical practice is still a novel process and likely to remain so for some time in ambulatory care, where evidence of effectiveness is more difficult to come by than in acute hospital care. Thus careful consideration of the aims and objectives of an outcomes assessment, of the availability of outcome instruments and of the organisational and logistical complexity is crucial to the success of a first attempt.

OUTCOMES ASSESSMENT: CHOOSING THE MEASURES

Practical experience of these concepts has been gained by the Outcome Measures for Ambulatory Care project which was designed and undertaken from 1991 to 1994 at a time when British clinical practice was beginning to espouse the principles of clinical audit (McColl *et al.*, 1995). Its aim was to assist clinicians to examine the impact of their care in a more structured manner, by providing practical tools which could be used in regular clinical practice; if not during the consultation then at a point in time close to it, in order to provide timely information to the clinician.

Experience in medical audit methods and early attempts at outcome measurement (North of England Study of Standards and Performance in General Practice, 1992b) had given the research team some insight into the difficulty of choosing a starting point for a substantial outcome assessment initiative. In particular our experience mirrored that of Davies *et al.* (1994) in highlighting that decisions concerned with choice of clinical topic and availability of suitable outcome measures are the most complex aspect of the project.

Therefore we knew that if a more extensive outcomes initiative were to be established, with the potential for use across the UK NHS, in both primary care and out-patient care, some means of prioritising topics would be required.

We chose to approach this problem by seeking the views of practising clinicians. Over 100 family doctors were asked to consider areas of clinical practice for which they wished to see outcome measures developed (Hutchinson and Fowler, 1992). As Table 2.1 shows, the doctors tended to choose the chronic illnesses which form an important and long-term component of the work of doctors in general practice, office specialist practice and hospital out-patient care.

Table 2.1   Ten most common clinical problems for which outcome measures were desired

---

Conditions are listed in descending order of priority

Asthma
Diabetes
Hypertension
Anxiety or depression
Heart disease
Terminal illness
Back pain
Cervical dysplasia
Smoking
Epilepsy

Number of respondents = 98

Through the use of the Delphi technique (Goodman, 1987), a methodology designed to achieve a structured consensus of opinion among groups of experts, it was also possible to demonstrate that the doctors were interested not only in what might be termed the traditional, biomedical, measures of health outcome but that they also wanted to have information on both functional and psychosocial health status. Respondents tended towards a holistic view of the requirements· for measuring the health of their patients. Moreover, the focus of concern proved to be condition-specific, with different domains of health being given priority according to disease. For example, in the care of people with asthma, respondents were particularly interested in assessing physical function while in diabetes the prime concerns were with complications and in hypertension iatrogenic problems were paramount.

This notion of using a combination of condition-specific domains together with more generic measures of health is one which was supported at the time by Steinwachs (1989) and reinforced more recently by Fitzpatrick and colleagues (Fitzpatrick *et al.*, 1992).

Choosing the right indicators and measures is not a straightforward exercise (Hutchinson *et al.*, 1995). If an outcomes assessment initiative is intended to describe health status at a point in time then it calls for the use of outcome indicators and under these circumstances the depth of information required may be quite limited. For instance, in the developing British initiative on population health outcome indicators for larger populations approaching 500,000 people, outlined by Lakhani in Chapter 9, there may be a requirement for only one or two clinical indicators per individual exhibiting the clinical problem of interest. If the concern is to describe aspects of teenage sexual health in a population, for example, it may only be important to record pregnancy rates in young women, for comparison against similar populations.

An indicator of this type may be derived from epidemiological data (McColl and Gulliford, 1993), or from a structured consensus such as a Delphi technique, or by identifying a key indicator through the further analysis of data used to derive more sensitive measures such as those developed by Steen and colleagues in their construction of symptom-based asthma outcome measures (Steen *et al.*, 1994).

However, when outcome assessment instruments are required to measure quality of care for smaller groups of patients in hospitals or in office-based practice (or even for individuals), then the instruments require a greater level of sensitivity and therefore a greater number of questions (Fitzpatrick *et al.*, 1992).

For small populations an outcome *indicator* may be an already validated health status measure, for which the attributes of validity and reliability have already been established, for which there is no need for the attribute of responsiveness to change to have been established and which has already been used in the population of interest. An example of such an instrument might be the Hospital Anxiety and Depression scale (Zigmond and Snaith, 1983), of proven usefulness in the assessment of psychological morbidity. Additional condition-specific information may then be required to put the results into context, for instance data on respiratory function if outcome is being measured in people with chronic respiratory disease.

A number of authors have reviewed the problem of availability of appropriate instruments (for instance, Wilkin *et al.*, 1992) and up to date information has now become available from institutions such as the NHS Clearing House on Health Outcomes (see address below). But access to appropriate outcome instruments remains one of the limiting factors to the process of assessment.

This problem was addressed in the Outcome Measures for Ambulatory Care study by reviewing a number of health status measures of relevance to the chronic diseases under study (asthma and diabetes), with the object of determining whether they had been used under similar circumstances to our project. Then selected measures were used in field studies to derive the domains for multidimensional health outcome instruments which would, in combination with a symptom measure and clinical indicators, act both as outcome indicators for cross-sectional assessment and as outcome measures for monitoring the effect of care in longitudinal or intervention studies.

The health status measures included in the study were:

Generic measures
Functional Limitations Profile (Patrick and Peach, 1989)
MOS SF-36 (Ware and Sherborne, 1992)
Duke-17 (Parkerson *et al.*, 1991)
Dartmouth COOP Charts (Nelson *et al.*, 1987)
EuroQol (EuroQol Group, 1990)
Hospital Anxiety and Depression scale (Zigmond and Snaith, 1983)

Condition-specific measures
Living with Asthma (Hyland *et al.*, 1991)
Diabetes Health Profile (Meadows *et al.*, 1988)

These were used together with newly derived symptom-based measures for asthma and diabetes (see Steen and McColl, Chapter 3).

More details of the methods of analysis used to derive the final measures are to be found in the publication of McColl *et al.* (1995). The resulting health outcome indicators for asthma and diabetes each have a number of domains and comprise approximately 40 items in total. The domains and their origins of the current (1995) versions of the measures are reproduced in Table 2.2 but, in the interests of brevity, the actual questions and the scaling and scoring systems are omitted. Further details of the scales and the population norms are available from the authors.

Assessment of health outcome may require the use of health outcome measures to evaluate the effect of a specific intervention. It is in the nature of such evaluations that they are very specific to a circumstance, thereby sometimes requiring additional information to that provided by a standard measure. This requirement proved to be the case in the Outcome Measures project when we attempted to investigate the impact of placing patients with asthma on inhaled steroid treatment for the first time. In addition to the outcomes instrument outlined in Table 2.2, specific questions on change in symptoms were required to meet the circumstances of the intervention. It is important to recognise the need to establish the reliability of any such additional questions before use, although pragmatic decisions often have to be taken as to the extent of the need to re-test the whole instrument.

Table 2.2   *Domains of the Outcome Measures for Ambulatory Care Questionnaire*

Asthma

Section A - General Health
(Physical function and energy/vitality from SF-36)

Section B - Emotional Health
(Depression from HAD scale)

Section C - Asthma Symptoms
(from Newcastle asthma symptoms questionnaire)

Section D - Asthma and Lifestyle
(Sports and colds from Living with Asthma)

Non-Insulin-Requiring Diabetes

Section A - General Health
(Physical function and energy/vitality from SF-36)

Section B - Emotional Health
(Depression from HAD scale)

Section C - Diabetes Symptoms
(from Newcastle diabetes symptoms questionnaire)

Insulin-Requiring Diabetes

Section A - General Health
(Physical function and energy/vitality from SF-36)

Section B - Emotional Health
(Depression from HAD scale)

Section C - Diabetes Symptoms
(Lowered mood from Diabetes Health Profile)

TAKING A PRACTICAL APPROACH TO OUTCOME ASSESSMENT

For busy clinicians the current state of the art in outcome assessment presents both an opportunity and a problem. If it were possible to develop indicators and measures of health which were valid in the settings in which patients are seen - out-patient clinics, doctors' offices or in general practice - then clinicians would have a tool to measure the health of patients in the same manner as standardised laboratory tests are available. But, just as with laboratory tests, the testing and analysis process requires to be unobtrusive and not a burden on either the patient or the clinician.

This "rule" is not an immutable requirement, of course. A number of general practitioners are now reporting that they have been using Dartmouth COOP charts as a means of structuring the opening phase of a consultation by asking patients to complete a chart just before the consultation begins, particularly valuing the questions on social functioning and psychosocial health (Nelson *et al.*, 1987). However, under such circumstances the charts are often not being used as outcome assessment tools in the true sense because rarely are the scores calculated and compared with norm referenced values. Instead the patients' response to the charts is used to guide the direction of the consultation.

Experience to date of collecting routine multidimensional outcome data in British clinical practice is severely limited and has almost universally been gained as part of a research project rather than being, for instance, part of clinical audit. One of the principal problems of outcome assessment lies in the area of balancing the value of the information against the cost of providing it. In order to make the best use of the technology it is necessary to expend substantial effort to collect, analyse, interpret and use outcome data, at least in the start-up phase of work. Hence an outcome assessment initiative must take account of issues of utilisation, in addition to the scientific criteria, so that any system designed to collect information is efficient and user-friendly.

In the Outcome Measures in Ambulatory Care study (McColl *et al.*, 1995) criteria relating to the practical issues were recognised as important as the scientific issues and their development proved no less challenging. The project team started from the premise that if health outcome assessment is to become a routine part of clinical practice then the methods must:
1) depend on relatively cheap and simple methods of data capture
2) not be intrusive into patient care
3) provide clear feedback of analysed data in a timely manner
4) have appropriate scientific attributes.

These criteria are generally applicable to practical outcome assessment and must be taken into account in any outcome initiative. In fact, it is actually the acceptance of these principles which are sometimes the most difficult to achieve. It is very easy to become diverted from a practical approach into a process which becomes all consuming. Once the principles have been embraced by the project team then unobtrusive collection of data, and its analysis and feedback, can be managed through the use of patient-completed questionnaires on health, the use of personal computers to capture and analyse data, and new techniques enabling the implementation of clinical change.

Evidence from the North of England Study of Standards and Performance in General Practice suggested to the Ambulatory Care study team that outcome data could be collected by questionnaires posted to patients with an expected response rate in excess of 80% after one reminder (North of England Study, 1992b). Even the use of structured data collection from, and onto, paper records used by the

North of England study in the 1980s provided a database from which it was possible to demonstrate a change in intermediate health outcome for children (North of England Study, 1992a). The rapid changes in information technology should make it possible to capture data from medical records as part of outcome data sets in an efficient manner.

The above findings were replicated in the Outcomes Measures project where response rates of over 80% were achieved when questionnaires were handed to patients by their doctors and response rates were over 70% when questionnaires were posted to patients. It seems, therefore, that these methods of data collection are acceptable to patients and doctors alike. The next step that is needed in terms of newer approaches is to develop a form of feedback to clinicians by which they can easily compare individuals or groups of individuals with a reference database.

Although clinicians are used to having standardised results available when consulting patients they as yet have little experience of using outcome data. It is unreasonable to expect that outcome indicator data can be collected during a consultation or analysed during the relatively short period of time a patient is consulting, even if indicator data could be refined enough to be used on an individual patient basis. Two mechanisms are needed to support the outcome assessment. First, there is a need for a system for analysing the outcome data so that clinicians are not involved with the process unless they desire it. Second, a system of clear feedback of results which provides clinicians with an unobtrusive means of access to comparative data in respect of their patients and similar patient groups elsewhere is required. This process is now being refined in the Outcome Measures project in both general practice and hospital out-patient clinics and will provide norm referenced information in graphical format.

OUTCOMES MANAGEMENT: THE CHALLENGE

When the Outcome Measures for Ambulatory Care project was completed in 1994 it was clear to the research team that what had appeared to be the great challenge - developing sound indicators and measures - was in fact only the first step in a substantial programme of work. Discussions with clinicians both in the UK and, through the European Research Group on Health Outcomes, across Western Europe, now suggest that the outcomes management element of assessment is most important. Essentially, clinicians need to be convinced that there is a value to them and their patients and that the benefits outweigh the costs. We have addressed these issues by developing an analysis package which local groups of clinicians can use to derive their own feedback.

With the completion of the development phase of the project, the next stage is to implement a programme of field testing in order to gain experience of outcome assessment in everyday clinical practice. In particular, it is important to know what clinicians will do with the information when they have it. How will they use it to improve patient care? This stage of the work has now begun with data being collected on over 8000 patients with asthma or diabetes, providing a substantial database which will allow an analysis of the value of outcome assessment in British clinical practice.

Further Information

Information on health outcome measurement may be obtained from the NHS Clearing House on Health Outcomes, The Nuffield Institute for Health, 71-75 Clarendon Road, Leeds LS2 9PL.

REFERENCES

Davies, A.R., Doyle, M.A., Lansky, D., Rutt, W., Orsolits Stevic, M. and Doyle, J.B. (1994) Outcomes assessment in clinical settings: a consensus statement on principles and best practices in project management. *Joint Commission Journal on Quality Improvement*, **20(1)**, 6-16.

Department of Health (1993) *Population health outcome indicators for the NHS 1993: England. A consultation document.* Brighton: Institute of Public Health, University of Surrey.

EuroQol Group (1990) EuroQol: a new facility for the measurement of health related quality of life. *Health Policy*, **16**, 199-208.

Fitzpatrick, R., Fletcher, A., Gore, S., Jones, D., Spiegelhalter, D. and Cox, D. (1992) Quality of life measures in health care. I: Applications and issues in assessment. *British Medical Journal*, **305**, 1074-1077.

Goodman, C.M. (1987) The Delphi technique: a critique. *Journal of Advanced Nursing*, **12(6)**, 729-734.

Grol, R. (1992) Implementing guidelines in general practice care. *Quality in Health Care*, **1**, 184-191.

Hutchinson, A. and Fowler, P. (1992) Outcome measures for primary health care: what are the research priorities? *British Journal of General Practice*, **42**, 227-231.

Hutchinson, A., McColl, E., Meadows, K.A., Riccalton, C. and Fowler, P. (1995) *A health status measures guide for asthma and diabetes.* Hull: University of Hull.

Hyland, M.E., Finnis, S. and Irvine, S.H. (1991) A scale for assessing quality of life in adult asthma sufferers. *Journal of Psychosomatic Research*, **35**, 99-110.

McColl, E., Steen, I.N., Meadows, K.A., Hutchinson, A., Eccles, M.P., Hewison, J., Fowler, P. and Blades, S.M. (1995) Developing outcome measures for ambulatory care: an application to asthma and diabetes. *Social Science and Medicine* (in press).

Meadows, K.A., Brown, K., Hones, H., Thompson, C. and Wise, P.H. (1988). An instrument for screening psychosocial problems in IDDM patients: initial findings. *Diabetes Research in Clinical Practice*, **5 Supplement 1**.

Nelson, E., Wasson, J., Kirk, J., Keller, A., Clark, D., Dietrich, A., Stewart, A. and Zubkoff, M. (1987). Assessment of function in routine clinical practice: description of the COOP Chart method and preliminary findings. *Journal of Chronic Diseases*, **40**, 55S-69S.

North of England Study of Standards and Performance in General Practice (1992b) Medical audit in general practice. II: Effects on health of patients with common childhood conditions. *British Medical Journal*, **304**, 1484-1488.

North of England Study of Standards and Performance in General Practice (1992a) Medical audit in general practice. I: Effects on doctors' clinical behaviour for common childhood conditions. *British Medical Journal*, **304**, 1480-1484.

Oxman, A.D., Sackett, D.L. and Guyatt, G.H. (1993) Users' guide to the medical literature. I: How to get started. *Journal of the American Medical Association*, **270**, 2093-2095.

Parkerson, G.R., Broadhead, W.E. and Tse, C.K. (1991) Development of the 17-item Duke Health Profile. *Family Practice*, **8**, 396-401.

Patrick, D.L. and Peach, H. (1989) *Disablement in the community*. Oxford: Oxford Univerity Press.

Shanks, J. and Frater, A. (1993) Health status, outcome and attributability: is a red rose red in the dark? *Quality in Health Care*, **2**, 259-262.

Steen, N., Hutchinson, A., McColl, E., Eccles, M.P., Hewison, J., Meadows, K.A., Blades, S.M. and Fowler, P. (1994) Development of a symptom based outcome measure for asthma. *British Medical Journal*, **309**, 1065-1068.

Steinwachs, D.M. (1989) Application of health status measurement in policy research. *Medical Care*, **27**, S12-S26.

Ware, J.E., and Sherbourne C.D. (1992). The MOS 36-item Short-Form Health Survey (SF-36). I: Conceptual framework and item selection. *Medical Care*, **30**, 473-483.

Wilkin, D., Hallam, L. and Doggett, A-M. (1992). *Measures of need and outcome for primary health care*. Oxford: Oxford Medical Publications.

Zigmond, A.S. and Snaith R.P. (1983). The Hospital Anxiety and Depression scale. *Acta Psychiatrica Scandinavica*, **67**, 361-370.

Chapter 3

DEVELOPING AND TESTING SYMPTOM-BASED OUTCOME MEASURES

NICK STEEN AND ELAINE McCOLL

INTRODUCTION

Methods for developing and testing health status measures have been recorded in some detail elsewhere (see for example McDowell and Newell, 1987; Streiner and Norman, 1989). The desirable measurement properties of such measures depend upon the context in which they are to be used. Adequate validity and reliability are properties required in all contexts; the importance of other properties will depend upon the purpose of the instrument. If outcome measures are to be used to demonstrate the impact of the process of health care on patient well-being, responsiveness to change will be an essential property. In this chapter we illustrate how psychometric principles underpinned the development of symptom-based outcome measures.

The development of our symptom-based outcome measures formed part of a major research project aimed at the development of condition-specific outcome measures that could be used in an evaluation of the management of the care of asthma and diabetes within primary care and out-patient departments. Symptom-based outcome measures were included to complement functional and psychosocial outcome measures (collected from the patient) and biomedical indicators of outcome (collected from the clinicians). The development process involved collecting data from 604 patients with asthma and 715 patients with diabetes, of whom 235 (33%) were being treated with insulin. All patients were aged 18 or over: the measures have not been designed for use with children suffering from either of the diseases.

THE NEED FOR SYMPTOM-BASED OUTCOME MEASURES

For some diseases such as asthma, control of symptoms is an important clinical management objective. For other conditions, control of symptoms may not be a direct objective of care but symptom frequency and severity may be affected by treatment aimed at meeting other objectives. In the care of patients with diabetes, an improvement in the level of diabetic control is often a primary objective. For some patients with diabetes, blurred vision may be an indication of rapidly changing blood glucose levels. Improved diabetic control might result in a less frequent occurrence of this symptom with a corresponding change in quality of life for the patient.

CRITICAL REVIEW

As is the case with selecting and developing any outcome measure, a review of the literature to locate previously developed measures is essential in order to avoid possible duplication of effort. In our case, we were able to identify previous work on the measurement of symptoms of diabetes by Freund *et al.* (1986) and Given (1984). Previous work on the measurement of asthma symptoms included that done by Kinsman *et al.* (1973), Usherwood *et al.* (1990) and Juniper *et al.* (1992).

The next stage is a critical review of any potential measures that have been identified. Is there any information relating to their reliability and validity? On what populations have the measures been used? Measures that have been developed for quite different purposes or those that have not been tested in the populations of interest may not be suitable for use without further testing and refinement.

The two asthma symptoms questionnaires developed by Kinsman *et al.* and Usherwood *et al.* had many symptoms in common, the Kinsman questionnaire being the more extensive. The purposes of the two questionnaires were slightly different - the Kinsman measure asked about the intensity of symptoms during an asthma attack while Usherwood's instrument asked about the frequency of symptoms over a specific period of time. The former was designed for use with adults, the latter was designed to collect data from parents of children suffering from asthma. Both questionnaires had good internal reliability and evidence was also given in support of their validity. However neither questionnaire fully met our needs. In addition to questions relating to clinical symptoms both included questions relating to functional health status; for instance the Usherwood questionnaire asked about the extent to which asthma limited the child's life and general psychosocial health status was also covered (as in the Kinsman questionnaire which included the item "I am worried about myself"). These aspects of health status were already being measured by other instruments selected for use in our study. Our requirement was for a questionnaire that measured clinical symptoms only. Nevertheless, the two instruments provided a useful source of potential clinical symptoms which could be considered for inclusion in a new questionnaire.

Similarly neither of the diabetes symptoms questionnaires referenced above could be directly adopted for our purposes but each provided a useful checklist of symptoms.

SELECTION OF SYMPTOMS FOR A NEW QUESTIONNAIRE

Two of the most fruitful sources of symptoms are expert clinical opinion and the patients themselves. The project team adopted both approaches. Symptoms included in the two diabetes questionnaires reviewed above had been derived only from clinicians. It was felt that, in the interest of completeness and face validity, it would be appropriate to obtain the views of patients. A number of patients with diabetes were brought together to form a focus group. Using an unstructured format, they were asked to describe any symptoms which they felt were attributable to their disease. A potential pitfall here is that it may not be possible for a patient with a chronic disease to tell whether a symptom is due to that disease or due to some other cause. For example, some patients attributed their headaches to their diabetes but a number of clinicians expressed doubt as to whether the cause was actually the patient's diabetes. This problem of attributability is exacerbated in patients with a number of concurrent diseases. Despite these problems, a number of new symptoms were identified by patients and added to the pool of items obtained from the literature review.

For both conditions, a team of consultant physicians and general practitioners was asked to review the pool of items for completeness (to determine if any symptoms were missing) and appropriateness. That is, they were asked to ensure the *content validity* of the new questionnaire. For asthma, a number of symptoms (e.g. itchy skin) were dropped as they were felt to be too vague and open to misinterpretation. An extra question relating to nocturnal symptoms was included at this stage, since clinicians felt this to be a key feature of asthma. The task proved to be much more problematic for diabetes. There was much debate about which symptoms were specific to diabetes, which symptoms arose as a result of diabetic complications and which symptoms were non-specific. The final pool of symptoms for each condition is shown in Box 3.1.

If an outcome measure questionnaire is to be acceptable to respondents, simplicity is of paramount importance. Symptoms need to be expressed in a form that can be easily understood by the lay reader. Clinical terms such as nocturia are obviously not appropriate. Moreover, some of the symptoms obtained from the literature were expressed in American English and needed to be Anglicised. Patient focus groups and individual interviews provided an appropriate mechanism for piloting different forms of wording to determine what was unambiguous and easily understood by most patients. For example, the term that most patients preferred to describe perineal/genital itching was "itchy down below".

Box 3.1   Symptoms selected for inclusion in the first draft of the Newcastle symptoms questionnaires

Diabetes	Asthma
Headache	Breathless during exercise
Nocturia	Breathless during day when not exercising
Thirst	Wheezing during day
Blurred vision	Coughing during day
Polyuria during the day	Wheezing at night
Palpitations	Breathless at night
Perineal/genital itching	Coughing at night
Nausea	Disturbed sleep
Dizziness	Fear because of asthma
Vomiting	Feeling of tightness in chest
Exhaustion	
Hunger	
Feeling shaky	
Cold hands and feet	
Feeling sleepy	
Pain in limbs	
Pins and needles	
Feeling faint	
Hypoglycaemia	
Abnormal sweating	

CONSTRUCTION OF ITEMS

To a large extent, the precise wording of items depends upon the constructs that the questionnaire is intended to measure. In the case of a symptom questionnaire possible constructs might be "effect of symptoms on social function", "distress caused by the occurrence of symptoms" and "frequency with which symptoms occur". The most appropriate constructs in an outcome measure for a particular condition will depend upon the objectives of care for that condition. For example, in the management of asthma two clinical objectives might be to reduce the frequency with which asthma attacks occur and to minimise the severity of symptoms experienced during those attacks. A comprehensive evaluative tool should therefore measure both.

For our purposes, we set out to measure symptom frequency and symptom severity for both asthma and diabetes. Each construct presented its own problems. For symptom frequency the most problematic issue was that of choosing the time period to which the questions should refer. The main problem in obtaining data on symptom severity from the patient was the essentially subjective nature of the construct.

Symptom Frequency

A number of factors must be taken into account when deciding on the choice of time period. Recall over a short period of time in the recent past is likely to be more accurate than recall over a protracted period. Thus a questionnaire that asks about symptoms experienced in the previous week is likely to be more *reliable* than one that asks a patient about symptoms experienced during the preceeding three months. A second consideration is the prevalence of symptoms in the target population. If the prevalence of a particular symptom is low, very few patients may endorse a question relating to its occurrence if the recall period is too restricted, for example confined to the previous day. Low item endorsement may reduce the utility of the measure for purposes of detecting change in health status between individuals (Streiner and Norman, 1989). A further factor which has a direct bearing on this issue is that of the size of the population on which the questionnaire is intended to be used. Low item endorsement may be less of a problem if one is using the measure on very large samples to compare two populations, than if one is using the measure to evaluate care of a small population within a single general practice over a period of time.

If information relating to a protracted time period is required, an alternative approach is that of obtaining repeated observations from a patient where each relates to a relatively short period of time. This might take the form of a daily diary for example. However this approach is not without problems. Hyland *et al.* (1993) report that patients' enthusiasm for completing diary cards diminishes over time. This method may not, therefore, be as reliable as one might expect.

In our study, we aimed to strike a balance between a time-frame which was overlong, perhaps leading to recall bias, and too short a period, which might lead to low item endorsement. In coming to the decision about the optimum time period, we drew upon both the panels of clinicians and the patient focus groups. Patients could remember the occurrence of unusual adverse events (such as an emergency admission to hospital) over a long period of time but when asked about "routine" symptoms, one month seemed to be the longest period of time over which they could provide reliable data. For example, when questioned about how they worked out their responses to pilot questions relating to a three-month period, many patients reported that they estimated the frequency of symptoms in a single month and then extrapolated to three months to obtain their final answer. The clinicians felt that a one-month period was acceptable and was in line with previous work on measuring symptom level in chronic diseases.

Symptom Severity

The main problem in assessing symptom severity was that of finding suitable expressions that were acceptable to patients and clinicians. A number of clinicians felt that it would not be appropriate to ask patients to rate different symptoms (such as headache and occurrence of hypoglycaemic attacks) on a scale ranging from not severe to very severe. Clinical psychologists suggested that it was more important to try and determine the impact of the symptoms on the patients. It was felt that some patients with asthma, for example, might find a severe incidence of wheeze during the day slightly less of a problem than a slightly less severe attack during the night. Various forms of wording were considered. "How much distress does the symptom cause?" was rejected because the word distress was felt to be too emotive. "How much trouble does the symptom cause?" was also rejected. The final choice was, "How much bother does the symptom cause?".

Please circle the number that best describes how you have been in the last month

*In the **last month**, on how many **days** have you wheezed **during the day**?*

never	on one or a few days	on several days	on most days	every day
0	1	2	3	4

How much bother did the wheezing cause?

does not apply to me	no bother at all	not much bother	much bother	very much bother
8	0	1	2	3

Figure 3.1   Final format of questions included in the first draft of the Newcastle symptoms questionnaires

SCALING RESPONSES

Although each question measuring symptom frequency was of the form "On how many days in the last month have you experienced ....?", it was felt unreasonable to expect the patient to recall the exact number of days. Again we drew on the experience of other researchers (from our literature review), our panels of clinicians and the groups of patients. Figure 3.1 shows the final format of the questions. An ordered five-point scale ranging from "never" to "every day" was acceptable to both clinicians and patients. Bother was measured on a four-point scale ranging from "no bother at all" to "very much bother". We provided a "does not apply to me" category for those patients who had not experienced that particular symptom during the previous month.

TESTING THE QUESTIONNAIRES

Piloting

The development of a self-completion questionnaire is an iterative process of testing and modification. The first thing to test for is *interpretability*. The questions must be phrased in a way that can be easily understood and requires only low levels of reading ability. The wording must also be unambiguous. This testing is best done by administering the questionnaire to individual patients in the presence of a researcher. The researcher may observe problems as the questionnaire is being completed. Either at the end of each question or at the end of the questionnaire the patient should be asked to explain what they understood by each of the items and encouraged to describe any difficulties that they had experienced.

Item Endorsement

After the questionnaire has been tested for readability and absence of ambiguity, it should be given to a large group of subjects to test for other attributes including endorsement frequency. Items where the vast majority of patients endorse only one of the categories are usually rejected. Streiner and Norman (1989) suggest that if more than 95% of patients endorse a single response category, we can learn very little by knowing how a patient responded to that question (since we can predict what their response will be with 95% accuracy) and we should consider omitting that item. There would be grounds for retaining such a symptom, however, if it is known that its presence (or absence) would have a markedly greater impact on a patient's quality of life than the presence (or absence) of the remaining symptoms in the questionnaire.

Streiner and Norman suggest that 50 subjects should be regarded as an absolute minimum sample size for examining item endorsement. With a sample size of 50, there is a 12% chance of at least 95% of the sample endorsing a category even if only 90% of the population actually exhibit that trait. With a sample size of 100 (and the same population endorsement of 90%), the probability of at least 95% of the sample endorsing the category reduces to less than five percent.

Of the symptoms included in the asthma and diabetes symptoms questionnaires, there was only one symptom which required careful consideration based on the criterion of endorsement. Only three percent (95% confidence interval: 1.6%, 4.8%) of patients with non-insulin-treated diabetes recorded experiencing a hypoglycaemic attack during the three months preceding the administration of the questionnaire. This was probably because the question was only relevant to a small group of those patients on oral hypoglycaemic drugs. Many of the remaining patients reported that they did not understand the question. Thus there was a high risk of patients responding incorrectly. It was therefore decided to omit the question despite the potentially high impact hypoglycaemia is likely to have on the small group of patients for whom the question is relevant.

Discrimination

If the measure is intended for use in evaluating the care of a particular disease group, it is appropriate to include only those symptoms which result from having that disease. One would not expect a change in the management of asthma, for example, to affect symptoms that are not associated with that condition. Therefore, the questionnaire should be able to discriminate between patients with the disease and patients who do not have the disease. As described earlier, there was some doubt expressed by clinicians as to whether or not certain symptoms were attributable to the patient's diabetes. We therefore decided to administer the diabetes symptom questionnaire to a matched sample of diabetes controls (patients without diabetes but similar in age and gender to the diabetic patients). Although clinicians and patients were in very close agreement in their assessment of which symptoms resulted from having asthma, we also gave the asthma questionnaire to a group of controls. As a result of these comparisons, we were able to confirm that all symptoms on the asthma questionnaire discriminated between asthmatics and controls and we were able to eliminate approximately half of the diabetes symptoms.

Homogeneity of the Items

When constructing a measure it is desirable that all the items measure the same trait (in this case, the level of symptoms experienced by a patient due to their asthma or diabetes). One way of measuring the overall impact of symptoms is to scan the responses to the individual items to obtain a simple index. Such an index would not be easy to interpret if the constituent items measured different traits. Cronbach's alpha is a widely used measure of internal consistency (Cronbach, 1951). Low values of alpha indicate poor internal consistency; the items do not all measure the same trait. If alpha is very high there may be some redundancy in the items. In other words, the variables correlate so highly that we could probably obtain most of the information by asking only a subset of questions. There is no hard and fast rule as to what constitutes an optimum value of alpha but somewhere in the range 0.70 to 0.85 would seem reasonable. However, in some cases, for example when the main purpose of the instrument is to discriminate between two populations, internal consistency is not such a critical criterion and lower values of alpha are acceptable. The internal consistency of the ten item asthma symptoms questionnaire and the reduced (nine item) diabetes symptoms questionnaire were respectively 0.93 and 0.78. The very high coefficient for the asthma symptoms questionnaire suggests that some items may be redundant. Many of the symptoms correlate very highly. For example a patient who suffers from wheeze usually also suffers from breathlessness. This indicates that it may be possible to eliminate some items without losing too much information.

Dimensionality

In addition to determining the internal consistency of items we can investigate the dimensionality of the scale. If all the items measure the same trait one would expect the scale to be unidimensional. It was felt that most of the asthma symptoms identified arose from a common biomedical mechanism and the scale was therefore expected to be unidimensional. The mechanisms giving rise to diabetes symptoms, however, were less clear cut. The panel of clinicians identified four mechanisms whereby a patient's diabetes was manifested in symptoms. These were very high levels of blood sugar, very low levels of blood sugar, rapidly changing levels of blood sugar and complications of diabetes. Thus there was a suggestion that it might be possible to group the symptoms into a number of sub-scales; responses to items within these sub-scales could then be summed to give a number of indices that could be interpreted in terms of the biochemistry of the disease.

A number of approaches can be used to investigate dimensionality. In cases where a single dimension is expected tests for unidimensionality have been proposed (see for example Stout, 1987). However software for their implementation is not currently widely available. If theory suggests a more complex structure confirmatory factor analysis can be used (Long, 1983). The main problem of this technique at present is that the rigorous statistical comparison of different models is only possible if one is prepared to make the assumption that responses to the items follow a multivariate normal distribution. Methods requiring fewer assumptions are being developed (see for example Browne, 1984) but formal tests of hypotheses comparing different models have not yet been finalised. In the case of the diabetes symptoms, there was some disagreement among clinicians as to the mechanism giving rise to each of the symptoms. It was therefore felt appropriate to use exploratory factor analysis to investigate possible groupings. Assumptions of multivariate normality were not appropriate for items in the questionnaire for the diabetes symptoms, so a principal components analysis with orthogonal rotation of the components was carried out. Although there were two eigen values greater than one, the scree plot (Figure 3.2) suggested that a one factor solution might be appropriate. However, two and three factor solutions were examined to see whether they yielded meaningful clusters of variables. The three factor solution is shown in Figure 3.2 (the three factor solution was chosen in

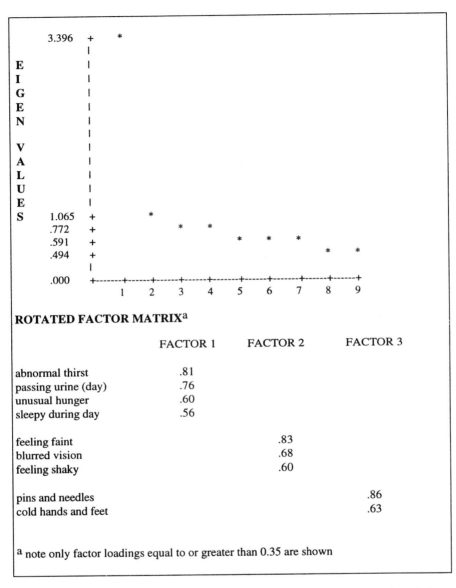

ROTATED FACTOR MATRIX[a]

	FACTOR 1	FACTOR 2	FACTOR 3
abnormal thirst	.81		
passing urine (day)	.76		
unusual hunger	.60		
sleepy during day	.56		
feeling faint		.83	
blurred vision		.68	
feeling shaky		.60	
pins and needles			.86
cold hands and feet			.63

[a] note only factor loadings equal to or greater than 0.35 are shown

Figure 3.2   Factor analysis of diabetes symptoms questionnaire: scree plot of eigen values and rotated three factor solution

preference to the two factor solution because there was much smaller cross-loading of items across factors). While some of the groupings of variables can be rationalised they are not those predicted by the clinicians. The symptoms of hunger and thirst load onto the same factor. Yet some clinicians identified excessive thirst as a symptom of hyperglycaemia and hunger as being a symptom of hypoglycaemia. The factors produced by the statistical analysis have little clinical meaning in the context of diabetes care. Putting this evidence together with the scree plot and the high level of internal consistency among all nine symptoms noted above, it is difficult to see any advantage in breaking the symptom questionnaire down into three sub-scales.

FROM ITEMS TO SCALES

If it is intended to combine responses from a set of items to form a single index, the way in which this is done should be carefully considered. The simplest method of combining the items is to simply sum the individual responses. In the case of the asthma symptoms questionnaire, each of the ten symptoms has a score of between zero and four; with simple addition the total score will lie between zero and 40. There are two assumptions implicit in this approach; first, that symptoms are being measured on an interval scale and second, that all symptoms have equal importance. Consider two symptoms, say breathlessness during exercise and wheezing at night. There are three ways of combining them to obtain a score of two. These are 2+0, 1+1, and 0+2, where the first number represents the score for breathlessness and the second for wheezing. The assumption is that these three combinations are equivalent. That is, scoring two on one symptom and zero on the other is equivalent to scoring two ones on separate symptoms, in other words, that being breathless on several days, but never wheezing, is equivalent to suffering both symptoms on one or a few days. This can only be the case if each of the following conditions apply: (i) the difference between a response of one and two is the same as the difference between a response of two and three, (or three and four or zero and one); and (ii) the two symptoms are equally important - a score of three for breathlessness has the same impact on the patient as a score of three for wheezing.

An alternative is to assign weights to each response category and/or weights to each symptom. Two approaches to this problem have been commonly adopted. The first is theoretical. Experts may be able to come to a consensus about the relative importance and impact of both symptoms and response categories. In the case of the asthma symptoms questionnaire clinicians may regard wheezing during the night as potentially causing more of a problem for a patient than coughing during the day. Greater weight can then be given to wheezing. The main problem with this approach is that it requires the derivation of value judgements which may not be reliable.

The second approach is empirical; the data are used to derive the weights. There are number of ways that this can be done. A purely statistical approach would be to use the coefficients of the first principal component. This will give the linear combination of symptoms which explains the greatest amount of the observed variation in the data. (A more complete explanation of principal components analysis will be found in Chatfield and Collins, 1980.) A similar method, described by Dunn (1989), is to select the weights so as to maximise the reliability of the final score. Dunn shows that, provided we can make some assumptions about the individual items, the weights required will be inversely proportional to the variance of the item scores. A variation on this method is to choose the weights so as to maximise the predictive accuracy of the scale score. Multiple regression can be used to generate coefficients when some dependent variable is regressed on the individual symptoms. In the case of asthma, the symptoms could be regressed against time off work or the number of unplanned consultations. The problem with this method is that the dependent variable is likely to depend on a number of other factors besides asthma symptoms.

Table 3.1   Mean bother for each symptom

Symptom	Response category (frequency)			
	On one or a few days	*On several days*	*On most days*	*Every day*
Breathless on exercise	0.9	1.3	1.6	2.1
Breathless during the day	1.0	1.3	1.7	2.4
Wheezing during the day	0.8	1.2	1.5	2.0
Coughing during the day	0.7	1.1	1.4	1.9
Wheezing at night	0.9	1.2	1.6	2.3
Breathless at night	0.9	1.5	1.7	2.5
Coughing at night	0.8	1.3	1.7	2.2
Disturbed sleep	1.0	1.4	1.9	2.3
Fear due to asthma	1.4	1.7	2.2	2.7
Chest feeling tight	0.9	1.3	1.7	2.1

Whichever method of weighting is adopted, the costs of the increased complexity should be assessed. A sophisticated scoring system means that it is not so easy to use the scale. In general, the weights will be derived from a sample of patients; the sample must be large enough so that the standard errors associated with the weights are small in comparison with the variation between the weights.

One would need to have a good idea about the reliability of the weights before advocating their use. Furthermore, it is not clear that weights derived for one population will be valid for use with another. It must be demonstrated that costs do not outweigh the benefits; the weighted index must clearly perform better than the unweighted one. Cox *et al.*(1992) give a more technical description of some of these issues.

In our research, we were interested in the impact of symptoms on the patient's quality of life. This was why we added the questions which asked about the amount of bother each symptom caused. It was felt appropriate to investigate weighting the symptoms using this information; symptoms that caused patients most bother could be given the highest weights. The mean level of bother corresponding to each response category is given in Table 3.1. The main problem is that if we are to make use of this data directly, again we have to make the assumption that bother is being measured on a scale that is at least interval. We could simply assign the values given in Table 3.1 as the weights corresponding to each response. Unfortunately the standard errors associated with the mean bother varies greatly from cell to cell (where a "cell" is an item-category combination). This is because the number of patients upon which the cell means are based varies from 11 to 185. A multiple regression analysis of the data indicated that there was a symptom effect (the mean level of bother varied from symptom to symptom), that there was a response category effect (the mean level of bother changed as patients reported higher symptom frequency), but that there was no symptom-response category interaction effect. That is, the way in which bother depends upon symptom frequency is the same for all symptoms. This implies that we are justified in adopting a simpler weighting system in which we adopt relative weights for each of the response categories and relative weights for each of the symptoms (Tables 3.2 and 3.3).

Table 3.2 Relative weights for symptoms

Symptom	Weight
Breathless on exercise	0.96
Breathless during the day	1.03
Wheezing during the day	0.88
Coughing during the day	0.81
Wheezing at night	0.96
Breathless at night	1.05
Coughing at night	0.95
Disturbed sleep	1.06
Fear due to asthma	1.30
Chest feeling tight	0.99

Table 3.3   Relative weights for symptom frequency response categories

Response category	Never	On one or a few days	On several days	On most days	Every day
Ordinal score	0	1	2	3	4
Weight	0	1.4	2.2	2.7	3.7

The weighted score was then compared with the unweighted score in terms of its reliability, validity and responsiveness using the techniques described in the following sections. The weighted score performed no better than the unweighted one and thus the final recommendation is that a complex weighting system is not required.

The last point about weighting relates to the choice of the items themselves. If a subset of items are highly correlated there is an implication that they are likely to be measuring the same aspect of the trait under consideration. Because more questions relate to this aspect, it is implicitly being given a higher weight for its contribution to the index. For example, in the above scale there are four items which apply specifically to the occurrence of symptoms during the day and four items that refer to symptoms that occur at night. It is therefore implicit in the unweighted scale that these aspects of asthma symptomology are equally important.

TRANSFORMATION OF THE FINAL SCORE

The final score can be transformed onto a scale from zero to 100 where zero represents no symptoms at all and 100 represents all symptoms occuring every day. This sort of transformation might be appropriate if a range of measures is being used. For any individual measure, the patient's score in relation to the end points of the scale is easily assessed without having to check the possible range for that scale. The real issue, however, is one of clinical meaningfulness. What does a score of 40 represent? What change in score represents a clinically significant improvement? These sorts of questions can only be answered slowly as the scale is used in practice and results can be put into context.

STANDARDISED SCORES, POPULATION NORMS

The derivation of standardised scores and population norms is really an issue of utility. The scores obtained from a symptoms questionnaire will be of most use if we have some knowledge of the distribution of scores for the whole population of patients with the particular disease. Standardising scores based on the standard deviation of a sample will give some indication of how particular individuals compare with others in that sample only. If the population standard deviation is used we will be able to interpret all individual scores in a wider context. We would be able to compare, for example, scores of patients with asthma in a particular general practice against all patients with asthma. To do this the standard deviation of scores in the population must first be estimated. This necessarily involves taking a large random sample from the population, which obviously requires substantial resources. Further, if scores depend on other factors such as age of patient, gender or seasonal effects, the utility of the symptoms questionnaires will be enhanced with the availability of population norms corresponding to these variables.

A major advantage of this approach is that, if a range of measures is available, it is possible to compare different aspects of a patient's health status. It might be possible to identify particular problem areas such as abnormal levels of depression in comparison with scores in other domains such as symptom frequency.

RELIABILITY

Having developed a new measure, it is important to assess its reliability; that is, whether it can give reliable and consistent results. If the measure is administered to an individual twice under identical conditions, how good is the agreement between the two sets of responses? However, there are practical difficulties in assessing test-retest reliability in this way. If a questionnaire is given on two occasions to the same patient, the time between the two administrations should be sufficiently long that patients cannot remember their initial responses. The problem is that the longer time gap, the more likely things are to have changed. This is particularly true for symptom-based outcome measures for a condition such as asthma where there may be wide natural variation from day to day and month to month in the level of symptoms experienced. Nevertheless, if the measures are to be used in an evaluation of care delivered, it is important to gain some insight into reliability even though it may not be possible to determine precisely the loss of reliability that is due to a change in the underlying condition.

A preliminary assessment of reliability of these measures has been based on two administrations of the symptoms questionnaire, three months apart. This is much longer than the two to fourteen days recommended by Streiner and Norman (1989) for assessment of test-retest reliability. However, the data should provide a conservative estimate - some of the observed differences will be due to change in health status rather than poor reliability of the questionnaire. The variability in the total score obtained from the diabetes symptoms questionnaire are summarised in Table 3.4, a standard analysis of variance table.

Table 3.4   Analysis of variance summary table for total diabetes symptoms score

Source of variance	Sum of squares	Degrees of freedom	Mean square	F
Between parties	12288.9	207	59.4	11.8
Between tests	1.9	1	1.9	0.4
Residual error	1045.1	207	5.0	
Total	13335.9	415	32.135	

VALIDITY

Criterion Validity
A scale is valid if it actually measures what it claims to measure. The best way of assessing validity is to judge the measure against some external criteria. Ideally this will be a "gold standard", a definitive way of measuring the trait. This form of validity is known as criterion validity and is usually broken down into two components, concurrent validity and predictive validity. Concurrent validity is assessed when the standard is used at the same time as the measure which is being judged. (The usual technique is to see how closely the two measures correlate.) In predictive validity the criterion is measured at a later time. How well does the measure of the trait made at one point in time predict future events? The predictive validity may also give some indication of the utility of the scale.

Unfortunately, in the field of health status measurement there are few gold standards. This is certainly the case with symptom-based outcome measures. Often, expert clinical opinion is substituted for a gold standard but the problem with asking clinicians about patients' symptoms is that the information probably came from the patient in the first place. For a condition such as asthma, the patient may have had the symptoms some time prior to seeing the doctor and may even be symptom-free at the time of the consultation. Thus data about symptoms provided by doctors may suffer from two sources of variability - a patient effect and a doctor effect. In fact there is evidence from our study that data about symptoms collected from doctors is less reliable than data collected directly from patients (Steen *et al.*, 1994).

Table 3.5   Concurrent and predictive validity of the ten item asthma symptoms questionnaire

| | Spearman Rank Correlation Coefficients[a] | | | |
| | Ten item asthma symptoms scale | | SF-36 general health perception scale | |
Criteria	concurrent validity[b]	predictive validity[c]	concurrent validity[b]	predictive validity[c]
Number of asthma attacks	0.45	0.44	0.35	0.48
Chest infections	0.47	0.37	0.42	0.30
Routine consultations	0.53	0.57	0.40	0.47
Unplanned consultations	0.36	0.53	0.33	0.41
Impaired activity	0.56	0.53	0.67	0.59

a   Correlation coefficients are based on a sample of 107 patients who responded to all items in the two questionnaires. All correlations are significant at the 0.1% level.

b   In assessing concurrent validity, scale scores were correlated with the adverse occurrences (the criteria) which occurred during the three months prior to the completion of the questionnaire.

c   In assessing predictive validity, scale scores were correlated with the adverse occurrences which occurred in the three months following the completion of the questionnaire.

The panels of clinicians were therefore asked to consider what other criteria might be appropriate to assess concurrent and predictive validity. The panels felt that a high level of symptoms would be associated with a higher frequency of consultations and time off work (or impairment of other activities) due to asthma. Clearly these can in no way be regarded as measures of the same trait. There are factors other than disease symptoms that influence whether a patient makes an appointment to see a doctor or whether the patient takes time off work. Thus, although we would expect the correlations to be high, we would not expect them to be perfect. Table 3.5 allows us to assess how well the total asthma symptom score correlates with the criteria identified by the panel of experts. To provide context, correlations are supplied for a much used and well-validated general health status scale - the general health perception scale from the Medical Outcomes Study SF-36 (Brazier *et al.,* 1992). The correlations are very similar (in the context of 107 patients) across all the criteria and for both the asthma questionnaire and the generic health status measure. What we are observing is the influence of a chronic disease. It is the disease which is causing the symptoms and the adverse occurrences and it is the disease which is having an effect on the general health perception of the patient.

RESPONSIVENESS TO CHANGE

Perhaps the most important requisite for an outcome measure is that it should be able to detect change in health status over time. If they cannot detect such changes, the questionnaires will not be suitable for assessing patient outcome. The degree of responsiveness required will depend upon the purpose of the measure. A measure intended to assess outcome for a single patient will need to be more responsive than one intended to assess outcome for groups of patients.

Responsiveness to change of an instrument is one of the most difficult properties to assess. Once again the major problem is the lack of a gold standard. If the measure is administered to a group of patients at two points in time, it is probable that differences will be observed. Some patients may show an improvement, others may show a deterioration in health status. But are these differences due to genuine changes in the patients' health status or are they due to the poor reliability of the instrument? One approach that could be adopted to try and answer this question is to administer the measure at two points in time to a large group of patients and then somehow try, by other means, to identify those patients for whom there has been a substantial change in health status. The performance of the measure on those patients can then be assessed. For chronic diseases such as asthma or diabetes, only a fairly small proportion of patients are likely to experience substantial change in their condition in say a three month period. Thus a very large number of patients must be identified to provide sufficient numbers for the assessment.

The ten item asthma symptoms questionnaire was administered twice to 250 patients three months apart. The patients were also asked directly about how they thought their asthma had changed during that three month period. It was hoped that in this way we could identify patients for whom there had been a change in condition. However, there are problems inherent in this sort of exercise. Patients have to recall how their asthma was three months ago (which may not be easy) and then make a subjective assessment of how things have changed. They often tend towards being optimistic. This is a form of positive response (or acquiescence) bias (Streiner and Norman, 1989). This seemed to apply to our sample. Twenty-six patients reported that their asthma was much better; only five patients recorded it was much worse. Application of the binomial test (Siegel and Castellan, 1988) indicates that this difference is significant at the one percent level. (There are other possible explanations for such a difference - such as some sort of seasonal effect - but the evidence is inconclusive.)

Table 3.6   Change in total symptoms score for patients reporting much improvement in their asthma: summary statistics and paired t-test

Variable	Number of cases	Mean score	Standard deviation	Standard error
Baseline score	26	14.5	9.1	1.8
Follow-up score	26	8.5	6.8	1.3

(Difference) Mean	Standard deviation	Standard error	t value	Degrees of freedom	2-tail prob.
6.0	8.4	1.6	3.65	25	.001

For the purposes of assessing responsiveness, perhaps the most important finding was that most of patients (88%) felt that their asthma was about the same or that there had been only a little change. Thus even a comparatively large sample of 250 patients is barely adequate for assessing responsiveness to change. The twenty-six patients who did indicate a significant improvement in their asthma have allowed a provisional assessment of responsiveness (Table 3.6).

The paired t-test is significant at the 0.1% level. There has been a significant change in the total symptom score for patients who have reported much improvement in their asthmatic health.

In order to assess responsiveness two other statistics are often computed. These are effect size (Kazis *et al.*, 1989; Deyo *et al.*, 1991) and Guyatt's responsiveness statistic (Guyatt *et al.*, 1987). The effect size is given by:

$$\text{Effect size} = \frac{\text{Mean score at follow-up} - \text{Mean score at baseline}}{\text{Standard deviation of baseline scores}}$$

For the data given in Table 3.6, it has the value of 0.72. The corresponding effect size for change in the general health perception sub-scale of the SF-36 is only 0.22*. The corresponding paired t-test for the SF-36 sub-scale was not significant. Thus there is some preliminary evidence to suggest that, for asthma at least, the symptom-based outcome measure is much more responsive to change in the asthmatic health of the patient than a generic measure.

Effect size is most useful when there are a range of scales to be compared. To make most use of Guyatt's responsiveness statistic, it is desirable to define the smallest clinically important change for the scale score. It may be possible for clinicians to come to some sort of consensus about significant changes in biomedical indicators such as peak flow rates or glycosylated haemoglobin but it is very difficult to achieve such a consensus for a total symptom score.

The number of patients needed for a responsiveness study might be reduced if it is possible to identify a group of patients who are likely to experience a significant change in their health status. This will most often be patients who are about to undergo some form of treatment intervention. The diabetes symptoms questionnaire is currently being tested on patients with diabetes who are being put on insulin for the first time. It is of course by no means certain that such patients will all undergo significant changes in health status. It is still therefore important to try and find other evidence to identify those patients who do.

CONCLUSION

The steps involved in the developing and testing of symptom-based outcome measures have been described; each step has been illustrated using the example of symptom-based measures developed for asthma and diabetes. The point has been made that much time and effort can be saved by drawing on the work of those who have previously carried out research in this field of interest. Then if new symptom-based measures need to be further developed, they must have the same attributes of reliability and validity as all other forms of outcome measure. Above all, if the measures are to be used to evaluate care, they should be responsive to change. The work reported here demonstrates that it is possible to develop symptom-based outcome measures that have these desirable properties. There is also some evidence that the measures may be more responsive to change than generic measures, a point which further reinforces the need for such condition-specific outcome measures. The role of a symptom-based outcome measure is clearly

---

* Effect size for the change in the SF-36 general health perception scale was based on a sub-sample of 13 patients. (In the experimental design all patients received the asthma specific instruments but patients only received a selection of the generic scales being tested.) The corresponding paired t-test statistic was $t_{12} = 0.79$ which is not significant.

defined in symptomatic conditions such as asthma but the utility of such measures in diseases such as diabetes is less clear. The work has identified higher levels of certain symptoms in a diabetic population than was expected by the clinical experts. This is clearly of intrinsic interest but how do we relate this information to the measurement of outcome?

The next phase of the development will be to focus on their clinical utility. What is the clinical significance that is associated with a particular change in scale score? One strand of work will be to determine the magnitude of change associated with seasonal effects, socio-economic and demographic effects and treatment effects. The signs are optimistic that the symptoms questionnaires will be useful audit tools; they may be used alongside other outcome measures to help evaluate care within a given site (such as a general practice or out-patient department) - the intended function of the measures. It is also possible that the questionnaires may have some utility in assessing outcome for individuals. We are currently assessing whether they can form part of a patient profile that will assist the clinician in the management of the condition for an individual patient.

REFERENCES

Brazier, J.E., Harper, R., Jones, N.M.B., O'Cathain, A., Thomas, K.J., Usherwood, T. and Westlake, L. (1992) Validating the SF-36 Health Survey Questionnaire: new outcome measure for primary care. *British Medical Journal*, **305**, 160-164.

Browne, M.W. (1984) Asymptomatically distribution-free methods for the analysis of covariance structures. *British Journal of Mathematical and Statistical Psychology*, **37**, 62-83.

Chatfield, C. and Collins, A.J. (1980) *Introduction to multivariate analysis*. London: Chapman and Hall.

Cox, D.R., Fitzpatrick, R., Fletcher, A.E., Gore, S.M., Spiegelhalter, D.J. and Jones, D.R. (1992) Quality of life assessment: can we keep it simple? *Journal of the Royal Statistical Society, Series A*, **115**, 353-393.

Cronbach, L.J. (1951) Coefficient alpha and the internal structure of tests. *Psychometrika*, **16**, 297-334.

Deyo, R.A., Diehr, P. and Patrick, D.L. (1991) Reproducibility and responsiveness of health status measures: statistics and strategies for evaluation. *Controlled Clinical Trials*, **12**, 142S-158S.

Dunn, G. (1989) *Design and analysis of reliability studies: the statistical evaluation of measurement errors*. Oxford: Oxford University Press.

Freund, A., Johnson, S.B., Rosenbloom, A., Alexander, B. and Hansen, C.A. (1986) Subjective symptoms, blood glucose estimation, and blood glucose concentrations in adolescents with diabetes. *Diabetes Care*, **9**, 236-243.

Given, C.W. (1984) Measuring the social psychological health states of ambulatory chronically ill patients: hypertension and diabetes as tracer conditions. *Journal of Community Health*, **9**, 179-195.

Guyatt, G., Walter, S. and Norman, G. (1987) Measuring change over time: assessing the usefulness of evaluative instruments. *Journal of Chronic Diseases*, **40**, 171-178.

Hyland, M.E., Kenyon, C.A., Allen, R. and Howarth, P. (1993) Diary keeping in asthma: comparison of written and electronic methods. *British Medical Journal*, **306**, 487-489.

Juniper, E.F., Guyatt, G.H., Epstein, R.S., Ferrie, P.J., Jaeschke, R. and Hiller, T.K. (1992) Evaluation of impairment of health related quality of life in asthma: development of a questionnaire for use in clinical trials. *Thorax*, **47**, 76-83.

Kazis, L.E., Anderson, J.J. and Meenan, R.F. (1989) Effect sizes for interpreting changes in health status. *Medical Care*, **27**, S178-S189.

Kinsman, R.A., Luparello, T., O'Banion, K. and Spector, S. (1973) Multidimensional analysis of the subjective symptomatology of asthma. *Psychosomatic Medicine*, **35**, 250-267.

Long, J.S. (1983) *Confirmatory factor analysis*. London: Sage Publications.

McDowell, I. and Newell, C. (1987) *Measuring health: a guide to rating scales and questionnaires*. Oxford: Oxford University Press.

Siegel, S. and Castellan, N.J. (1988) *Nonparametric statistics for the behavioral sciences*. London: McGraw-Hill.

Steen, N., Hutchinson, A., McColl, E., Eccles, M.P., Hewison, J., Meadows, K.A., Blades, S.M. and Fowler, P. (1994) Development of a symptom-based outcome measure for asthma. *British Medical Journal*, **309**, 1065-1068.

Stout, W. (1987) A nonparametric approach for assessing latent trait unidimensionality. *Psychometrika*, **52**, 589-617.

Streiner, D.L. and Norman, G.R. (1989) *Health measurement scales: a practical guide to their development and use*. Oxford: Oxford University Press.

Usherwood, T.P., Scrimgeour, A. and Barber, J.H. (1990) Questionnaire to measure perceived symptoms and disability in asthma. *Archives of Disease in Children*, **65**, 779-781.

Chapter 4 _____

DEVELOPING OUTCOME MEASURES FOR CHILDREN: "QUALITY OF LIFE" ASSESSMENT FOR PAEDIATRIC ASTHMA

DAVINA FRENCH AND MARGARET CHRISTIE

INTRODUCTION

Management of Paediatric Asthma

As the title indicates, this chapter is concerned with measuring the quality of life experienced by a child who has asthma; it is therefore concerned with measurements of response to the disease and its management which go beyond the physical outcome indicators such as peak flow and into more "holistic" appraisals of psychosocial factors. Attempts at measurement of quality of life are evident in a range of contexts: ours was initiated when evaluation of a paediatric, longer-acting β_2-agonist (Brittain, 1990) was being planned and attempts were made to go beyond assessments of safety and efficacy and into a more comprehensive evaluation (Upchurch and McCullough, 1995).

Technological and pharmaceutical developments have made feasible the more effective clinical control of chronic diseases such as diabetes and asthma. But clinicians' perceptions of optimal management may not always include awareness of the psychosocial burdens which self-management can impose on patients. Included within outcome measurement, therefore, one finds evidence of "quality of life" assessments which attempt a more comprehensive evaluation of management effectiveness. Literature from the diabetes field is beginning to reflect this (Shillitoe, 1988; Bradley et al., 1991), but asthma lags behind. Yet technological and pharmaceutical developments have been particularly evident within asthma management over the past two decades. Bronchodilation can be effective, with an inhaled selective β_2-agonist and longer-acting preparations now available. Anti-inflammatory medication, such as sodium cromoglycate and corticosteroids, are also available as inhaled preparations, though the former is recommended for use four times per day. A range of delivery systems is available, and peak-flow meters are on prescription in the United Kingdom (UK).

For the child and the family, however, there may be the need to change aspects of their lifestyle. They need to recognise allergic trigger factors such as seasonal pollen, animal dander and house dust, or such non-allergic triggers as emotional arousal, rhinoviral infections or cigarette smoke. They need, also, to adjust their lives as far as possible to avoid these, but with minimal limitation of the normal "quality of life". Asthma management, then, is a fine balance between a regimen which targets biological benefits but jeopardizes a child's normal psychosocial development, and the neglect of good management practice, which may result in adverse outcomes such as hospital admissions, or broken nights disturbed by coughing, or school absence.

Hilton (1995) suggests that such comprehensive appraisals of patients' responses to chronic disease and its management are emphasised within the United Kingdom's postgraduate vocational training for general practice. But while this training "aims to instil ability to make intuitive assessments on matters such as quality of life", Hilton observes that more formal appraisals are rarely made. One obvious reason this is the case within paediatric asthma management may be the dearth of appropriate measurement tools.

Quality of Life with Paediatric Asthma

Our work was aimed at the development of disease-specific, evaluative questionnaires, designed for the three age ranges of four to seven, eight to eleven and 12-16 years. These are child-centred, being derived from children's own perceptions of asthma and its management as an ambulatory condition, in contrast to American (Staudenmayer, 1982) and British (Usherwood *et al.*, 1990) instruments which were developed from clinicians' views of the child's life with asthma.

The view that the family's rather than the asthmatic child's quality of life should be evaluated has been put forward by Hyland (1991b), but Jones (1991) has expressed a contrary view that children's perceptions should be taken into account. These discussions followed Hyland's report of work on a disease-specific, patient-centred questionnaire for assessments of adults' views of Living with Asthma (Hyland, 1991a; Hyland *et al.*, 1991), developed from material gathered during patients' discussions in focus groups. This approach was adopted in the early stages of our work with groups of children, in schools, homes and health care settings.

Recent publications have emphasized the difficulties of producing paediatric instruments, for the "moving target" of a developing organism (Rosenbaum *et al.*, 1990), and also the time, effort and expertise needed (Johnson, 1991). In the context of optimal care for paediatric asthma, Gillespie (1990) has expressed her belief that listening to the children could result in clinicians being able to "more fully and successfully treat the whole patient...win compliance...do more than alleviate symptoms...change the course of the disease itself." As we have indicated however, such "holism" for chronic disease management, in the current climate of health care evaluation, "demands hard data" (Shillitoe and Christie, 1988). Given the costs of developing the means for such measurement in paediatric disorder, do the potential benefits outweigh the costs?

Policy Issues
The UK's national consultative document (Department of Health, 1991) noted the substantial morbidity caused by asthma and suggested that self-management protocols agreed between patient and doctor should "have a favourable impact on the burden imposed by asthma on the individual and the community." Contemporary literature (e.g. Pearson, 1990; Bevis and Taylor, 1990) is indicating the contribution toward self-management of asthma which can be expected of a child from the age of eight years. The impact on relatively normal quality of living for school-age children with asthma is also beginning to be reported (Eiser and Havermans, 1995). We would argue, then, that the "self-management protocols agreed between patient and doctor" should, from the age of eight onwards, explore the child's perception of its chronic disease/management and should include a holistic evaluation of the outcome of any management changes.

Methodological and Developmental Considerations for Paediatric Outcome Measures

In developing our outcome measures, we drew heavily on theory and empirical research in the educational, developmental and psychometric sectors, as well as the clinical paediatric literature.

Given the current emphasis on involving children in the management of their asthma, and the increasingly frequent calls for children's self-reports to be included in paediatric assessments in a variety of fields (e.g. Beitchman and Corradini, 1988; La Greca, 1990), it is pertinent to ask whether children's self-reports are capable of meeting the psychometric standards normally required of outcome measures, in particular whether the reports reach the usually accepted criteria for reliability and validity. Our view echoes that of Flanery (1990), that children's self-report measures are "subject to the same standards that apply to all diagnostic, prognostic and evaluative devices". In fact, in some respects these requirements assume even greater importance than usual, since child respondents may be particularly prone to miscomprehension or lapses in attention.

Methodological considerations

Reliability, or the consistency of reporting, must be examined both temporally, as test-retest reliability, using correlations between reports on two different occasions, and internally, using coefficients such as Cronbach's alpha which are based on mean inter-item correlations. These reliability checks will ensure that the child understands that the items all refer to a specific dimension, e.g. their own activities and not those of others, and that this interpretation does not change over time.

Where the behaviour or activity is directly observable, e.g. frequency of school absence, the objective accuracy of reports should also be checked. The validity of reports, that is whether the instrument is measuring what it claims to measure, can only be assessed by the accrual of relevant data (Johnson, 1991), and will be particularly difficult where the symptom or state of interest is not directly observable. Likely sources of information on validity include differences in scores between clinician-defined "cases" and "non-cases", or between those suffering different levels of severity, as well as longitudinal evidence of changes in disease state being accompanied by corresponding changes in scores on the outcome measure.

The lack of self-report measures of quality of life for children with asthma has already been noted, but psychometric evidence drawn from comparable cases such as childhood depression, functional disability and children's behavioural problems is encouraging. Martini and colleagues (1990) describe the development of a self-report measure of depressive symptoms for pre-school children. They obtained high levels of test-retest reliability and internal consistency in the reports of three to five year olds, but did not find significant levels of agreement between the children and their parents. This pattern, of consistent reports that differ from those of adult observers, recurs in a review of findings concerning child behavioural and emotional problems (Achenbach *et al.*, 1987) where one might expect any problems to be more overtly observable and therefore, perhaps, observer and self-reports to be more closely related. The figures that emerge from their meta-analysis of more than 100 studies indicate a weighted mean correlation between parents and children of 0.25, and between teachers and children of 0.20. In contrast the mean level of test-retest reliability was 0.74. Finally, in the field of functional disability, Walker and Green (1991) report satisfactory levels of test-retest reliability, internal consistency and concurrent validity for eight to 16 year olds reporting on how much trouble they had experienced doing everyday tasks. These findings and those of other studies suggest that children are potentially reliable reporters of both internal states and functional limitations.

In many patient care settings, particularly for a symptom-dominated condition such as asthma, it would also be desirable to ask about the occurence of symptoms. Since children are at school for part of the day and at home for the rest, they are the only ones to have 24 hour-a-day access to such information. The problem here is not so much one of reliability as accuracy. If the child's answers can be assessed against those of an adult, or by some other observable criteria, and the child is shown to be reasonably accurate, it becomes feasible to ask for the child's reports of the frequency of behaviours or symptoms to complement the incomplete reports of adult observers. However, evidence on this point is difficult to assimilate. As Achenbach *et al.* (1987) point out, if the phenomenon in question varies across situations, e.g. if symptoms are more frequent at certain times of the day, low correlations between the reports of different informants may reflect inconsistency in the phenomenon rather than unreliability of reporting.

One study that sheds light on the accuracy of children's reports is Johnson *et al.*'s (1986) study on children's recall of their diabetes management behaviour. However, even here the authors note that complete consistency cannot be expected since "few parents are able to observe all of their child's activities". Ten to fifteen year olds showed good levels of agreement with parents over all aspects of diabetes management behaviour, including types of food eaten, frequency of eating and timing of injections and blood glucose monitoring. Six to nine year olds were also reliable reporters of frequency data, but were somewhat less accurate for measures involving time. In a study on asthma symptoms, using peak expiratory flow rates (PEFRs) as the criterion for accuracy, Fritz *et al.* (1990) found that accuracy varied widely but it was not associated with age or other demographic variables. These findings suggest that whilst it may be useful to include symptom reports in outcome measures for children, it would be wise to complement them with the reports of adult observers and/or objective clinical measures, such as PEFR for patients with asthma.

Developmental considerations

The achievements of some of the studies reviewed above suggest that the successful production of paediatric outcome measures is dependent upon more than traditional psychometric expertise. Because of the unique characteristics of children as respondents - their limited literacy and communication skills in the early years, as well as their changing understanding of the self and its internal states - it is essential that the body of knowledge accumulated by developmental and educational psychologists is brought to bear upon the process of measure construction. It is helpful in this context to think of the process as having three distinct elements: the determination of the content of the items, the format of both the questions and their response options, and the structure of the test as a whole, that is whether it is to be unidimensional or composed of a number of sub-scales.

Considerations related to the content of a questionnaire or interview tend to be specific to the measures in question. The format, however, is a more general issue encompassing concerns about the way in which questions are asked and whether the required responses fall within the cognitive capabilities of the children being investigated.

With respect to inner states, there is clear evidence that by the age of three years children spontaneously refer to their own emotional states - "happy", "sad", "afraid" and "mad" - perhaps "cross" would be a British equivalent to "mad" (Smiley and Huttenlocher 1989). Smiley and Hutterlocher also report that three and a half to four year olds reliably discriminate between the facial expressions that usually portray these emotions. The use of visual stimuli to help young children to think about their feelings is indicated by the success of Martini *et al.*'s (1990) study, where picture cues helped them to achieve a test-retest reliability coefficient of 0.85 and internal consistency (Cronbach's alpha) of 0.89, and in the findings of Culross (1985) whose measure of self-concept for children with hearing impairment, which used picture stimuli with four- to eight-year-olds, also showed adequate psychometric properties. This line of argument is consistent with the views of Stone and Lemanek (1990) who suggest that below the age of about eight children use external cues such as facial expressions, rather than internal ones, to identify their own feelings. It therefore follows that showing children pictures, against which they can compare their self-perceptions, has a higher chance of success with four- to eight-year-olds than using verbal enquiries alone. Investigations of children's understanding of time concepts can also help the researcher to design tools that will elicit meaningful responses from children. For instance, it has been shown that children as young as three to four years understand the passage of time to some extent and know about the usual duration of everyday activities (Friedman, 1990). They also use language indicative of this knowledge, such as "yesterday", "tomorrow", "before" and "after" (Weist, 1989). This concrete knowledge is not, however, accompanied by an abstract concept of time until a little later. The concept of time has been addressed by Piaget (1969) where it is claimed that the passage of time is inferred from information about speed and distance travelled, and thus the concept is not acquired until these inferential skills develop, at the age of about eight years. Recent studies, using more meaningful situations, such as Westman (1989), also show that young children do not have an abstract concept of time, but by the age of seven years they readily discriminate real from apparent duration, thus indicating a sophisticated concept of time which is not necessarily dependent upon inference. It therefore seems likely that the very young child, of four to five years, is unlikely to give reliable information about frequency, unless it is of the most rudimentary kind, whilst children who are a little older may be able to do so.

Continuing with the process of test construction, the psychometric structure of the whole measure - the number of sub-scales and the relationships between them - should also be considered in the light of developmental findings. Pertinent findings in this respect are those on the structure of children's self-concept at different ages, since this is likely to limit the ways in which children can think about themselves and their illness. Harter and Pike (1984) have found that four- to seven-year-olds use at least four self-evaluative dimensions - cognitive competence, physical competence, social competence and behavioural conduct - whilst at around eight years children can recognise that these dimensions may also vary with situations (Harter, 1990). By adolescence the self-concept has acquired further dimensions, such as a differentiation between popularity with peers and specifically romantic appeal.

Since in a measure of a new construct, such as quality of life, the major adult dimensions are still unclear (Schipper *et al.*, 1990), quite apart from how these may develop and differentiate through childhood and adolescence, we strongly recommend the use of exploratory factor analysis during test construction. The use of factor analysis in this way, to identify the dimensionality of perceptions at various ages, would be expected to show, in line with the developmental literature, progressively more complex perceptions of quality of life with increasing age. Similarly, developmental considerations suggest that the format of the measure itself should become more complex as respondents develop. Implicit in this conclusion is the fact that, just as a child is not a small adult, so a six year old is not like a twelve-year-old, thus different outcome measures are likely to be needed for children of different ages.

THE CHILDHOOD ASTHMA QUESTIONNAIRES

Development of the Childhood Asthma Questionnaires

The recent development of the Childhood Asthma Questionnaires (CAQs) as outcome measures in paediatric asthma will be used to illustrate the points raised above. Following from our earlier arguments, three forms of the CAQ have been developed: Form A (CAQA) uses picture items to ask about feelings but does not ask about frequency or duration; Form B (CAQB) uses more advanced pictures and includes items about the frequency of activities and symptoms; Form C (CAQC) requires numerical responses to questions about feelings and frequency. CAQA is designed to be read by a child and parent together; it is suitable for children aged four to seven years whose reading is not yet independent. CAQB can be completed by eight to eleven year olds, able to read without help from an adult. CAQC, for 12- to 16-year-olds, stresses confidentiality and should be completed independently. Forms B and C are also suitable for group administration, for example in a classroom. Although the general format for the CAQs takes account of previous research, the content is based on a more empirical approach. In order to ensure both face validity (acceptability to the respondents) and content validity (adequate representation of the components of quality of life) in an area as subjective as this, field work was carried out with children, to find out what they thought were the important influences on and indicators of their day-to-day well-being.

Groups of eight- to eleven-year-olds stressed that their ability to take part in physical activities with their friends, especially running and ball games, and their pastimes at home, including play with pets, were the main areas where having asthma had a potential impact on their happiness. They also experienced a good deal of anxiety or apprehension over the likelihood of having an asthma attack and their ability to deal with it, for instance if their relief medication was in the care of an adult who was temporarily unavailable. Older children were also concerned about these things but chiefly in terms of how others would view their limitations. In the mid-teen years youngsters felt more in control of their illness but distressed about looking different, or being treated differently from others.

These findings were used to generate items for the CAQs, resulting in patient-centred, rather than clinician-centred, questionnaires. Although the perceptions of clinicians, and also of parents (e.g. Usherwood *et al.*, 1990), have their role in paediatric outcome assessment, they cannot substitute for the views of the child. In the field of paediatric asthma, Eiser *et al.* (1987) have found no agreement between mothers and children about what precipitates their asthma attacks and in more diverse fields Kazdin and Petti (1982) and Achenbach *et al.* (1987) have stressed the lack of agreement between children's reports and their parents' assessments. These authors all consider that discrepant reports may result from differing access to information and that the views of both groups of informants are therefore valuable. Finally, Lomas *et al.* (1987) have shown, in the context of a quality of life measure for adult aphasics, that patients and clinicians generate different items and conclude that "clinician-generated items are not fully representative of patient values."

The CAQs are representative of patients' values and the methods used take full consideration of the cognitive capabilities of the respondents. Figures 4.1 to 4.3 indicate the way in which the questions are expressed - children completing Forms A and B colour in the box or face that represents their answer, whilst respondents to Form C select the appropriate face then enter the number associated with it into the box - all are simple Likert scales with different degrees of pictorial assistance. In all three forms the first section of the questionnaire booklet contains items about daily activities, for instance, running around outside and listening to stories for four- to seven-year-olds, PE and games lessons and reading books for older children; this section can be completed by children who don't have asthma as well as those who do. A second section, for asthmatic children only, asks about asthma, beginning with questions about coughing, wheezing and asthma attacks and going on, for 12- to 16-year-olds, to ask about the social impact of asthma, as shown in Figure 4.3. Forms A and B have been used in school settings to gain quality of life data from non-asthmatic reference groups, by asking them to complete the first section of the questionnaire.

12a. Do you cough?
      Colour in **one** box

      Yes

      No

12b. Which face is **you** when you cough?
      Colour in **one** face

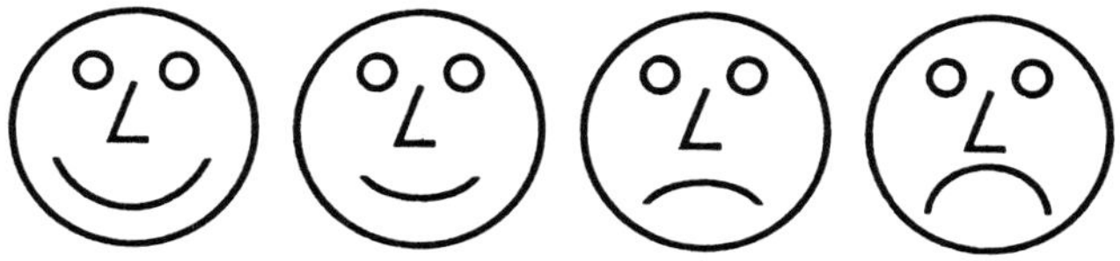

Figure 4.1   Sample item from CAQA

17a. How much have you been coughing recently?

      A lot

      Sometimes

      Hardly ever

      Not at all

17b. Which picture describes how you feel when you cough?

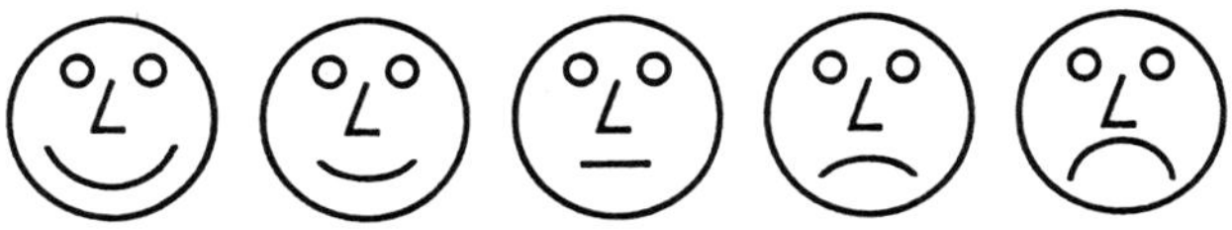

Figure 4.2   Sample item from CAQB

How do you feel?

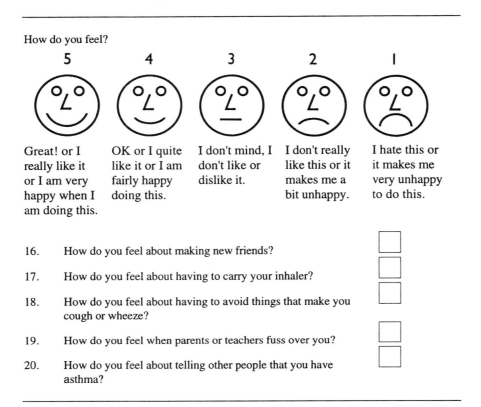

5	4	3	2	I
Great! or I really like it or I am very happy when I am doing this.	OK or I quite like it or I am fairly happy doing this.	I don't mind, I don't like or dislike it.	I don't really like this or it makes me a bit unhappy.	I hate this or it makes me very unhappy to do this.

16.   How do you feel about making new friends?

17.   How do you feel about having to carry your inhaler?

18.   How do you feel about having to avoid things that make you cough or wheeze?

19.   How do you feel when parents or teachers fuss over you?

20.   How do you feel about telling other people that you have asthma?

Figure 4.3   Sample items from CAQC

The Structure of the CAQs

Exploratory factor analysis of the CAQs has revealed the dimensionality of quality of life for differing age groups, and for children of differing health status. In all cases an oblique rotation technique was used to relax the constraints of independence between the factors and to explore the extent of inter-correlations between factors. Table 4.1 summarizes the sub-scales of the CAQs.

The fourteen items of CAQA yield two factors - the first ten items about enjoyment of daily activities load on a factor interpreted as Quality of Living whilst the remaining four items form an asthma-specific factor indicating distress about symptoms. In a recent sample of 80 children the two sub-scales derived from summing these items showed a negative correlation of -0.34, $p < 0.05$. Distress scores also correlated positively with the parent's rating of severity of asthma, r=0.42, p<0.01. Both Distress and Quality of Living correlated with parents' reports of how much the rest of the family was being affected by their child's asthma; multiple regression showed these relationships to be independent, with β coefficients of 0.26 (p<0.05) between each sub-scale and effects on the family.

Table 4.1   The sub-scales of the Childhood Asthma Questionnaires (CAQs)

CAQA	CAQB	CAQC
Quality of Living - enjoyment of all daily activities	Active Quality of Living - enjoyment of running, swimming, P.E. etc.	Active Quality of Living - enjoyment of sports, swimming, P.E. etc.
	Passive Quality of Living - enjoyment of reading, watching T.V. etc.	Teenage Quality of Living - enjoyment of teenage social activities
Distress - feelings about asthma	Distress - feelings about asthma symptoms	Distress - feelings about asthma symptoms and social impact
	Severity - frequency of asthma symptoms	Severity - frequency of asthma symptoms
		Reactivity - awareness of environmental triggers

As shown in Table 4.1, CAQB is comprised of four sub-scales, derived from the factor analysis of 23 items. The items in the Quality of Living scales all ask how children feel; the items asking "how often?", effectively asking about functional disability, do not contribute to the assessment of quality of living since for many children with mild asthma there is little activity reduction and for all children variance in the frequency of activities such as swimming and physical education is largely accounted for by factors other than asthma. The frequency items have been retained, since they provide useful orientation for the respondents but they are not scored; the score for Active Quality of Living (AQoL) is the sum of responses to how children feel about active pastimes - those with the potential to induce asthma - whilst Passive Quality of Living (PQoL) reflects how children feel during sedentary pastimes such as reading, drawing and watching TV. CAQB also has two sub-scales asking directly about asthma; Severity (SEV) is the sum of children's reports of the frequency of symptoms such as coughing, wheezing and waking at night and Distress (DIS) is how children feel about these experiences.

In a sample of 127 children with mild asthma AQoL was correlated with both DIS and SEV, and multiple regression showed these two asthma-related scores to be independent predictors of AQoL, β = -0.19 and -0.21 respectively, p<0.05. Scores on all three sub-scales showed the significant correlations with parents' ratings of the effect of their child's asthma on the rest of the family seen in Table 4.2. SEV scores also showed a positive correlation with parents' ratings of severity, r=0.44, p<0.001.

Table 4.2   Correlations between the sub-scales of CAQB and parents' ratings of the effect of asthma on the rest of the family

	Severity	Distress	Active QoL
Effect on the family	r = 0.45 p< 0.001	r = 0.41 p = 0.001	r = -0.26 p< 0.025

The relationships between children's perceptions of their asthma and parents' perceptions of how much the rest of the family is affected occur in both age groups and serve to indicate that disruption to family life may also be a useful outcome measure, provided that it is not regarded as a substitute for gaining the child's views. The effect of a child's asthma on the rest of the family is assessed by one question at the end of CAQs A and B; we are not currently aware of alternative instruments that treat this area in greater depth.

In a sample of 242 children clinicians' ratings of severity of asthma were available. Two hundred and twelve non-asthmatic children also completed the first section of the questionnaire to give estimates of asthma-free levels of quality of life. The mean scores for children with mild, moderate and severe asthma and from the non-asthmatic sample are shown in Figure 4.4. Statistical analysis indicates that moderate to severe asthma significantly reduces QoL, although the scores from those with mild asthma do not differ significantly from those of non-asthmatic children.

Perhaps even more revealing, with respect to the impact of asthma on the child, is the finding that factor analysis of the item responses of healthy children does not yield a two factor solution. For the child without asthma the enjoyment of everyday life is a single construct whereas the experience of having asthma causes children to think of their activities as falling into two distinct groups - those that may induce symptoms and those that are unlikely to.

CAQC is somewhat longer, with 41 items entering the factor analysis. The most clearly interpretable solution yields five factors, broadly similar to those found in the younger sample. AQoL is again the items about sports, swimming etc, whilst Teenage Quality of Living (TQoL) is a factor made up of the items asking how youngsters feel about the usual social activities of this age group, such as going to dances and meeting friends. Distress and severity are clearly identifiable as the same psychological constructs in this age group as they are in the junior school sample, although the situations in which the distress is manifested are more widespread, reflecting the increasing concern of these youngsters about the impact of their asthma on their social relationships. High scores on the fifth factor (Reactivity) have been interpreted as reflecting increased reactivity to environmental triggers, being identified by items about smoking and cigarette smoke, cold air and distress at being without relief medication. This interpretation is further supported by the pattern of correlations between scores on Reactivity and responses concerning the frequency of symptoms. Table 4.3 shows that Reactivity is associated with the frequency of environmentally induced symptoms, but not with symptoms in general.

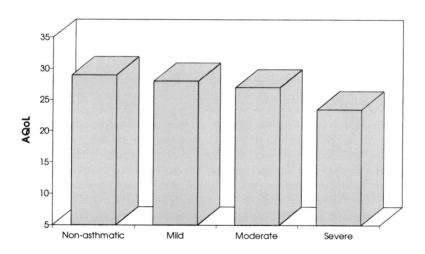

Figure 4.4   Score on CAQB-AQoL for three levels of asthma severity and non-asthmatic children

Again DIS and SEV were significantly negatively correlated with AQoL in the pilot sample of 229 teenagers. TQoL was not correlated with any of the asthma-related sub-scales. Since the young people in this age group stressed their desire for confidentiality and independence there were no questions for parents in CAQC, and thus no information is available regarding the correlations between patients' scores on CAQC and ratings supplied by other informants.

Table 4.3 Correlations between Reactivity and other items of CAQC

		Frequency of:		
	wheeze	*asthma attacks*	*animal-induced symptoms*	*exercise-induced symptoms*
Reactivity	r = 0.06 n.s.	r = 0.06 n.s.	r = 0.23 p < 0.01	r 0.22 p < 0.01

Evaluation of the CAQs
Test-retest reliability

Test-retest reliability trials have revealed the stability of scores over time in all three age-groups; for forms A and B this information is available for asthmatic and non-asthmatic samples.

The interval between administrations was crucial in this instance since the symptoms of childhood asthma are so episodic, frequently varying with the peak seasons for various allergens. Children's responses may also undergo permanent changes over fairly short periods of time, reflecting changes in their preferences and activities brought about by developmental progression. For instance the child who has just learned to swim may suddenly feel much more positive about trips to the swimming pool, whilst the girl who has just entered puberty may suddenly become acutely self-conscious about using an inhaler in public; neither change is related to the child's asthma as such but both may contribute to variability in scores over time. The retest intervals selected were therefore as short as possible to avoid this variability, whilst long enough to ensure that the children had forgotten their previous responses and were basing their answers on perceptions formed on two separate occasions. The intervals selected were one week for CAQA and three weeks for CAQB and CAQC, with the non-asthmatic samples providing estimates of the stability of quality of life scores in the absence of potentially variable symptoms.

The test-retest reliability coefficients obtained in this way, with some children receiving the questionnaires by post at appropriate intervals whilst others were visited in their schools, are shown in Table 4.4, which also indicates the number of children in each sample and their mean age. The reliability is in all cases adequate, increasing with age to adult levels on CAQC and being comparable in asthmatic and non-asthmatic samples. This suggests that the coefficients obtained are true estimates of reliability, or at least unlikely to have been lowered by fluctuations in the children's asthma symptoms. The coefficients are also similar to those obtained in the comparable studies cited earlier in this chapter e.g. Culross (1985); Walker and Green (1991). Values of Cronbach's alpha obtained at the first administration of the test-retest reliability trials also show a similar pattern of internal consistency increasing with age and being comparable with other paediatric instruments of similar length.

Table 4.4   Test-retest reliability of the CAQs

| | *CAQA* | | | | *CAQB* | | | *CAQC* |
	asthma	*non-asthma*			*asthma*	*non-asthma*		*asthma*
N	80	103			103	153		96
mean age	5.5 years	5.5 years			9.8 years	9.5 years		13.8 years
QoL	0.68	0.63	*AQoL*		0.74	0.74	*AQoL*	0.81
			PQoL		0.75	0.70	*TQoL*	0.83
Distress	0.63		*Distress*		0.75		*Distress*	0.73
			Severity		0.73		*Severity*	0.73
							Reactivity	0.84

Accuracy

The accuracy of children's reports may be addressed by considering the relationships between the children's reports and those of their doctors and parents. As was noted earlier, different informants have access to different perspectives on any situation so perfect agreement would not be expected, especially in an area such as quality of life, where the outside observer's access is clearly limited. Nevertheless, one should expect at least significant levels of correlation between children and adults on measures such as symptom severity.

On CAQB, the form where child and parent responses are most clearly comparable, the fact that the two informants agree about severity of illness has already been noted. In fact, in the sample of mild asthmatics cited earlier there was 88% agreement between child and parent in response to a question about severity, reported on a simple three-point scale. In a further sample of 61 children with moderate to severe asthma the correlation between scores on SEV and parents' ratings of severity was 0.43, p=0.001, remarkably similar to the earlier sample. Although concordance on the simple severity rating was poor at 47%, there was good agreement on specific events observable by both informants, such as school absences, r=0.78, p<0.001, and disturbed nights, r=0.43, p=0.001.

Sensitivity

Data on the accuracy of children's self-reports of severity and the relationship between quality of life reports and objective measures such as peak expiratory flow rates (PEFRs) are clearly important elements of the questionnaire evaluation procedure. Current data on forms A and B suggest that children's quality of life, although related to their own reports of severity (SEV) and distress (DIS), is not related to their parents' estimates of severity. Since DIS scores on CAQA and SEV scores on CAQB are moderately correlated with both parents' severity ratings and quality of life scores, it seems likely that children's responses to questions about asthma symptoms incorporate more information than other symptom scores - the children are thinking not only of whether symptoms occurred, but how limiting they were. To this extent children's scores on SEV will be moderately correlated with PEFR, and more so than quality of life, which is affected by so much more than the experience of having asthma. SEV is more than just the frequency of symptoms, it is how bad the asthma feels to the patient. Figure 4.5 represents this line of argument in diagrammatic form; whereas an observer's rating of severity is influenced just by the occurence of symptoms, the child's report of SEV also takes the resulting limitations into account. DIS scores are determined by these limitations and the unhappiness brought about by symptoms and their effects, but also by more general psychological variables such as anxiety and depression. Quality of life as an outcome measure, in this case the AQoL score, is influenced by the illness itself, psychological response to it and many non-health-related aspects of the quality of the child's life.

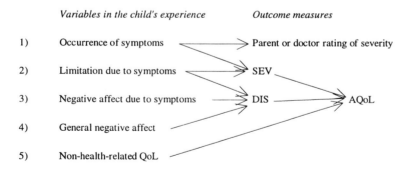

Figure 4.5 Model of variables underlying outcome measures

It is anticipated that in the near future data from clinical trials will become available to test the strength of these relationships. Variables 1) and 2) should improve with medical intervention, 3) may also do so but is more likely to change with educational intervention, 4) and 5) are not asthma-specific and therefore unlikely to change in a clinical trial. It is therefore likely that SEV, being the purest and most complete measure of those variables likely to change with a pharmaceutical intervention, will be the most sensitive measure in a clinical trial whilst DIS, less suitable in the former context owing to its potential sensitivity to a placebo effect, is potentially useful in evaluating more psychological interventions. AQoL, whilst providing important information about individual children, may vary with too many other, uncontrollable variations to be useful in clinical evaluation.

DISCUSSION

The use of the CAQs has helped the authors to clarify their ideas about the way that children perceive their asthma. These perceptions also vary with age, justifying our approach of producing three separate questionnaires. For instance, the extent to which having asthma impacts on self-image varies, with the teenagers feeling that their illness affects their social relationships whereas the younger children do not. This methodology has been associated with the generation of reliable self-reports, the validity and accuracy of which, although still under investigation, appear promising. It has also revealed important influences in the way that children's experiences are reflected in paediatric outcome measures, thus providing insight for researchers studying a wide variety of illnesses and interventions.

What, though, of the relevance for health professionals involved in the day-to-day management of paediatric asthma, seeing patients and their parents in general practice or out-patient clinic? The relevance of hard data for evaluation of the comprehensive approach to chronic disease management, taking account of interactions between biological, psychological and social factors, was noted in our opening paragraphs. It is, we would argue, just as relevant for the clinician to be able to evaluate the effects of intervention along dimensions beyond the one which reflects asthma severity. High distress scores in a youngster whose asthma is apparently well-controlled signal the need for exploration of difficulties. One source of problems for the junior school age child may be the contrast between the clinician's aim of supporting self-management and barriers to this in a school which requires medications to be held by an adult. Evidence that many teachers lack awareness of contemporary management of asthma - especially its prophylactic aspects - is now reported (Bevis and Taylor, 1990; Brookes and Jones, 1992). A junior school age child prescribed sodium cromoglycate, four times per day, in a school which restricts access to the inhaler - which may even be in a locked office in the lunch break - is anxious. And reluctance to challenge the "powerful adults" (Eiser and Havermans, 1993) may well result in an apparent lack of adherence to management plans.

Teenage asthma is notoriously difficult to deal with and recently reported audit data from a UK general practice (Hilton, 1991) indicated that 12% of its diagnosed asthmatic youngsters in the 13-16 age range were taking no medication, while, in comparison with the practice average of 50%, only 27% were taking preventative treatment. Our experience with developing the CAQC has indicated the shift in attitudes to asthma which accompany youngsters' development toward adulthood. There is evidence of greater confidence in managing (or choosing not to!) their medication, but emergent anxieties about the impact of asthma on their self-image. It matters to teenagers that an inhaler bulges in the jeans pocket, that use of it on the school bus causes comment - that they are "different". Again, a higher than expected distress score may signal the need to explore potential barriers to optimal self-management, to follow up with suggested adjustments to the regimen. The outcome from such adjustments needs to be assessed in terms of the psychosocial as well as the biomedical benefits - reductions in the distress associated with managing chronic disease, as well as increases in the benefit from recent decades' advances in medication.

The problems of developing paediatric outcome measures have been indicated above, but the benefits are, we suggest, potentially substantial. Our own work has crossed a number of professional boundaries and drawn upon a range of expertise. Central to the production of the CAQs has been the input from developmental, educational and cognitive psychology, coupled with skills of psychometrics. Further, we have had continuous support from health professionals, both those at the coal-face of paediatric asthma management and clinical practice, and those involved in the management of clinical research. Such skill-mix and collaboration can overcome the difficulties associated with developing comprehensive paediatric outcome measurement which is "not only a critical building block for good science, it is a critical component in good patient care" (Johnson, 1991).

REFERENCES

Achenbach, T.M., McConaughy, S.H. and Howell, C.T. (1987) Child/adolescent behavioural and emotional problems: implications of cross-informant correlations for situational specificity. *Psychological Bulletin,* **101,** 213-232.

Beitchman, J.H. and Corradini, A. (1988) Self-report measures for use with children: a review and comment. *Journal of Clinical Psychology,* **44,** 477-490.

Bevis, M. and Taylor, B. (1990) What do school teachers know about asthma? *Archives of Disease in Childhood,* **65,** 622-625.

Bradley, C., Home, P. and Christie, M.J. (1991) Evaluating new technologies: psychological issues in research design and measurement. In: Bradley, C., Home, P. and Christie, M.J. (Eds.), *The technology of diabetes care: converging medical and psychosocial perspectives*. Chur: Harwood.

Brittain, R.T. (1990) Approaches to a long-acting, selective β_2-adrenoceptor stimulant. *Lung*, **168 (suppl)**, 111-114.

Brookes, J. and Jones, K. (1992) Schoolteachers' perceptions and knowledge of asthma in primary school children. *British Journal of General Practice*, **42**, 504-507.

Culross, R.R. (1985) Adaptation of the Pictorial Self-Concept Scale to measure self-concept in young hearing-impaired children. *Language, Speech, and Hearing Services in Schools*, **16**, 132-134.

Department of Health (1991) *The health of the nation: a consultative document for health in England*. London: HMSO.

Eiser, C. and Havermans, T. (1995) Knowledge and attitudes as determinants of "quality of life" in children with asthma. In: Christie, M.J. and French, D.J. (Eds.), *The assessment of quality of life in childhood asthma*. Chur: Harwood.

Eiser, C., Town, C. and Tripp, J.H. (1987) Mother's understanding of allergen induced asthma. *Early Child Development and Care*, **28**, 13-20.

Flanery, R.C. (1990) Methodological and psychometric considerations in child reports. In: La Greca, A.M. (Ed.), *Through the eyes of the child: obtaining self-reports from children and adolescents*. Boston: Allyn and Bacon.

Friedman, W.J. (1990) Children's representations of the pattern of daily activities. *Child Development*, **61**, 1399-1412.

Fritz, G.K., Klein, R.B. and Overholser, J.C. (1990) Accuracy of symptom perception in childhood asthma. *Developmental and Behavioral Pediatrics*, **11**, 69-72.

Gillespie, D. (1990) Let's listen to the children! National Asthma Campaign Henry Blair Prize Essay. *Asthma News*, **23**, 5.

Harter, S. (1990) Issues in the assessment of the self-concept of children and adolescents. In: La Greca, A.M. (Ed.), *Through the eyes of the child: obtaining self-reports from children and adolescents*. Boston: Allyn and Bacon.

Harter, S. and Pike, R. (1984) The pictorial scale of perceived competence and social acceptance for young children. *Child Development*, **55**, 1969-1982.

Hilton, S. (1991) Report on National Asthma Campaign 'Asthma in Teenagers' Workshop. 2-3.

Hilton, S. (1995) Management of childhood asthma in general practice. In: Christie, M.J. and French, D.J. (Eds.), *The assessment of quality of life in childhood asthma*. Chur: Harwood.

Hyland, M. (1991a) The Living with Asthma questionnaire. *Respiratory Medicine*, **85 (Suppl B)**, 13-16.

Hyland, M. (1991b) Panel discussant. *Respiratory Medicine*, **85 (Suppl B)**, 34.

Hyland, M., Finnis, S. and Irvine, S.H. (1991) A scale for assessing quality of life in adult asthma sufferers. *Journal of Psychosomatic Research*, **35**, 99-110.

Johnson, S.B. (1991) Methodological considerations in pediatric behavioral research: measurement. *Developmental and Behavioral Pediatrics*, **12**, 361-369.

Johnson, S.B., Silverstein, J., Rosenbloom, A., Carter, R. and Cunningham, W. (1986) Assessing daily management in childhood diabetes. *Health Psychology*, **5**, 545-564.

Jones, P.W. (1991) Panel discussant. *Respiratory Medicine*, **85 (Suppl B)**, 34.

Kazdin, A.E. and Petti, T.A. (1982) Self-report and interview measures of childhood and adolescent depression. *Journal of Child Psychology and Psychiatry*, **23**, 437-457.

La Greca, A.M. (1990) Issues and perspectives on the child assessment process. In: La Greca, A.M. (Ed.), *Through the eyes of the child: obtaining self-reports from children and adolescents*. Boston: Allyn and Bacon.

Lomas, J., Pickard, L. and Mohide, A. (1987) Patient versus clinician item generation for quality of life measures. *Medical Care*, **25**, 764-769.

Martini, D.R., Strayhorn, J.M. and Puig-Antich, J. (1990) A symptom self-report measure for preschool children. *Journal of the American Academy of Child and Adolescent Psychiatry*, **29**, 594-600.

Piaget, J. (1969) *The child's conception of time*. London: RKP.

Pearson, R. (1990) *Asthma management in primary care*. Oxford: Radcliffe.

Rosenbaum, P., Cadman, D. and Kirpalani, H. (1990) Pediatrics: assessing quality of life. In: Spilker, B. (Ed.), *Quality of life assessments in clinical trials*. New York: Raven.

Schipper, H., Clinch, J. and Powell, V. (1990) Definitions and conceptual issues. In: Spiker, B. (Ed.), *Quality of life assessments in clinical trials*. New York: Raven.

Shillitoe, R.W. (1988) *Psychology and diabetes: psychosocial factors in management and control*. London: Chapman and Hall.

Shillitoe, R.W. and Christie, M.J. (1988) Psychosocial and biomedical contributions to the holistic management of diabetes mellitus. *Holistic Medicine*, **3**, 205-211.

Smiley, P. and Huttenlocher, J. (1989). Young children's acquisition of emotion concepts. In: Saarni, C. and Harris, P.L. (Eds.), *Children's understanding of emotion*. Cambridge: Cambridge University Press.

Staudenmayer, H. (1982) Medical manageability and psychosocial factors in childhood asthma. *Journal of Chronic Disease*, **35**, 183-198.

Stone, W.L. and Lemanek, K.L. (1990) Developmental issues in children's self-reports. In: La Greca, A.M. (Ed.), *Through the eyes of the child: obtaining self-reports from children and adolescents*. Boston: Allyn and Bacon.

Upchurch, F. and McCullough, S. (1995) Measurement of inputs and outcomes: an industry perspective. In: Christie, M.J. and French, D.J. (Eds) *The assessment of quality of life in childhood asthma*. Chur: Harwood.

Usherwood, T.P., Scrimgeour, A. and Barber, J.H. (1990) Questionnaire to measure perceived symptoms and disability in asthma. *Archives of Disease in Childhood*, **65**, 779-781.

Walker, L.S. and Green, J.W. (1991) The Functional Disability Inventory: measuring a neglected dimension of child health status. *Journal of Pediatric Psychology*, **16**, 39-58.

Weist, R.M. (1989) Time concepts in language and thought: filling the Piagetian void from two to five years. In: Levin, I. and Zakay, D. (Eds) *Time and human cognition: a life-span perspective*. Amsterdam: Elsevier Science Publishers.

Westman, A.S. (1989) Development of time concepts: differentiating clock and calendar from apparent durations. *Journal of Genetic Psychology*, **148**, 259-270.

Chapter 5 _____

AN ECONOMIC PERSPECTIVE ON HEALTH OUTCOME MEASUREMENT

JOHN BRAZIER AND JOHN CAIRNS

INTRODUCTION

The measurement and valuation of changes in the quantity and quality of individuals' lives is a central concern of health economics. Such information is an important element in health care decision-making, not only at the aggregate level for purchasers and providers but also at the individual level for patients and clinicians. The development of formal purchasing through contracts in the United Kingdom (UK) National Health Service (NHS) and elsewhere, and the increased emphasis on the importance of a patient-centred approach to decision-making, has been particularly important in contributing to the interest in measuring health outcomes. It is, however, a controversial area, partly because of concerns over the use to which such information might be put by those making choices in resource allocation, and partly because of the complex and largely subjective nature of the concept of "quality of life".

Our aim is to promote dialogue with other disciplines and with potential users of health outcomes information. To this end, we set out the reason for the economists' interest in outcome assessment and the characteristics which are required for economic evaluation. A critical review of the appropriateness for use in economic evaluation of two existing measures (Barthel Rating Scale and Medical Outcomes Study SF-36) explains economists' dissatisfaction with many existing measures. The conventional psychometric notions of reliability and validity are assessed from an economic perspective. Economists have been associated particularly with Quality Adjusted Life Years (QALYs), but in this chapter we show that the contribution of economics to health outcome measurement extends far beyond this one particular concept.

THE INTEREST IN MEASURING HEALTH OUTCOMES

For Patients

Economics involves making decisions. Decisions to pursue one course of action invariably result in a sacrifice of other actions, thus, for example, the decision to jog for 20 minutes a day will leave less time for pursuing other activities. This weighing up of costs and benefits involves very personal judgements, which in the case of jogging will include the value of any supposed health benefits against the risks and the discomfort of the activity. Decisions about the consumption of most goods and services including time spent jogging are usually left to individuals to choose, since they are regarded as being in the best position to judge the costs and benefits to themselves. For health care, this assumption is questioned since consumers (patients) have inadequate information on the benefits and risks of health care (Mooney, 1986). An important role for measures of health outcome is to provide information in order to help people make these choices. Economists seek explicitly to build outcome measures which are rooted in individuals' preferences.

For Clinicians

Professionals play an important part in health care decision-making. They are concerned with the effectiveness of a treatment, which is often determined by its effects on biomedical indicators, such as blood pressure and respiratory function, and symptoms. Their main interest is in establishing efficacy and therefore they require measures which are reliable and sensitive to "clinically" significant health change across individuals or groups within a clinical trial (Guyatt *et al.*, 1987). They tend to be less interested in the values underlying such measures, and are often ill-equipped to trade-off the risks and costs with the benefits of treatment.

For Policy Makers

All health care systems are faced with the problem of scarce resources, and thus choices have to be made. For instance, decisions are made whether to prioritise patients waiting for treatment on the basis of first-come, first-served, on the ability to benefit, or even on the ability to pay (via private health insurance). This is not exclusively a problem for governments. In the United States, insurance companies and large businesses (the main payers of premiums) have also been concerned with cost containment. Benefit to the patient or effectiveness of treatment are becoming important criteria for funding services, and an important constituent of these would be improvements in health and survival. In the NHS, purchasers of health care in the form of District Health Authorities and fundholding family doctors are seeking to promote the health gain of their residential or practice population (Department of Health, 1992).

While the techniques developed by economists have been utilised in patient and clinical decision-making, health outcome measurement in economics has focused on conducting economic evaluations to inform decisions about resource allocation, such as choices between alternative treatments, or choices between different areas of spending.

HEALTH OUTCOMES IN ECONOMIC EVALUATION

Economic evaluation assesses the value for money from different interventions or, to be more technical, economists attempt to assess the efficiency of an intervention and its consequences for equity (Drummond, 1980 and Drummond *et al.*, 1987). There are two distinct forms of efficiency:

1) *Operational efficiency*, or *technical efficiency*, refers to the way in which different inputs are combined to produce a given output. An efficient allocation of resources is one which minimises the cost of producing a specified outcome or a given objective. For example, the efficiency of alternative methods of screening can be compared in terms of costs per breast cancer case detected, or costs per life year saved. This type of assessment is called cost-effectiveness analysis (CEA). A related technique which has been developed specifically to evaluate health care interventions is cost-utility analysis (CUA); this involves the evaluation and comparison of the relative costs of interventions (usually in money terms) and their relative utility. Neither CEA nor CUA question whether the activity is worthwhile compared with other uses of the resources.

2) *Allocative efficiency*, on the other hand, concerns the mix of outputs. It is achieved when it is impossible (with a given level of resources) to produce a mix of outputs which is more highly valued than the current one. Thus information is required on the value of the benefits as well as cost. Such an assessment is undertaken in cost-benefit analysis (CBA), where all the benefits of an intervention are valued in money terms so as to make them comparable with costs.

We now consider in more detail the requirements of these three techniques (CEA, CUA and CBA) with respect to outcome measures.

Cost-Effectiveness Analysis (CEA)

The simplest cases are where the interventions have a single and readily measurable outcome so that interventions can then be compared in terms of cost per unit of outcome. Typically, the analyst would choose an outcome measured in "natural" units, such as the number of cases of breast cancer detected or life years saved, where there has been no valuation of the outcome. It would be possible to use a measure of health status, such as the Barthel Rating Scale, and derive a cost per score improvement, but an economist would be extremely cautious of using such a measure in this way without testing the values which underlie it. (We look critically at the Barthel Rating Scale from an economic perspective in the next section.)

One particular problem is that for economic purposes measures of outcome should be at a minimum *ordinal,* and ideally should be *interval scales.* In this context, ordinality implies that a higher score would always indicate a less desirable health state and a lower score would always indicate a more desirable one (where zero or a low score indicates the absence of ill health, symptoms, disability etc.). Interval scales, in addition to being ordinal, have the attribute that the differences between points on the scale can be meaningfully compared. For example, using the Fahrenheit scale of temperature, the difference between 80° and 70° is half the difference between 80° and 60°. Note, however, that it is not the case that 80° is twice as hot as 40°. The latter comparison requires a scale with *ratio* properties where the zero point denotes absence of the quality being measured; length or temperature in degrees Kelvin are good examples. For allocative purposes, economists generally require an interval measure of health so that different improvements in health can be related to their cost and then compared with one another.

A more complex comparison is between interventions which perform differently across a range of health outcomes, for example symptom control, functional health status and magnitude of side-effects. There is no problem if one intervention clearly dominates another, for instance, where an intervention costs less, but achieves the same or greater improvements across all the health outcomes; or when it costs the same but achieves more on at least one health outcome while the others are not affected adversely. Nonetheless, even in these cases of dominance, the health outcome measures must have ordinal properties.

In practice, however, one intervention will not dominate all others, or if it does, it will also cost more. In the treatment of many common conditions, for example, there is often a choice between surgical and medical interventions. Surgery may alleviate the adverse symptoms of a condition for most individuals, but may entail the risk of complications and even mortality, and can be very debilitating in the short-term for all patients. In contrast, medical interventions may be less effective in terms of symptom relief but may be associated with less risk. There is a trade-off not only between different aspects of quality of life, such as the short-term consequences of surgery for physical mobility and pain and its greater long-term effectiveness, but also its risk of mortality. For the patient, this can be a difficult choice, and for the purchaser of health care, these factors should influence the overall value of treatment by surgery compared with medicine. To address these questions requires a different form of analysis; a means whereby the different dimensions of outcome can be aggregated to a single measure (with interval properties). This brings us to the approach of Cost-Utility Analysis.

Cost-Utility Analysis (CUA)

The use of monetary valuations of outcomes in the health care field has generally not been popular with economists, at least in the UK. This is partly a result of the absence of meaningful price data in situations when health care is free at the point of use. Health economists have therefore developed CUA where the benefits are assessed solely in terms of health, and are measured on a single scale which combines improvements in survival with health-related quality of life. CUA seeks to combine these different health consequences into a single scale in order to compare interventions in terms of cost per Quality Adjusted Life Year (QALY) or other unit of "utility". Although the term CUA suggests that the outcome of interest is change in utility as a result of an intervention, most QALYs do not measure utility *per se* but rather the health improvement from health care. Some economists have advocated using the cost per QALY of health care programmes as a guide to resource allocation (Williams, 1985). However, there are a number of criticisms of QALYs as measures of health benefit.

There are many techniques used in economics for deriving QALYs, which attempt to estimate peoples' preferences for different states of health (see Torrance, 1986 for review), and these costs yield different results. There are important ethical questions about whose values should be sought, and how they should be weighted in deriving the overall QALY. The requirements for such a measure include the conventional psychometric concerns of reliability, and its possession of interval properties. When comparing treatments for the same condition it might be appropriate to have a condition-specific measure of health gain, but comparisons of the benefits of treatment between conditions requires a single-index generic measure of health.[*]

In order to measure the consequences of an intervention in terms of utility it would be necessary to take individuals' risk and time preferences into account. For example, consider two treatments with the same expected outcome for a terminally ill patient; treatment A has a 90% chance of extending survival by two years and with treatment B there is a 20% chance of an extra nine years. The expected outcome of the two treatments is 1.8 years of extra life, but they need not be viewed as being equally desirable in the eyes of the patient (or anyone else), since the patient's preference between the two will depend on their attitude to risk.

In clinical trials, the conventional analyses of quality of life data assume that the value of health is independent of time. Time preference is an important factor since people usually prefer to have benefits sooner rather than later and, it has been argued, this applies to health as much as to other more tangible benefits. The conventional way of treating this time preference is by discounting future benefits

---

[*]Readers interested in examining the techniques which have been used by economists are referred to Torrance, 1986 for a general review, and on specific instruments to Torrance, 1976; Williams, 1985; EuroQol, 1990; Kaplan and Anderson, 1990; and Mehrez and Gafni, 1991.

(as well as costs) at a particular rate such as 6% per annum (Drummond, 1980). The appropriateness of this procedure for health, however, has been questioned, since a person's time preference for health and money may be quite different. Time can also affect the value of health via duration of experience (Torrance, 1986). It has been suggested that people adapt to health-related difficulties, and this can offset some of the disability. In contrast, it has been found that, in the case of haemodialysis, utility declines with duration (Sackett and Torrance, 1978). There are obviously important empirical concerns to resolve.

Cost-Benefit Analysis (CBA)

When the question of interest concerns the worth of one activity compared with alternative uses of the resources, a different form of analysis is required. QALY "league tables" have sometimes been used as a guide to allocating resources between competing health care programmes. However, this approach is subject to the criticisms set out above. CBA permits an explicit weighing of the costs and all the benefits of an activity. It is relevant where there are a range of different benefits associated with an intervention, since it tries to value all benefits, including health gain, on a single dimension (money).

Because of the absence of markets in health care, or more precisely, the absence of markets where transactions take place at prices indicating the marginal value of the health care to the consumer, it is difficult to place monetary valuations on the health or other benefits resulting from different interventions. One technique which has yet to be widely used, but which is increasing in popularity, is willingness-to-pay. Its use does not eliminate the need for descriptions of health outcomes but it may offer a means of incorporating a wider range of benefits into the analysis.

A REVIEW OF TWO MEASURES FOR ECONOMIC EVALUATION

To demonstrate the problems of using existing health measures in an economic evaluation we have chosen two well-known and widely used measures, the Barthel Rating Scale, which is a measure of disability, and a generic health profile measure, the Medical Outcomes Study SF-36.

Barthel Rating Scale (BRS)

The Barthel Index was developed in 1965 (Mahoney and Barthel) and was modified by Granger et al. (1979) to comprise the Barthel Rating Scale. It was originally intended for use in clinical practice to assess independence in patients with neuromuscular or musculoskeletal disorders; more recently, its target population has been extended to a wider range of patients and it has been used to assess needs for services, predict outcome, and evaluate services. It is a measure of disability, and has ten items covering activities such as continence, grooming, mobility and dressing. Patients are rated by health professionals on each item using detailed instructions provided by the developers of the measure (Mahoney and Barthel, 1965; Granger *et al.*, 1979). The scoring system is intended to reflect the time given to assist patients in each of the disabilities, and scores range from 0 (worst possible state) to 100. There have been numerous revisions, but the basic method has remained unchanged.

This index is not well suited for use in economic evaluation. It covers only one dimension of health (i.e. disability) and unless other aspects of health are unaffected by the interventions it will not describe overall effects on health. The use of professional assessment can create problems of bias unless the observers are independent. The derivation of the scoring system is a further limitation. The scores reflect the consequences for care, not the impact and importance of different disabilities to the patient. Independent in walking scores 15, whilst bathing scores only 5 because it is a less frequent activity and overall takes up less time for staff (Wilkin *et al.*, 1992). However, to a patient, being independent in bathing may be regarded as a more important ability. This raises major doubts about the ordinal properties of this measure in terms of patient preference. To be used in economic evaluation, the original unscored response data would need to be entirely revalued.

But even such a revalued scale would be of limited usefulness in that the BRS will only ever be applicable to a subset of conditions and thus could not be used generally to inform decision-making between different areas of health care.

Medical Outcomes Study SF-36
The SF-36 is a standardised, generic health status measure, designed for self-completion (Ware and Sherbourne, 1992). It contains 36 items, which cover eight dimensions of health (including physical functioning, pain and mental health). Each dimension is scored separately. The scoring of items assumes an equal interval between each potential response (e.g. not limited at all is 3, limited a little is 2 and limited a lot is 1). These item scores are summed so that each is given an equal weight, and the result is transformed to yield a scale from 0 (worst health) to 100 (best health) for each dimension.

To be used in CEA, the scales must at least be ordinal. In the case of some dimensions, such as pain and social functioning, this seems to be achieved because they have only two items and there is little scope for conflict. In the larger and more complex dimensions, such as physical functioning (5 items) and mental health (5 items), the case for ordinality is less convincing. For example, in the physical functioning dimension, a person "limited a lot in lifting or carrying groceries" receives the same score as another person "limited a lot in climbing several flights of stairs". Yet patients may regard one as far more disabling than another. SF-36 dimension scores must therefore be interpreted with caution in the context of economic evaluations.

Situations where changes in the dimension scores are in conflict present further problems of interpretation. A ten-point change in one dimension is not comparable with another dimension, since the scores do not have any obvious intuitive meaning. A simple question on whether a patient's health (in their view) has improved following treatment would be easier to interpret. The scores could be combined into a single index using arbitrary weights, as has been done for the Nottingham Health Profile (O'Brien *et al.*, 1987). However, this is not a valid procedure for use in CEA or CUA. The required single index will not have interval properties and may not even be ordinal if it has been constructed using arbitrary weights. Explicit valuation procedures should be used in order to ensure a scale has the necessary measurement properties.

The SF-36 is not designed to derive a single measure of health. The main problem is a lack of ordinality between the items within each dimension, and as a result it is extremely difficult to apply conventional valuation techniques (Brazier, 1993). As a consequence, most economists have preferred to develop their own instruments.

ECONOMICS AND PSYCHOMETRICS

This discussion of the Barthel Rating Scale and the SF-36 reflects the focus of economic research: the values underpinning different measures. In contrast, the psychometric literature has often been primarily concerned with item response patterns and correlation (Streiner and Norman, 1989). There are well established tests to examine the reliability of an instrument in terms of its repeatability between observers, methods of administration and responsiveness to change. These are important measurement characteristics which have sometimes been neglected in economics research (Carr-Hill and Morris, 1991).

The health descriptions used in QALYs have been rightly criticised for their insensitivity and irrelevance for many diseases (Carr-Hill and Morris, 1991; Wilkin *et al.*, 1992). However, testing the "validity" of the values or scores generated by an instrument is more problematic. It is generally accepted that there is no "gold standard" for measuring health. In psychometrics, one approach is to examine *construct* validity; that is, a measure is judged by its ability to produce an expected distribution of scores, such as by age, income or diagnostic category. Economists have been reluctant to examine many of the usual forms of construct validity, such as those based on agreement with clinical diagnosis. Using clinical judgements implies a degree of circularity, when the purpose of assessing the quality of life consequences of treatments is to introduce values other than those of doctors. Another test in psychometrics is the ability of a measure to predict health service use. While the use of health care may be correlated to some extent with health-related quality of life (HRQL), the relationship tends to be weak due to variations both on the demand and supply side (e.g. attendance at Accident and Emergency has been found to be closely related to accessibility).

Validity, in economists' terms, is concerned with whether values in a measure truly reflect the preferences of patients, society or whoever's values are regarded as relevant. The valuation techniques used by economists have been criticised for being too hypothetical and out of context (e.g. interview). One approach to testing the validity of valuations elicited in a hypothetical setting is assessed by whether these stated preferences correspond with those revealed by observable choices. Therefore, if a HRQL instrument suggests one treatment would be preferred to another (assuming all else is constant) then this could be tested by examining the informed decision of patients facing the choice between treatments. In willingness to pay, the hypothetical values for injury states would be compared with, for example, the money spent on safety devices for cars. In practice, it can be difficult to find market decisions where health consequences are the only consideration.

Many of these concerns about validity are raised by other health measures such as the SF-36. Simply ignoring valuation issues does not mean they have been avoided. For example, the focus on the mean score changes, and not the distribution of those outcomes (except for the estimation of statistical significance), involves an overly narrow perspective when evaluating, say, high risk surgical procedures.

CONCLUSION

The reasons for patients', clinicians' and purchasers' need for measures of outcome are very different, but for all of them values play a central role. Throughout, we have tried to emphasise the central role of individuals' preference in the economist's approach. The fundamental criticism of many measures of health is that they fail to be explicit regarding their underlying values. Condition-specific measures such as the BRS and generic profile measures such as the SF-36 have only limited roles in economic evaluation. The values underlying these measures are not based on patient and societal values. The scores are in units of measurement which are difficult to interpret since there is no numeraire for comparing between dimensions or between measures.

Economists have tended to focus on the use of outcome measures in resource allocation and purchasing through the application of economic evaluation. At the simplest level, the operational efficiency of treatment A can be assessed on whether it is able to dominate treatment B in terms of health outcomes and cost. But even this requires that the scores generated by a measure be at least ordinal, which has not been demonstrated for many existing measures. More commonly, decision-making requires a measure to have an interval scale, which combines the different dimensions into a single index, otherwise there is no basis for establishing whether treatment A is better overall than treatment B. For this reason economists have tended to develop their own measures. Nonetheless, for economists to make the most of existing research, they need to consider ways of using the data generated by measures such as the BRS and SF-36.

The contribution of economics extends beyond QALYs, to provide a critical perspective which can be applied to the whole field of outcome measurement. To make significant progress in this area requires a multi-disciplinary approach. We hope by highlighting the economic perspective to encourage such work.

REFERENCES

Brazier, J.E. (1993) The SF-36 Health Survey Questionnaire: a tool for economists. *Health Economics*, **2**, 213-215.

Carr-Hill, R. and Morris, J. (1991) Current practice in obtaining the "Q" in QALYs: a cautionary note. *British Medical Journal*, **303**, 699-701.

Department of Health (1992) *The health of the nation: a strategy for health in England.* London: HMSO. (Cm. 1986)

Drummond, M.F. (1980) *Principles of economic appraisal in health care.* Oxford: Oxford University Press.

Drummond, M.F., Stoddart, G.L. and Torrance, G.W. (1987) *Methods for the economic evaluation of health care programmes.* Oxford: Oxford Medical Publications.

The EuroQol Group (1990) EuroQol: a new facility for the measurement of health related quality of life. *Health Policy*, **16** (3), 199-208.

Granger, C.V., Dewis, L.G., Peter, N.C., Sherwood, C.C. and Barrett, J.E. (1979) Stroke rehabilitation: analysis of repeated Barthel Index Measures. *Archives of Physical Medicine and Rehabilitation*, **60**, 14-17.

Guyatt, G., Walter, S. and Norman, G. (1987) Measuring change over time: assessing the usefulness of evaluative instruments. *Journal of Chronic Diseases*, **40**, 171-178.

Kaplan, R.M. and Anderson, J.P. (1990) The General Health Policy Model: an integrated approach. In: Spilker, B. (Ed), *Quality of life assessments in clinical trials.* New York: Raven Press Ltd.

Mahoney, F.I. and Barthel, D.W. (1965) Functional evaluation: the Barthel Index. *Maryland State Medical Journal*, **14**, 61-5.

Mehrez, A. and Gafni, A. (1991) The healthy-years equivalent: how to measure them using the standard gamble approach. *Medical Decision Making*, **11**, 140-146.

Mooney, G.H. (1986) *Economics, medicine and health care.* Brighton: Wheatsheaf Books.

O'Brien, B.J., Buxton, M.J. and Ferguson, B.A. (1987) Measuring the effectiveness of heart transplant programmes: quality of life data and their relationship to survival analysis. *Journal of Chronic Diseases*, **40**, 137S-153S.

Sackett, D.L. and Torrance, G.W. (1978) The utility of different health states as perceived by the general public. *Journal of Chronic Diseases*, **31** (**11**), 697-709.

Streiner, D.L. and Norman, G.R. (1989) *Health measurement scales: a practical guide to their development and use.* Oxford: Oxford University Press.

Torrance, G.W. (1986) Measurement of health state utilities for economic appraisal. *Journal of Health Economics*, **5**, 1-30.

Torrance, G.W. (1976) Social preferences for health states: an empirical evaluation of three measurement techniques. *Socio-Economic Planning Sciences*, **10** (3), 128-136.

Ware, J.E., Jr. and Sherbourne, C.D. (1992) The MOS 36-Item Short-Form Health Status Survey. I: Conceptual framework and item selection. *Medical Care,* **30**, 473-483.

Wilkin, D., Hallam, L. and Doggett, M.A. (1992) *Measures of need and outcome for primary health care*. Oxford: Oxford Medical Publications.

Williams, A. (1985) Economics of coronary artery bypass grafting. *British Medical Journal*, **291**, 326-329.

Chapter 6

TAKING A PATIENT-CENTRED APPROACH TO OUTCOME MEASUREMENT

ANDREW M GARRATT AND DANNY A RUTA

INTRODUCTION

Improving quality of life has become a main focus of interest in clinical research. In most studies, however, instruments purporting to measure quality of life fail to provide any underpining definition or conceptual basis for the construct; they usually comprise a number of dimensions that have been criticised for being much narrower than quality of life (van Dam *et al.*, 1981; Bergner, 1989; Siegrist and Junge, 1989). Although the term "quality of life measure" is used in the literature, the vast majority of instruments actually measure health status or health-related quality of life.

The measures that are available often share similar dimensions of interest including, for example, physical functioning, role limitations, symptoms, and general perceptions of health (Bergner *et al.*, 1981; Hunt *et al.*, 1985; Ware and Sherbourne, 1992). The choice of dimensions and the values attached to them are imposed on the individual. Not only will these different dimensions have different meanings to individuals but the values they place on changes in them will differ as well. A high level of physical functioning, for example, while of great importance to a marathon runner, may have little value for someone with a sedentary lifestyle. Similarly, an improvement in physical function could mean the difference between a silver and a gold medal for the former while the latter may not even notice this improvement. Quality of life, then, could be said to mean different things to different people (Bulpitt and Fletcher, 1990) or, as Ziller (1974) has suggested, quality of life is in the eye of the beholder.

Calman (1984) has also suggested that quality of life can only be measured in individual terms. He defines quality of life as "the extent to which our hopes and ambitions are matched by experience" and suggests that a key aim of medical care should be "to narrow the gap between a patient's hopes and expectations and what actually happens." According to this definition, quality of life is a dynamic concept that can be enhanced by bringing reality and expectations closer together. This definition of quality of life has been employed before in the field of clinical research (Cohen, 1982; Presant, 1984; Dupuis, 1988; Nordenfelt, 1989).

In this chapter, Calman's definition of quality of life is used to form the conceptual basis for a patient-centred measure of outcome, the Patient Generated Index (PGI) of quality of life. The development of the PGI is described along with some examples of how an individualised quality of life assessment is derived from patients. Finally, the findings of a large study in which the PGI was administered to patients with low back pain are reported and the implications for its use in the evaluation of medical care are discussed.

MEASURING QUALITY OF LIFE: THE PATIENT GENERATED INDEX

Building on Calman's definition, we produced a measure that attempts to quantify the difference between individuals' hopes and expectations and reality in a way that has meaning and relevance in the context of their daily lives. Such a measure must possess three properties. First, it must allow individuals to *choose* the areas of their lives that they consider to be of the greatest importance. Secondly, it should allow individuals to *quantify* the extent to which reality matches expectations in their chosen areas. Thirdly, it must allow individuals to *assess* the relative importance of their chosen areas. In addition, if the measure is to have practical application, it must be acceptable and satisfy the psychometric criteria of validity and reliability (Streiner and Norman, 1989). Finally, if the measure is to have the evaluative potential of an outcome measure, it must also be responsive to changes in quality of life over time, and staying within our overall construct of quality of life, it should allow individuals to value those changes. In developing the PGI we hoped to devise a measure of quality of life specific to the individual while still retaining the attributes identified above.

The PGI was derived from two techniques developed in unrelated fields. In developing a condition-specific measure for clinical trials in chronic respiratory disease, Guyatt *et al.* (1987a) observed that the activities affected by dyspnoea varied widely among patients. To produce a measure that had relevance to the individual, patients were asked to list important aspects of their lives affected by their breathing difficulties, with the aid of a trigger list to assist recall. From these they were then asked to choose the five most important aspects, which constituted the domains for measuring the effect of dyspnoea on quality of life, and to rate how badly affected they were in each area. The second technique, the Priority Evaluator Method, was developed by Hoinville (1977) and has been used by town planners to take account of the preferences of future residents. Subjects are faced with a set of features, such as garden size, parking facilities and shopping amenities, and are asked to choose between them by performing trade-offs. For example, some subjects may be willing to forego a large garden in order to have a parking space for their car.

The PGI can be self- or interview-administered and is completed in three stages. These are shown in Table 6.1 using the responses of a 30-year-old man with low back pain as an example. Following Guyatt's method (1987a), in stage one a. patient is asked to specify the five most important areas of his life affected by the index condition, in this case low back pain. Respondents are told that these aspects might be small and personal to themselves; for example, they may have difficulty playing with their children or the pain might be a continual worry in the back of their mind. If a patient is unable to think of five areas of his/her life affected by his/her condition, a trigger list of the aspects most frequently mentioned by other sufferers of the same condition is provided; the triggers will have been derived through a series of interviews with patients. If a respondent feels that less than five aspects of his/her life are affected by the index condition, the instructions are to write "none" in the remaining boxes.

In stage two, the respondent is asked to rate how badly affected he/she is in each of the nominated areas; a scale of zero to 100 is used, where zero represents the worst state that the patient can imagine for him/herself and 100 represents exactly as he/she would like to be (Table 6.1). A sixth box is provided to enable him/her to rate all other aspects of his/her life affected by the index condition but not important enough to be included in the top five boxes, as well as areas of life which might be unrelated to that condition or even to his/her health in general. The second column of Table 6.1 shows that this respondent's five nominated areas, particularly his work, are considerably affected by his back pain; however, he has few complaints about the remainder of his life which is quite close to how he would like it to be.

In the third and final stage, using Hoinville's approach (1977), the respondent is asked to imagine that he/she can improve some or all of the chosen aspects of his/her life. Sixty "points" are supplied and the respondent is invited to "spend" these on those aspects of his/her life that he/she would most like to improve. The points can be allocated to one or more of the six listed areas (i.e. the five nominated aspects of life affected by the index condition and "the rest"). Patients are asked to imagine that areas receiving no points remain the same. The points given to each aspect are taken to represent the relative importance of potential improvements in that area. In Table 6.1, although the respondent's ability to play with his children is less affected than his work, he places greater value on an improvement in the former and hence gives this area more points. To generate the index, the ratings for each aspect of life are multiplied by the proportion of points given to that aspect and totalled, resulting in a score between zero and 100 (in this case, 45). Following Calman's definition, this score is designed to represent the extent to which reality falls short of patients' hopes and expectations, especially in those aspects of life that are affected by the index condition and in which they would most value an improvement.

Table 6.1 Stages in the completion of the Patient Generated Index

			Stage 1 *Area of activity*	*Stage 2* *Score* *out of* *100*		*Stage 3* *Spend* *your* *points*	*Stage 4* *Total* *score*
100	Exactly as you would like to be	1	Work suffers	10	X	10/60	= 1.7
90	Close to how you would like to be	2	Makes me moody	30	X	10/60	= 5.0
80	Very good but not how you would like to be	3	Always thinking	30	X	5/60	= 2.5
70	Good but not how you would like to be	4	Can't play with kids	50	X	20/60	= 16.7
60	Between fair and good	5	My sex life suffers	70	X	10/60	= 11.7
50	Fair	6	ALL OTHER ASPECTS OF	90	X	5/60	= 7.5
40	Between fair and poor		YOUR LIFE NOT MENTIONED				
30	Poor but not the worst you could imagine		ABOVE				
20	Very poor but not the worst you could imagine						
10	Close to the worst you could imagine						
0	The worst you could imagine						45.0

Figure 6.1 shows a breakdown of the PGI for two women suffering from varicose veins, aged 30 and 37 respectively. Although both patients achieve the same PGI score of 40, the bar chart serves to highlight the differences in the aspects affected by their varicose veins, the extent to which they are affected, and the values that they attach to improving each area. The two patients share certain areas, such as feeling tired, but even here are affected to a different extent. Patient

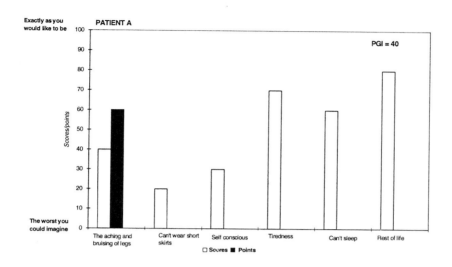

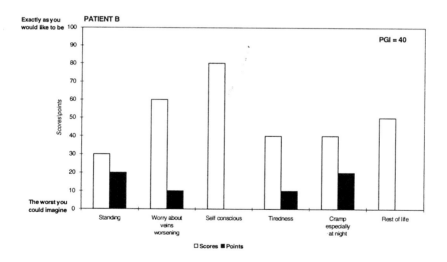

Figure 6.1   Quality of life for two varicose veins patients

A allocates a score of 70 to "tiredness", while patient B allocates a score of 40, suggesting that patient B is further from her personal ideal in this aspect of life. They also have different priorities with respect to desired improvements, as indicated by differences in allocation of points to potential improvements. Patient A allocates all of her 60 points to removing the aching and bruising of her legs, while patient B distributes her points more evenly across her chosen aspects.

Figure 6.2 shows the PGI for a 64-year-old woman with low back pain when she first presented to her general practitioner, and again after one year. At baseline, she assigns low scores to all aspects of life, both the areas nominated as being affected by the index condition and the rest of her life. She distributes points across all six aspects of life, giving the greatest share (one third of her points) to improving her tiredness; this results in a total score of 27.5. After a year, two of her nominated aspects remain the same, namely "gardening" and "lifting her grandchild"; however, her scores out of 100 for these aspects have more than doubled, suggesting that she is less badly affected in these areas than previously. At baseline, this patient had indicated that she "cannot go out much"; one year later she identifies "dancing" and "walking far" as areas affected by her back pain. It could well be that she no longer has the same difficulties "going out" and has been able to change her lifestyle to encompass new pursuits, albeit activities that are badly affected by her back pain. Initially, this patient valued an improvement in her tiredness most highly, giving it a third of her 60 points. After a year this no longer represents an important area; indeed it is not even nominated as one of the five areas affected by her back pain. Moreover, an improvement in the area replacing "tiredness" in her second PGI - i.e. "dancing" - is not valued at all and hence is not allocated any points. Instead, despite the improvement in the patient's ability to play with her grandchild and to do the gardening, she allocates these activities an extra 15 points. These changes have the net effect of increasing the patient's PGI score from 27.5 to 49.2 over the year; in other words the gap between expectations and reality has narrowed.

ASSESSING THE PGI IN LOW BACK PAIN PATIENTS

The acceptability, validity, reliability and responsiveness of the PGI was assessed by administering it through a postal questionnaire to low back pain patients identified in general practices and hospital out-patient departments within Grampian. The questionnaire was sent out to patients in general practice within two weeks of their initial consultation and to the referred patients before their first out-patient appointment. At the same time, family doctors were asked to assess their patients on a four point scale of symptom severity - none, mild, moderate and severe. The questionnaire contained, in addition to the PGI, the Medical Outcomes

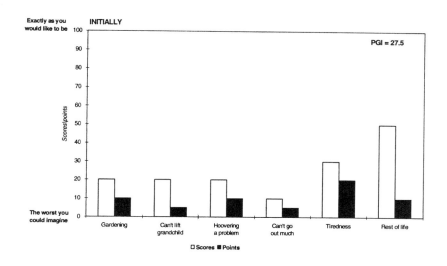

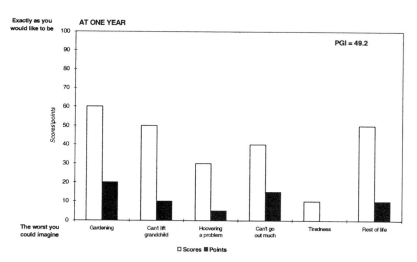

Figure 6.2   Quality of life for a low back pain patient initially and at one year

Study SF-36 (Ware and Sherbourne, 1992), the Aberdeen Back Pain Scale (Ruta *et al.*, 1994b), some questions on medication, and a series of socio-demographic questions. The SF-36 is designed to measure health across three dimensions using eight separate scales (e.g. physical functioning, mental health, pain) and has been validated in the United States (McHorney *et al.*, 1992; McHorney *et al.*, 1993) and in the UK (Brazier *et al.*, 1992; Garratt *et al.*, 1993; Jenkinson *et al.*, 1993). The Aberdeen Back Pain Scale is a 19 item questionnaire devised from questions commonly used in the clinical assessment of patients presenting with low back pain. Out of the 777 patients who were identified with low back pain, 571 returned a questionnaire following two reminders. Of these, 359 (63%) had correctly completed the PGI, giving an overall response rate of 46%. The validity of a new measure is often assessed by comparing it with some established measure of the concept under study, in this case quality of life. In attempting to validate the PGI the following question is posed: is the PGI measuring what it purports to measure, i.e. the gap between expectations and reality in those areas in which subjects most value an improvement? Without some "gold standard" measure of quality of life employing the same underlying definition with which to compare the PGI, it is very difficult to answer this question. A compromise solution is to correlate the PGI with a "gold standard" measure of a concept that is closely related to quality of life - health status (Ruta *et al.*, 1994b). To the extent that health contributes to our ability to perform daily activities that enhance perceived quality of life, one would expect subjects with poor health to score lower on the PGI than subjects in good health. It is recognised, however, that certain socio-demographic characteristics may also influence quality of life, for example, employment status, income and marital status.

In assessing validity, patients' PGI scores were correlated with their scores on the eight SF-36 scales and the Aberdeen Back Pain Scale (Ruta *et al.*, 1994a). Known-group validity was assessed by setting up several hypotheses; namely, PGI scores should be:

a) higher in non-referred than referred patients
b) related to family doctor's ratings of symptom severity
c) lower in patients taking analgesics and strong analgesics
d) higher in patients owning their own homes
e) higher in patients who are married
f) lower in unemployed patients.

As shown in Table 6.2, PGI scores are highly correlated with the low back pain clinical scores, and six of the SF-36 scales (P < 0.001). Correlations with role limitations due to emotional problems and general health perception are weaker. Table 6.3 shows the results of the remainder of the validity testing. Referred patients have significantly lower mean scores than patients being managed solely within general practice. In all but the severe category, PGI scores tend to decrease with increasing symptom severity as assessed by the general practitioner. Mean

PGI scores are lower in patients taking analgesics than those not taking drugs; patients taking stronger analgesics have lower mean PGI scores than those taking milder drugs. Similarly, our hypotheses are not rejected for the socio-demographic variables. Patients with privately-owned houses have higher mean scores than those living in rented accommodation; single patients have lower scores than married patients; and unemployed patients have lower scores than those in work.

Table 6.2 Validity: correlation between PGI score, the low back pain clinical score, and the eight scales of the SF-36 health profile

	Measure	Correlation with the PGI score
A	Low back pain clinical score	0.42 [a]
B	SF-36 health profile scores:	
	Physical functioning	0.26 [a]
	Social functioning	0.38 [a]
	Role limitations due to physical problems	0.27 [a]
	Role limitations due to emotional problems	0.18 [a]
	General mental health	0.23 [a]
	Energy/vitality	0.27 [a]
	Bodily pain	0.47 [a]
	General health perceptions	0.13 [b]

[a] Significant at the 0.1% level
[b] Significant at the 1% level

Source: Ruta et al., 1994a

The reliability of measures of outcome should be assessed by the test-retest method (Kirshner and Guyatt, 1985). To assess the test-retest reliability of the PGI, a subset of 167 patients who completed the PGI correctly were mailed a second questionnaire two weeks later (Ruta et al., 1994a). This questionnaire contained an additional question asking patients if their health had changed since they had completed the first questionnaire. Of the 111 patients who returned a questionnaire with the PGI correctly completed, 69 stated that their health had remained the same since they returned the initial questionnaire. Correlating the two sets of scores for the 69 patients resulted in a Pearson coefficient of 0.7 ($P < 0.0001$). This is acceptable for comparisons between groups of patients.

Table 6.3 Validity: PGI score by referral, severity, medication, housing, marital status and employment

Variable	Number of patients	PGI score
Patient referred to hospital:		
No	206	34.7 [b]
Yes	153	29.2
GP severity rating:		
None	6	44.7
Mild	81	37.0
Moderate	105	32.5
Severe	12	36.0
Analgesic medication being taken:		
No	64	35.9
Yes	295	31.6
Analgesic strength [a.]		
Mild - moderate	58	36.1
Moderate - severe	172	33.1
Housing tenure:		
Privately owned	255	33.4
Rented accommodation	104	29.7
Marital status:		
Married	278	32.6
Single	78	31.4
Employment status:		
Part or full-time employment	234	33.4
Unemployed	8	28.0

[a] BNF classification of analgesic strength
[b] Difference significant at the 1% level

Source: Ruta *et al.*, 1994a

Given that the goal of most treatments is to improve patients' quality of life, if the PGI is to have clinical relevance it must be responsive to changes in quality of life.   A number of different methods have been proposed for assessing the responsiveness of measures of outcome (Guyatt *et al.*, 1987b; Kazis *et al.*, 1989; Katz *et al.*, 1992). One such method, the Standardised Response Mean (SRM), has the advantage of enabling comparisons to be made in terms of responsiveness across different measures (Katz *et al.*, 1992). SRMs are calculated by dividing the mean change in scores over two points in time by the standard deviation of the score differences. SRMs of 0.2, 0.5, and 0.8 indicate small, moderate and large changes respectively.

The responsiveness of the PGI was assessed by mailing patients a follow-up questionnaire at 12 months. One hundred and thirty-six patients completed a questionnaire at both one year and baseline. The distributions of the two sets of scores are shown in Figure 6.3. The difference between the initial mean scores of 30.6 and the mean score at 12 months of 41.1 is significant ($P < 0.01$). Dividing the mean difference in PGI scores by the standard deviation of the differences produces an SRM of 0.46, which represents a small to moderate change.

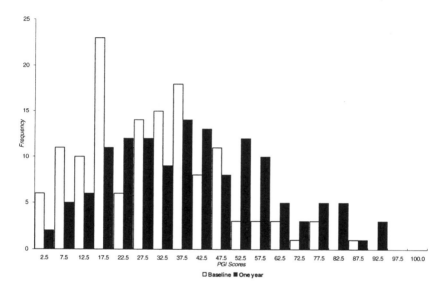

Figure 6.3 Change in PGI scores over time for low back pain patients

CONCLUSION

Of the few measures available that actually purport to measure quality of life, even fewer provide any underlying definition of the construct, let alone go on to measure it. Typically the measures available to researchers and health care professionals focus on something much narrower - for example, clinical signs and symptoms or health status. The domains covered by such instruments, along with weights or values attached, will rarely coincide with the preferences of the individual patient.

Calman's definition that quality of life represents the gap between an individual's expectations and reality has provided the basis for a quality of life measure that asks the individual patient to rate how badly affected they are by a particular condition in up to five aspects of their lives. The Patient Generated Index (PGI) allows patients to express the aspects of their lives affected by their condition and to attach values to improving them.

In a sample of low back pain patients, the PGI has satisfied validity and reliability criteria and was found to be responsive to changes in perceived quality of life when patients were followed up at one year. Health is not valued for its own sake but for its contribution to our daily lives insofar as it enables us to take part in the activities which are important to us. This is supported in validity testing by the strong correlation between patients' PGI scores, the SF-36 and the Aberdeen Back Pain Scale. Similarly, referred patients were found to have a poorer perceived quality of life than patients being managed solely by their GP. A cause for concern, however, is the completion rate for the PGI, with just over 37% of respondents who returned a questionnaire failing to complete it. These patients were found to be significantly older, had a lower age on leaving full-time education and were more likely to be divorced or separated (Ruta *et al.*, 1994a). A series of interviews with these patients has been conducted to try and ascertain particular areas of difficulty encountered in completing the PGI, with a view to producing a simplified version that retains the required attributes of validity, reliability and responsiveness. Although the PGI is still being developed, we believe it offers a promising new approach to the problem of measuring quality of life.

REERENCES

Bergner, M. (1989) Quality of life, health status, and clinical research. *Medical Care*, **27**, S148-S156.

Bergner, M., Bobbitt, R.A., Carter, W. and Gilson, B.S. (1981) The Sickness Impact Profile: development and final revision of a health status measure. *Medical Care*, **19**, 787-805.

Brazier, J.E., Harper, R., Jones, N.M.B., O'Cathain, A., Thomas, K.J., Usherwood, T. and Westlake, L. (1992) Validating the SF-36 Health Survey Questionnaire: new outcome measure for primary care. *British Medical Journal*, **305**, 160-164.

Bulpitt, C.J. and Fletcher, A.E. (1990) The measurement of quality of life in hypertensive patients: a practical approach. *British Journal of Clinical Pharmacology*, **30**, 353-364.

Calman, K.C. (1984) Quality of life in cancer patients: a hypothesis. *Journal of Medical Ethics*, **10**, 124-127.

Cohen, C. (1982) On the quality of life: some philosophical reflections. *Circulation*, **66 (5 pt 2)**, III29-III33.

Dupuis, G. (1988) *International perspectives on quality of life and cardiovascular disease: the quality of life systemic inventory*. Presented at the workshop on quality of life in cardiovascular disease. Winston-Salem, NC.

Garratt, A.M., Ruta, D.A., Abdalla, M.I., Buckingham, J.K. and Russell, I.T. (1993) The SF-36 Health Survey Questionnaire: an outcome measure suitable for routine use within the NHS? *British Medical Journal*, **306**, 1440-1444.

Guyatt, G.H., Berman, L.B., Townsend, M., Pugsley, S.O. and Chambers, L.W. (1987a) A measure of quality of life for clinical trials in chronic lung disease. *Thorax*, **42**, 773-778.

Guyatt, G.H., Walter, S. and Norman, G. (1987b) Measuring change over time: assessing the usefulness of evaluative instruments. *Journal of Chronic Diseases*, **40**, 171-178.

Hoinville, G. (1977) *The Priority Evaluator Method*. London: Department of Social and Community Planning and Research, London University. (Methodological Working Paper 3)

Hunt, S.M., McEwen, J. and McKenna, S.P. (1985) Measuring health status: a new tool for clinicians and epidemiologists. *Journal of the Royal College of General Practitioners*, **35**, 185-188.

Jenkinson, C., Coulter, A. and Wright, L. (1993) Short-Form 36 (SF-36) Health Survey Questionnaire: normative data for adults of working age. *British Medical Journal*, **306**, 1437-1440.

Katz, J.N., Larson, M.G., Phillips, C.B, Fossel, A.H. and Liang, M.H. (1992) Comparative measurement sensitivity of short and longer form health status instruments. *Medical Care*, **30**, 917-925.

Kazis, L.E., Anderson, J.J. and Meenan, R.F. (1989) Effect sizes for interpreting changes in health status. *Medical Care*, **27**, S178-S189.

Kirshner, B. and Guyatt, G. (1985) A methodological framework for assessing health indices. *Journal of Chronic Diseases*, **38**, 27-36.

McHorney, C.A., Ware, J.E., Jr., Rogers, W., Raczek, A.E. and Lu, J.F. (1992) The validity and relative precision of MOS Short- and Long-Form Health Status Scales and Dartmouth COOP Charts: results from the Medical Outcomes Study. *Medical Care*, **30**, MS253-MS265.

McHorney, C.A., Ware, J.E., Jr. and Raczek, A.E. (1993) The MOS 36-Item Short-Form Health Survey (SF-36). II: Psychometric and clinical tests of validity in measuring physical and mental health constructs. *Medical Care*, **31**, 247-263.

Nordenfelt, L. (1989) Quality of life and happiness. In: Bjork, S. and Vang, J. (Eds.), *Assessing quality of life*. Linkoping: Samhall Klintland.

Presant, C.A. (1984) Quality of life in cancer patients: who measures what? *American Journal of Clinical Oncology*, **7**, 571-573.

Ruta, D.A., Garratt, A.M. and Leng, M. (1994a). A new approach to the measurement of quality of life: the patient generated index (PGI). *Medical Care*, **32**, 1109-1126.

Ruta, D.A., Garratt, A.M., Wardlaw, D. and Russell, I.T. (1994b) Developing a valid and reliable measure of health outcome for patients with low back pain. *Spine*, **19**, 1887-1896.

Siegrist, J. and Junge, A. (1989) Conceptual and methodological problems in research on the quality of life in clinical medicine. *Social Science and Medicine*, **29**, 463-468.

Streiner, D.L. and Norman, G.R. (1989) *Health measurement scales: a practical guide to their development and use*. Oxford: Oxford University Press.

van Dam, F.S., Somers, R. and van Beck-Couzijn, A.L. (1981) Quality of life: some theoretical issues. *Journal of Clinical Pharmacology*, **21**, 166S-168S.

Ware, J.E., Jr. and Sherbourne, C.D. (1992). The MOS 36-Item Short-Form Health Survey (SF-36). I: Conceptual framework and item selection. *Medical Care*, **30**, 473-483.

Ziller, R.C. (1974) Self orientation and quality of life. *Social Indicators Research*, **1**, 301-327.

Chapter 7 _____

MEASURING PATIENT OUTCOMES OF NURSING

SENGA BOND

INTRODUCTION

In this chapter, we turn our attention to nursing. We consider some aspects of current attention to patient outcomes of nursing, recognising nursing as one contributor to the production of health and the provision of health care. The chapter is organised into three main sections. The first section places outcomes within the broader framework of the assessment of quality in health care and of nursing services in particular. What follows is an examination of some of the problems facing outcomes measurement in nursing, including the identification of what should be measured, the availability or otherwise of appropriate measures, and the attribution of outcomes to nursing. The state of the science of outcome assessment in nursing is considered. In the final section some suggestions are made about ways in which outcomes research in nursing may be advanced.

WHY MEASURE OUTCOMES OF NURSING?

The quest for effective and efficient health care which has gained prominence internationally over the last twenty years and which is addressed to other aspects of the production of health in this book applies in equal measure to nursing. Donabedian's (1966) work has attracted attention from all health professions and his contention that following the principles of good *medical* practice is insufficient to guarantee improvement in health became associated with a movement towards the systematic evaluation of health care quality by nurses also. In the United Kingdom (UK), further impetus was provided by Cochrane (1972) whose monograph, *Effectiveness and Efficiency,* focused particularly on medical interventions but also considered the need for evaluations of the outcomes of physiotherapy and social work. Cochrane drew attention to the virtual absence of work in evaluating the entire package of "care" provided within the UK National Health Service (NHS) compared with "medical care" encompassing cure-related activities. Attention to the quality of health care inevitably has concentrated on the activities of medical care givers. Because it is all too easy to regard health care and medical care as synonymous, increasingly other professional groups such as nurses have recognised the need to assert their particular contributions to health and health care, and to attend to the quality of the care they provide.

Donabedian's (1980) approach to separating out the components of health care into structure, process and outcome has become a convenient way in which to consider aspects of quality. This framework was applied to nursing by Bloch (1975) who proposed extensive testing of process-outcome relationships in nursing practice while cautioning about the difficulties of doing so. Donabedian's categorisation has been adopted subsequently in much of the standard-setting and quality assurance activities of the Royal College of Nursing (Kitson, 1993). However, examination of the various standards produced show that there has been a tendency to focus on elements of nursing which fall within the structure of care (the staffing and other resources, skills and infrastructure) and the process of care (what nurses should actually do and how patients may respond) than to identify health outcomes in the short or longer term. As the Audit Commission (1992) observed, "In the absence of reliable outcome measures for nursing, discussions about the quality of nursing services have tended to concentrate on the process of care and on organisational audit." But to consider the quality of nursing as processes, that is *what* nurses do, without considering its effects on patients has long been recognised as an incomplete assessment (Haussman and Hegyvary, 1977).

Interest in patient outcomes of nursing, more particularly the use of patient outcomes to measure the effectiveness of health care, is not new to nursing. Florence Nightingale was probably the earliest proponent of outcome evaluation and used mortality and morbidity statistics to describe the effects of hospitals in the Crimea (Nightingale, 1858). She also collected data which allowed her to describe the state of patients discharged from the hospitals in London as "recovered or relieved", "discharged incurable, unrelieved, for irregularities, or at their own request", or "died" (Nightingale, 1862) which is more informative than routine data about the condition of patients discharged today.

A consistent thrust to the quest for measures of nursing effectiveness and efficiency relates to questions of nurse staffing. Because the 167,000 nurses employed in the NHS represent the largest single occupational category in the service (Department of Health, 1993a) and consume the largest slice of the NHS revenue budget (some 46% of the salaries budget and 29% of the total revenue annually), they are an easy target for reduction. The repeated quest for efficiency through attention to the number, grades, rostering, and workload of nursing staff led the Audit Commission to offer, as a preliminary to detailed conclusions of its enquiry into making the best use of nursing resources, that "more large scale research is needed into nursing outcomes and how they are affected both by the number and mix of ward staff and by changes in nursing practice and the organisation of care." Such large-scale research is rare in British nursing but one early example is found in the minority report of the working party on the recruitment and training of nurses submitted to the Ministry of Health in 1948 (Ministry of Health, 1948). In it Cohen wrote:

> "The problem as it appears to a psychologist is one of measuring efficiency by evaluating, on some acceptable criterion, the performance of nursing duties. I have taken as the criterion of nursing effectiveness in hospital the patient's duration of stay, which is assumed to be an index of sickness."

While Cohen recognised that length of hospital stay is only a proxy measure of patient health and is influenced by many variables over and above nursing, he nonetheless demonstrated in acute care voluntary nurse training hospitals a consistent and inverse relationship between the number of qualified nurses and the length of patients' hospital stay. This relationship did not hold for medical staff. He advanced an economic argument, setting the costs of additional nurses against days of work, and hence output achieved due to earlier discharge, and concluded that employing more qualified nurses made economic sense.

Cohen's analysis, while crude and open to criticism, nevertheless exemplifies one of the few consistent findings in nursing research, namely that there is a direct relationship between patient output and outcomes and the quality of the nursing workforce as measured by qualifications and/or grade (Buchan and Ball, 1991). Identifying direct indices of nursing effectiveness in terms of measurable patient outcomes is poorly developed. Consequently most of the assessments of quality have focused on output rather than outcome, and on process and structure-process relationships rather than on process-outcome relationships. The point has been made elsewhere of the need for strong structure-process-outcome studies which enable the development of models to clarify and explain relationships (Bond and Thomas, 1991) and which assess all three components in a scientifically credible manner (Russell and Wilson, 1992).

Since measures of structure and process are easier to obtain, the emphasis in the United Kingdom has been on developing instruments by which the care provided to patients, particularly in hospital, and by whom it is provided, can be described. Scales developed in the USA, such as Qualpacs (Wandelt and Aager, 1974) and the Phaneuf audit (Phaneuf, 1976), and adapted for use in the United Kingdom (Goldstone et al., 1983), have been widely adopted for routine use in audits of nursing care (Kitson, 1993). Despite their dubious validity and reliability as audit tools (Whelan, 1987; Balogh, 1992; Norman et al., 1992; Redfern et al., 1992) they have also been used in research which has attempted to relate structures to process and outcomes (Pearson *et al.,* 1989; Carr-Hill *et al.,* 1992). Because they are relatively blunt instruments and are not related to specific conditions but to broad aspects of care, relating data collected using these audit tools to patient outcomes is a long shot.

Current questions posed to and by nursing continue to seek answers not only about the optimum workforce, but also about its organisation, and, more specifically, the value for patients of the interventions that nurses make. Large-scale macro-level studies of the kind envisaged by Cohen in the 1940s are not yet feasible in the United Kingdom. In part this is because the data which would enable such studies to be undertaken are not routinely collected and it would be prohibitively expensive to do so. While recent atlases have been created of the morbidity and mortality associated with some conditions, based on the areas covered by health authorities (Department of Health, 1993b), and while these show variations across the country, we are a long way from being able to relate these data to specific features of nursing. The databases necessary to collect process and outcome data have not been developed as yet. In the United States, the necessity for patient-based and Diagnosis Related Group costings for billing purposes, and information necessary for the accreditation of hospitals and other health care facilities, have led to developments in information technology to produce large data sets. Yet even these systems have not at this time "sufficient breadth and depth to even begin to answer questions on outcomes associated with non-physician providers" (Stevic, 1992). The major need is to unravel the nature of the cause-effect relationship in more modest studies and to focus attention on creating knowledge of the effectiveness and appropriateness of well-delineated nursing interventions applied to specific patient groups.

There exists a tension between the state of the science and the demand for outcome measures and information. Demand has been given impetus by the NHS reforms described in *Working for Patients* (Department of Health, 1989). Health authorities are required to purchase health care and to monitor the extent to which needs for appropriate and effective services are met. Similarly the introduction of audit into service provider units means that nursing services as well as nurses, as part of clinical services, face increasing pressure to identify appropriate outcome measures for their activities. The establishment of a Clinical Outcomes Group co-chaired by the Chief Medical and Nursing Officers, with nursing among its constituencies, adds impetus. Further impetus is enshrined in the current national strategy for nursing, *A Vision for the Future* (Department of Health, 1993d), which sets as a target for its first year that all provider units in the NHS "should have identified three outcome indicators responsive to nursing, midwifery or health visiting practice." Identification presents one challenge; obtaining the data to meet it yet another.

SOME PROBLEMS OF MEASURING PATIENT OUTCOMES

Types of Outcome

Despite the recognised need for patient outcome measures to describe nursing quality, there is little consensus about what these should be. Outcome measurement takes place at four levels: the individual, groups with a common condition, groups with dissimilar conditions being cared for in the same environment, and populations. Reasons for undertaking outcome measurement range from audit and quality assessment through needs assessment and resource allocation to research in order to determine effectiveness and efficiency. Given the extent of this agenda, consensus is a pious hope.

The case of infant mortality, an easy outcome to measure, points up the need for different kinds and levels of analysis. At the individual level, infant mortality can be reduced through appropriate antenatal care, targeted at the identification and amelioration of specific problems. However, social factors including female literacy, income, level of education and minority ethnic status, also correlate with infant mortality at a population level (World Bank, 1989). Somehow nursing must locate itself within this multiplicity of perspectives.

There is no shortage of studies which have posed questions of nursing effectiveness, and classifications of outcomes used in nursing studies have been developed (Lang and Marek, 1990). Waltz and Strickland (1988) offered a whole volume of research about measuring patient outcomes of nursing, but there has been relatively little debate in the United Kingdom about what would comprise appropriate patient outcome measures for nursing in specific situations (Tierney, 1992). In part this reflects the rudimentary stage in the development of a theoretical basis for outcomes of nursing, as well as the diffuse nature of the concepts being grappled with.

Health and Nursing Functions

Nursing has transferred its focus to creating health rather than only to ameliorating ill health. This is consistent with an international paradigm shift (World Health Organisation, 1983). As Lohr (1988) observed, definitions of "medical outcomes" have shifted from the classic definition of the five Ds (death, disease, disability, discomfort, and dissatisfaction) towards more positive aspects of health including survival rates, states of physiological, physical and emotional health, and satisfaction with health services. This being the case, outcomes of nursing needs to encompass some definition of health and to address its various dimensions. But what is the picture of health that nursing might adhere to and how can it develop indices of positive health? Donabedian (1966) wrote that "what is included in the category of 'outcomes' depends .... on how narrowly or broadly one defines 'health' and corresponding responsibilities of individual practitioners, or of the health care system as a whole." This agenda needs to be addressed in specific settings.

Table 7.1 Major clinical functions and short-term outcomes

	Maternity	Medical/ Surgical	Paediatric	Psychiatric	Critical care
Patient/ family education	Patient is able to demonstrate care of infant's umbilical cord	Patient is able to demonstrate proper insulin administration	Patient/family able to identify signs and symptoms of sickle cell crisis and when to seek medical attention	Family members able to identify alcohol co-dependency behaviours	Patient/family comprehend and co-operate with post-PTCA orders of strict bedrest for 18 hours
Facilitation of self-care	Caesarean section patients are able to ambulate the length of the hall with assistance by the second post-op day	Hypertensive patient monitors and maintains blood pressure within normal limits	Juvenile-onset diabetic monitors blood sugar and administers own insulin	Anorexic patient is able to gain weight and/or maintain weight within normal limits	While confined to strict bedrest, patient begins to work on range-of-motion exercises with nursing and physical therapy
Symptom distress management	Labour pains are effectively relieved	Post-operative pain is relieved through use of pharmacological agents and comfort measures	Patient's non-verbal cues of pain are assessed and pain is relieved	Patient is able to partially relieve anxiety through use of relaxation therapy	Patient's difficulty in breathing is assessed and relieved
Provision for patient safety	Labouring patients are properly placed and maintained in stirrups without injury	Absence of hospital-acquired pressure sores	Absence of patient falls from cots	Absence of suicide attempts	Absence of infection from central line
Enhancement of patient satisfaction	All patients feel that they were offered adequate comfort measures	Families of terminally ill patients feel that they were treated with dignity and respect	Parents perceive that they are included in the patient's plan of care	Patients were satisfied with the quality of the various group therapies	Family satisfied with the degree of information from the ICU staff regarding patient's condition

Adapted from Gillette and Jenko, 1991.

One attempt to offer a unifying framework for outcomes, based on identification of nursing responsibilities, is to establish the major clinical functions of nursing in a particular setting and to devise measures appropriate to the setting. Gillette and Jenko (1991) identified five such functions: patient/family education, facilitation of self-care, symptom distress management, provision of patient safety, and enhancement of patient satisfaction. Short-term outcomes were specified for each of these in relation to patients in hospital (Table 7.1). This analysis would present some difficulties to those who espouse a more holistic basis for nursing and aim to meet a comprehensive range of patient needs associated with broad notions of caring (Watson, 1985). While there has been research which has assessed caring in relation to both nurse-defined and patient-defined outcomes, including satisfaction and post-operative recovery, attempts to measure patient outcomes defined in specific domains meets with claims of reductionism (Greenwood, 1984). These are often associated with debates about epistemology and methodology - positivism versus phenomenology, quantitative versus qualitative, as if only one approach is acceptable (Greenwood, 1984; Lyne, 1990). Some, like Hegyvary (1992), call for synthetic research including different levels of analysis and different research methods which attend to the complexities of the contexts in which patients are cared for.

While applauding the vision, and agreeing that "studies that investigate the actions of a single provider group, be they nurses, physicians or others, run the risk of ignoring the context" (Hegyvary, 1992), without studies of specific interventions which account for context, then progress in relating outcomes to antecedents will be severely inhibited. An analysis of the nursing research literature on outcomes shows that most studies (59%) were condition-specific and the interventions being assessed were mostly physiological (41%) or psychosocial (42%). Studies of interventions at the physiological level tended to rely only on physiological outcome measures and psychosocial interventions generally ignored possible physiological outcomes (Abraham et al., 1992).

Sensitivity to Nursing
One interpretation of this narrow focus is that nursing's view of health and health gain remain limited. Another is that the investigators are being over cautious in the conceptual linkages between intervention and outcome. Why should intervention X have an effect on outcome Y? Relatively unspecific measures, for example general quality of life measures, may be considered too removed in concept from the care-giving intervention to be responsive to its effects. Moreover, quality of life may be influenced by many factors other than the intervention. Generalised measures of health or quality of life may therefore prove less sensitive to nursing interventions and less successful than outcome indicators which are more meaningful to the subject under investigation. Guyatt (1988) assessed treatment effectiveness in chronic respiratory disease by basing the outcome measures on the

five most important activities that the subject identified. Similarly Toseland *et al.* (1989) evaluated the effectiveness of support to family care givers by changes in individually identified problems. This line of work is likely to be attractive to nurses who have pressed for the need to individualise inputs to patient care but have provided little research evidence to show either that or how it is done or its effectiveness in terms of patient outcomes. There should be value in considering patient-specific as well as condition- and input-specific outcomes. The need to individualise and to expect different outcomes of medical interventions has been expressed by Wennberg (1990) who wrote:

"I predict, that for most conditions, rational choices among treatments require that the individual patients understand the predicaments they face. The predicaments arise because there is seldom a single correct answer to a medical problem. Most conditions and illnesses entail a number of morbidities, symptoms, and disabilities. Outcomes research will clarify the probabilities of the various outcomes for the various treatments, showing many to be effective in some respects that are important to patients."

Similarly, the appropriateness of nursing interventions and their effectiveness are likely to vary according to patients' social and psychological factors, physiological needs, and their interpretations of their situation related to desired outcomes.

Attribution to Nursing

The analysis of nursing outcomes by Abraham *et al.* (1992) was confined to nursing journals and to interventions described as "nursing or nursing related". This throws a rigidity around what may be encompassed within the ambit of nursing. Some antecedents in the form of specific interventions may not be the province of a single professional group. Continuing with the example of childbirth, in our own culture no one professional group provides antenatal care. Similarly, while it is usually the prerogative of midwives to supervise the second stage of uncomplicated births, assessing the outcome of whether women are instructed to push or not push during the second stage of labour is related to the effects of the specified intervention on the defined population rather than to the health professional who is assisting the labour. There have been studies which have considered the outcome of a specific intervention by different professionals, for example comparing general practitioners and psychiatric nurses (Marks, 1985). However, the care that patients receive and how that care is provided is arguably more important than who provides it. Nonetheless, there are economic implications since nurses cost less than medical staff. The status of the provider is apt to relate more to political considerations and to efficiency rather than effectiveness. Witness current developments in the blurring of professional boundaries in "patient-focused hospitals" and changes in nursing work to accommodate a reduction in junior hospital doctors' hours and the expansion of treatments in family medicine, such as nurse-prescribing.

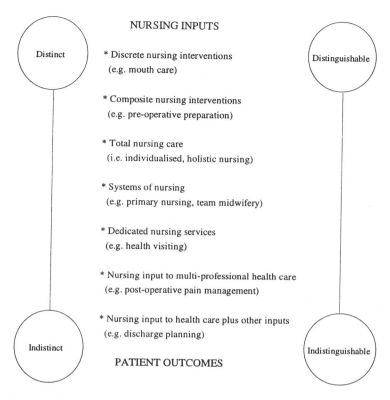

NURSING INPUTS

Distinct

Distinguishable

* Discrete nursing interventions
  (e.g. mouth care)

* Composite nursing interventions
  (e.g. pre-operative preparation)

* Total nursing care
  (i.e. individualised, holistic nursing)

* Systems of nursing
  (e.g. primary nursing, team midwifery)

* Dedicated nursing services
  (e.g. health visiting)

* Nursing input to multi-professional health care
  (e.g. post-operative pain management)

* Nursing input to health care plus other inputs
  (e.g. discharge planning)

Indistinct

Indistinguishable

PATIENT OUTCOMES

Source: Tierney, 1992.

Figure 7.1 Range of interventions

As Tierney (1991) has commented however, and shown in Figure 7.1, the less specific the intervention and associated outcomes, the greater the difficulty in attributing it to a single provider group rather than to a wider group of participants. Certainly this is the case in some interventions, for example the relative success of nursing homes over long-stay wards involves nurses as the major care giving group, but cannot be attributed solely to nursing (Bond and Bond, 1990). This does not mean that outcomes that can be attributed to nursing must remain associated with highly specific small-scale interventions, although such interventions, when associated with frequently occurring episodes, cumulatively will have enormous impact. There are examples of service innovation, for example for home care to enable the earlier discharge of low-birth-weight babies with both health and cost advantages (Brooton, 1986). Clear attribution of effectiveness, assessed by outcomes, to a wide-ranging and complex nursing service intervention is due to the study design which employed random allocation to alternative treatments. Major attention is being given to randomised studies in health care through the Cochrane Collaboration (Chalmers, 1992), and the importance of such designs is acknowledged. However, they are not always feasible, not least because of the little control nurses exert in service provision designed for medical purposes.

HOW SHOULD NURSING PROGRESS?

The need to assess nursing quality and effectiveness by outcomes for patients and some of the difficulties in doing so have been discussed. Outcomes measurement, an essential aspect of health services research as well as integral to clinical audit and health purchasing activities, has claimed a good deal of the limelight in advancing the quest for improved quality. It is in the interests of nursing to be a significant player in this activity and to be recognised as contributing to health gain. While there is a need for this contribution to be recognised as part of the whole, this holds the attendant possibility that the specific contribution of nursing will be lost. There are, therefore, two platforms of activity that need to be advanced. First, nursing needs to be recognised as an integral element of the whole health care provision. Secondly, if nursing is not to be subsumed into "health care", which by fiat will become "medical care" and hence render nursing invisible, its unique contribution needs to be delineated and defined and its cost-effectiveness made clear.

To do so requires both the development of theory and of the technology to enable nursing inputs as well as patient outcomes of nursing to be measured. Unless there is clear articulation of what nursing is aiming to achieve and what nursing inputs are involved, then there is no basis for the development of technology to capture the data required. Similarly, clear delineation of outcomes must precede technological development. Technology here applies to well-validated instruments which are sufficiently sensitive to detect nursing interventions as well as to adequately reflect patient characteristics. It also involves having a language and classification system which enables nursing to be identified and communicated. While information technology has for long held promise, we have yet to reap its benefits in these matters and in making data available in quantity as well as quality. In any case, no amount of computer hardware or software can compensate for the fundamental thinking that logically precedes their application.

There is a need to identify aspects of health need and focus on those conditions and nursing interventions which are likely to make significant contributions to health gain, however that is interpreted. While there are national and regional Research and Development priorities (Department of Health, 1993c), those aspects to which nurses make a significant contribution need to be identified, since it is here that new initiatives are likely to be funded. When the clinical conditions identified are likely to be influenced by nursing practice, then there should be specific elements addressed to nursing contributions within funded research studies or programmes. The contribution of nurses and midwives to genetic counselling is one case in point.

Of course, none of this is possible without strengthening the infrastructure and nursing's capability of carrying out the basic development and research work that underlies articulating nursing effectiveness. Here again there is much to be gained from working with other disciplines who have a great deal to contribute, but with the need to ensure that the agenda is a nursing agenda rather than one which is economic, sociological, psychological or whatever. While these disciplines offer much that can be applied in, to and for nursing, they are *not* nursing.

The national drive to a more explicit agenda and priority-driven Research and Development programme, and the recognition that there needs to be training in research to enable that programme to be carried, offers an opportunity never before presented to nursing. Whether we grasp the nettle remains to be seen.

REFERENCES

Abraham, I.L., Chalifoux, Z.L. and Evers, G.C.M. (1992) Conditions, interventions and outcomes: a quantitative analysis of nursing research (1981-1990). In: *Patient outcomes research: examining the effectiveness of nursing practice. Proceedings of a conference sponsored by the National Center for Nursing Research.* US: US Department of Health and Human Services, 93-3411.

Audit Commission (1992) *The virtue of patients: making best use of ward nursing resources.* London: HMSO.

Balogh, R. (1992) Audits of nursing care in Britain: a review and a critique of approaches to validating them. *International Journal of Nursing Studies*, **29(2)**, 119-133.

Berwick, D.M. (1989) Sounding board: continuous improvement as an ideal in health care. *New England Journal of Medicine,* **320,**53-56.

Bloch, D. (1975) Evaluation of nursing care in terms of process and outcome: issues in research and quality assurance. *Nursing Research,* **24 (4)**, 256-263.

Bond, S. (1992) *Outcomes of nursing: proceedings of an invitational developmental workshop.* Newcastle upon Tyne: Centre for Health Services Research (Report No 57)

Bond, S. and Bond, J. (1989) *Evaluation of continuing care accommodation for elderly people: a multiple-case study of NHS hospital wards and nursing homes: some aspects of structure and outcome.* Newcastle upon Tyne: Health Care Research Unit, University of Newcastle upon Tyne. (Report No. 38, Vol.3)

Bond, S. and Bond, J. (1990). Outcomes of care within a multiple-case study in the evaluation of the experimental National Health Service nursing homes. *Age and Ageing,* **19**, 11-18.

Bond, S. and Thomas, L.H. (1991) Issues in measuring outcomes of nursing. *Journal of Advanced Nursing,* **16**, 1492-1502.

Brooten, D., Kuman, S., Brown, L.P., Butts, P., Finkler, S.A., Bakewell-Sachs, S., Gibbons, A. and Delivoria-Papadopoulos, M. (1986) A randomised clinical trial of early hospital discharge and home follow-up of very-low-birth-weight infants. *New England Journal of Medicine,* **315**, 934-939.

Buchan, J. and Ball, J. (1991) *Caring costs. Nursing costs and benefits: a review for the Royal College of Nursing.* Brighton: Institute of Manpower services. (IMS Report No. 208)

Carr-Hill, R., Dixon, P., Griffiths, M., Higgins, M., McCaughan, D. and Wright, K. (1992) *Skill mix and the effectiveness of nursing care.* York: Centre for Health Economics.

Chalmers, I., Dickerson, K. and Chalmers, T.C. (1992) Getting to grips with Archie Cochrane's agenda. *British Medical Journal,* **305**, 786-788.

Cochrane, A. (1972) *Effectiveness and efficiency: random reflections on health services.* London: Nuffield Provincial Hospitals Trust.

Department of Health (1989) *Working for patients.* London: HMSO. (Cm. 555)

Department of Health (1993a) *Health and personal social services statistics for England.* London: HMSO.

Department of Health (1993b) *Population health outcome indicators for the NHS 1993: England. A consultation document.* Brighton: Institute of Public Health, University of Surrey.

Department of Health (1993c) *Research for health.* London: Department of Health.

Department of Health (1993d) *A vision for the future: the nursing, midwifery and health visiting contribution to health and health care.* London: Department of Health.

Donabedian, A. (1966) Evaluating the quality of medical care. *Milbank Quarterly,* **44** **(2)**,166-206.

Donabedian, A. (1980) *Explorations in quality assessment and monitoring. Vol. 1: The definition of quality and approaches to its assessment.* Ann Arbor, MI: Health Administration Press.

Gerst, M.S. and Moos, R.H. (1972) Social ecology of university student residences. *Journal of Educational Psychology,* **63 (6)**, 513-525.

Gillette, B. and Jenko, M. (1991) Major clinical functions: a unifying framework for measuring outcomes. *Journal of Nursing Care Quality,* **6 (1)**, 20-24.

Goldstone, L.A., Ball, J.A. and Collier, M.M. (1983) *Monitor: an index of the quality of nursing care for acute medical and surgical wards. North West Staffing Levels Project Report.* Newcastle upon Tyne: Newcastle upon Tyne, Polytechnic Products.

Greenwood, J. (1984) Nursing research: a position paper. *Journal of Advanced Nursing,* **9**, 77-82.

Guyatt, G. (1988) Measuring health status in chronic airflow limitation. *European Respiratory Journal,* **1**, 560-564.

Haussman, R.K.D. and Hegyvary, S.T. (1977) *Monitoring quality of nursing care. Part III: Professional review for nursing: an empirical investigation.* Hyattsville, Maryland: U.S. Department of Health, Education, and Welfare.

Hegyvary, S.T. (1992) Outcomes research: integrating nursing practice into the world view. In: *Patient outcomes research: examining the effectiveness of nursing practice. Proceedings of a conference sponsored by the National Center for Nursing Research.* US: US Department of Health and Human Services, No 93-3411.

Kitson, A. (1993) Quality assurance in nursing practice. *Proceedings of the Royal Society of Edinburgh*, **101B**, 143-163.

Lang, N.M. and Marek, K.D. (1990) The classification of patient outcomes. *Journal of Professional Nursing,* **6 (3)**, 158-163.

Lohr, K.N. (1988) Outcome measurement: concepts and questions. *Inquiry*, **25**, 37-50.

Lyne, P. (1990) The right questions about nursing care. *Nursing Standard*, **5**, 36-37.

Marks, I. (1985) Controlled trial of psychiatric nurse therapists in primary care. *British Medical Journal,* **290**, 1181-1184.

Ministry of Health (1948) *Working paper on the recruitment and training of nurses. Minority Report (The Cohen report).* London: HMSO.

Nightingale F. (1858) *Notes on matters affecting the health, efficiency, and hospital administration of the British Army.* London: Harrison & Sons.

Nightingale, F. (1862) *Hospital statistics and hospital plans* [Reprinted from the transactions of the National Association for the promotion of Social Science]. London: Emily Faithfull & Co, Victoria Press.

Norman, I., Redfern, S., Tomalin, D.A. and Oliver, S. (1992) Applying triangulation to the assessment of quality of nursing. *Nursing Times Occasional Paper*, **88**, 43-46.

Pearson, A., Durant, I. and Punton, S. (1989) Determining quality in a unit where nursing is the primary intervention. *Journal of Advanced Nursing*, **14**, 269-273.

Phaneuf, M. (1976) *The nursing audit: self-regulation in nursing practice.* New York: Appleton-Century-Crofts.

Redfern, S.J., Norman, I.J., Tomalin, D.A. and Oliver, S. (1992) The reliability and validity of quality assessment measures in nursing. *Journal of Clinical Nursing,* **1**, 47-51.

Russell, I.T. and Wilson, B.J. (1992) Audit: the third clinical science? *Quality in Health Care*, **1**, 51-55.

Stevic, M.O. (1992) Patient-linked data bases: implications for a nursing outcomes research agenda. In: *Patient outcomes research: examining the effectiveness of nursing practice. Proceedings of the State of the Science Conference sponsored by the National Center for Nursing Research.* US: Department of Health and Human Services.

Tierney, A.J. (1992) Outcomes that reflect nursing input. In: Bond, S. (Ed.), *Outcomes of nursing proceedings of an invitational developmental workshop.* Newcastle upon Tyne: Centre for Health Services Research, University of Newcastle. (Report No. 57)

Toseland, R.W., Rossiter, C.M. and Labrecque, M.S. (1989) The effectiveness of peer-led and professionally led groups to support family caregivers. *The Gerontologist*, **29**, 465-471.

Waltz, C.F. and Strickland, O.L. (1988) *Measurement of nursing outcomes.* New York: Springer Publishing Company.

Wandelt, M. and Aager, J. (1974) *Quality Patient Care Scale.* New York: Appleton-Century-Crofts.

Watson, J. (1985) *Nursing: human science and human care: a theory of nursing.* Washington: National League for Nursing.

Wennberg, J.E. (1990) Outcomes research, cost containment and the fear of health care rationing. *New England Journal of Medicine*, **323**, 1202-1204.

Whelan, J. (1987) Using monitor-observer bias. *Senior Nurse*, **7**, 8-10.

World Bank (1983) *World development report.* London: Oxford University Press.

World Health Organisation (1983) *1983 Constitution of the World Health Organisation.* Geneva: World Health Organisation.

Chapter 8 _____

USE OF OUTCOME MEASURES IN HEALTH CARE COMMISSIONING

MARTIN BARDSLEY

INTRODUCTION

In 1991 the United Kingdom (UK) Government brought about a radical change in the way the National Health Service (NHS) in England and Wales was organised (Department of Health, 1989). Among the changes was the development of a new role for statutory health authorities that divorced them from direct management of care and replaced that with a role of buying services from a range of providers in an "internal market". The health authorities were given the task of buying services to improve the health of defined geographical populations. This chapter considers the importance of outcome assessment in that commissioning process, the potential that exists and the problems that may be found.

Commissioning Health Care

Although changes in the organisation of the NHS are not uncommon, those introduced in 1991 were among the most radical ever seen. Figure 8.1 outlines the key elements of the resulting NHS structure. Despite further amendments (Department of Health, 1993a), the important division between health authorities who are given money to commission services (purchasers) and the providers of care looks set to remain.

The health service has been financed from two streams of money, mainly derived from general taxation. One of these, hospital and community health services (HCHS), has traditionally been a cash-limited grant to cover the costs of

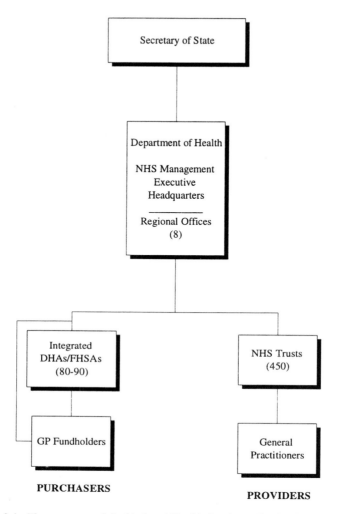

Figure 8.1   The structure of the National Health Service in England

acute hospitals and long-stay services as well as most community health services. The second stream of funding covers family practitioners and includes some non-cash-limited elements including general medical services (GMS) and costs of prescribed drugs. There are also a variety of cash-limited development funds.

HCHS money has been passed down to Regional Health Authorities (RHAs) and then to District Health Authorities (DHAs) as block allocations, usually based on some form of capitation formula with additional weighting factors. In 1991/92 this accounted for some £17,000 million compared to £6,500 million on family practice (see Figure 8.2). By far the largest block of expenditure is on hospitals. By 1994 almost all hospitals and community units will have an element of independence as self-governing trusts (although still firmly within the NHS).

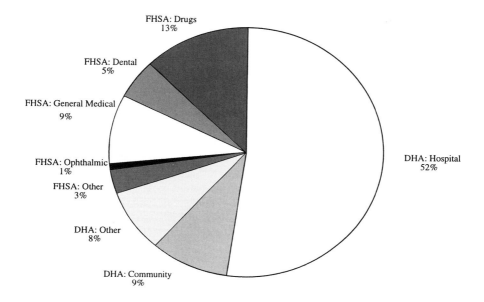

Source: Department of Health, 1992a

Figure 8.2   Health services expenditure 1991

District Health Authorities now contract with provider units or trusts for a given volume of services. They have the potential to move contracts between providers based on price or quality, and to ensure that the provider maintains certain standards. In theory, their power to dictate the pattern of services is great. In practice, they tend to be limited by policy constraints, historical associations and shared interests with local provider units. Contracts were originally in a block form, for example covering a full range of services in an acute hospital. Over time, contracting methods are becoming increasingly sophisticated and block contracts are being replaced by "cost and volume arrangements" or contracts based on certain case types (Ham, 1991). It is true to say that the process of commissioning services is undergoing a phase of rapid development (Mawhinney, 1993) and experiments in commissioning by case mix will soon be underway.

Another important arm of the health service concerns family doctors or general practitioners (GPs) and primary care. Family Health Service Authorities (FHSAs) are responsible for managing nationally agreed contracts with family practitioners (medical and dental practitioners, and retail pharmacists and opticians), assessing populations' needs for health care, planning services to meet those needs, and managing GP development funds (Ham, 1991). Funding of GPs is complex but the principle is that they are independent practitioners who receive payment based on the number of patients registered with their practice together with a variety of additional fees or grants. FHSAs have considerably less power than DHAs in dictating the pattern of service provision as so much is "demand led" by patients (Starey *et al.*, 1993). There are a number of discretionary grants available to FHSAs that can provide "levers" to shape local primary care provision. Since the NHS reforms, there has been a growing movement to combine the roles of DHAs and FHSAs into "health care commissions" that cover all local health services (Huntington, 1993). The government is committed to the legislative changes that are needed to do this completely by 1996 (Department of Health, 1993a). In the meantime, there is increasing cooperation locally between DHAs and FHSAs.

Finally, the 1989 White Paper introduced a third type of commissioner, the general practitioner fundholder. These are family doctors who have opted to control a local fund that is used to pay for some hospital and community services for their patients and to cover the costs of drugs (Glennerster *et al.*, 1992). Though the scale of funds is smaller than for DHAs and FHSAs, the services are in areas where the GP fundholder can exert an influence in shaping secondary care provision, though the extent to which they are doing this is unclear (Coulter and Bradlow, 1993). The number of such fundholders is increasing and the relationship between their purchasing and that of the DHAs and FHSAs is becoming increasingly important.

The Potential for Outcome Measurement
Though the scale and approach to commissioning can vary, all agencies aim to choose services based on their contribution to the health of a given population. In theory then, some appreciation of the outcome of the care is fundamental to that process. Yet in reality the ability of all these agencies to judge outcome is limited. Given the ever-present cost constraints on the health service, and the notion of competition between providers, there is the danger that services will be chosen on the basis of cost rather than of quality.

"The competitive market that is likely to be introduced when the White Paper is enacted means that, without adequate safeguards, performance within the contract is likely to be driven by price rather than quality." (Hopkins and Maxwell, 1990)

The information base for decisions about health care service provision is often very limited. Assessments of performance are typically based on measures of activity such as in-patient episodes or patient contacts, possibly expressed relative to costs. Such data, together with information on waiting lists, are being used throughout the health service in determining the levels of services that should be bought and in drives for greater "efficiency". There are some sophisticated mechanisms for comparative analyses of performance using such activity data and these demonstrate wide variations across the country (Ham, 1988; Jenkins *et al.*, 1988; Department of Health, 1992c). The problems of using information on input and throughput are well-known - the danger is of health services that become geared towards short-term gains in throughput yet with little impact on overall health. There have been calls to introduce outcome measurement in such comparisons (Birch and Maynard, 1986; Pollitt, 1989; Roberts, 1990) though the requirement to use only routinely collected data limits the progress that can be made. Nevertheless, there are moves towards a greater awareness of health outcome in decision-making. Later sections of this chapter discuss how this is becoming manifest within the health service.

PROBLEMS OF OUTCOME ASSESSMENT IN PRIMARY AND OUT-PATIENT CARE

There are a range of problems facing the application of outcome measurement in commissioning, especially in primary care and to some extent out-patient care.

Attribution: Identifying Responsibility for the Outcome
There are several ways to define outcomes (Donabedian, 1985; Liddell, 1992; Wilkin *et al.*, 1992). If the measures are to judge performance, then there must be some relationship between the activities of the health service and the resulting patient or population outcome. But the influences on health are many and uncertain. Is it possible to identify realistic improvements in health that can be attributed to a particular service? Are managers and clinicians willing to commit themselves to such an approach?

This problem of the uncertainty of the links between process and outcome is a recurrent one (Donabedian, 1988; Lohr, 1989) and the distinction can become blurred. As Donabedian has pointed out, "the process/outcome distinction divides rather arbitrarily into two: a continuous chain of means and ends."

If outcome measures are to work, there needs to be ways of dealing with this uncertainty, including some agreement between purchasers and providers on the range, definition and application of the outcome measures.

"No matter how carefully other contributory factors have been allowed for ... a large measure of doubt about the causes of the outcome persist. Outcomes are much more easily used ... only as cues that prompt and motivate the assessment of process and structure in a search for causes that can be remedied." (Donabedian, 1988)

Thus the outcome indicator should be a focal point of the dialogue between purchaser and provider and not seen in a legalistic technical way.

Identifying Objectives and Measures

An outcome measure must reflect the objectives of care (Wilkin, 1991). In primary care, there is a wide range of objectives reflecting a diverse client population. Metcalfe (1990) outlines seven distinct roles of general practice (Table 8.1). Each gives a slightly different view of the type of outcome measure that is appropriate. The commissioning process has to recognise this complexity when considering the standard of outcome by which services are to be judged.

As well as a range of different objectives, there may also be a variety of inputs, treatments or staff involved. For example, in an area such as childbirth, the health outcomes for a mother and baby can be the product of the work of family doctors, community midwives, health visitors, and the obstetrics team in the maternity hospital.

This makes it difficult to summarise outcomes into simple measures that are both meaningful to professionals and give a full reflection of the health benefits to the population or patients. It seems likely that the application of outcome measures will be based on specific selected conditions or roles rather than the totality of care.

Choosing the right type of outcome measure is a major issue (discussed in Chapter 11). In particular, issues of validity and responsiveness of the measure are important (Deyo and Inui, 1984; Brazier et al., 1992). There is only limited evidence on the performance characteristics of outcome measures in primary care or for chronic diseases, where health changes emerge over a longer time and tend to be less dramatic. Similarly, there are important choices to be made between generic and condition-specific measures (Patrick and Deyo, 1989) when thinking about the application of outcome measures to the commissioning process.

Identifying the Episode of Care

Evaluation of patient outcome must be made with respect to a particular time interval. For assessments of specific treatments, and in acute illness, this is considerably easier than for the general management of patients. The more time that elapses after care, the harder it becomes to identify the contribution of the care to that outcome.

Yet in primary and out-patient care, very often conditions are chronic and patient management continues over a long time period. Under these circumstances, evaluation of outcome has to be based on successive observations of changes over time rather than for a given end-point. Thus for example, the management of

Table 8.1   The range of tasks, objectives and outcomes in general practice

Tasks	Objectives	Outcome Measures
Prevention	Primary prevention by removal or neutralisation of causal factors Secondary prevention by early diagnosis	Primary: incidence in population Secondary: death rate or serious complication rate
Exclusion of illness	Reliable (i.e. safe) reassurance	Absence of subsequent disease serious for which complaint could have harbinger Subjective reduction in anxiety in the patient (where anxiety has been the reason for presentation)
Acute physical illness or trauma	Removal or correction of disease process; repair of trauma, restoration of function	Presence or absence of pathology Recovery or non-recovery of function
Chronic physical illness	Control of disease process Reduction of subjective distress Restoration or maintenance of function	Objective measures of pathophysiology Subjective measures of experience Objective measures of function
Psychological illness at psychosis level	Protection from self-harm Reduction of distress Support for family/carers	Self-harm happens or does not happen Distress estimated by observer or recorded by patient Family/carers' satisfaction with the extent to which their perceived needs were met
Psychological illness at neurosis level	Reduction of distress Restoration of self-management Improvement of self-image	Distress recorded by patient Personal and social function measurement Self-image assessed by observer
Terminal illness	Symptom control Maintenance of function Achievement of acceptance (peace of mind)	Symptom assessment by patient, principal carer or professional observer Assessment of daily living/social function by patient and carers Assessment of peace of mind by patient and carers

Modified from Metcalfe, 1990

diabetes could be based on changes between annual reviews (Bardsley and Coles, 1992). Yet this provides an incomplete picture of the long-term effects of good quality care as complications of poorly controlled diabetes can take decades to become manifest.

Organising Information
The numbers of patients and practitioners involved in primary and out-patient care creates its own problems in terms of handling information and ensuring consistency of definitions necessary for comparative analyses. Though there is an increasing recognition of the need, both to develop standard definitions of medical terms and consistent recording, we are yet some way from the ideal.

In out-patient clinics, basic computerisation of records or booking systems has tended to take second place to the development of computerised systems to support in-patient care. In addition, there are problems of the number of junior doctors that are involved in recording basic patient information. On the other hand, many British general practitioners have their systems computerised, general practice fundholders especially so.

Moving Towards Outcome Assessments in Practice
The vision of commissioning and monitoring health services based on specified outcomes is still some way off. Nonetheless, though there are many problems, there are also opportunities which are being taken to increase the awareness of considering outcomes in the commissioning process.

Using the Knowledge We Have
Though in general our knowledge of the effectiveness of health services is limited, there is a strong argument that we are still not making best use of the research evidence that is available.

The Management Executive of the NHS commissioned a series of studies in developing epidemiologically based needs assessments (for an example see Williams, 1992) which sought to compile the best information available on the incidence and prevalence of disease together with evidence of service effectiveness. This work was specifically designed to help health authorities in their new role of determining health needs as a basis for the commissioning process.

The Department of Health has also funded a series of effectiveness bulletins which attempt to summarise the research literature in a way that identifies the lessons for health authorities (Long and Sheldon, 1992). Box 8.1 gives an example of the type of advice that such a bulletin offers in relation to the treatment of depression in primary care (Effective Health Care, 1993).

Box 8.1   Example of recommendations in effective health care: advice for decision makers when considering services for the treatment of depression in primary care

---

Recommendations for decision makers

Clinical guidelines for depressed people will be influenced by the available services locally but should include:

- criteria for detection/recognition of major depression in primary care, based upon a reliable diagnostic classification such as DSMIII-R

- clear guidance on appropriate treatment packages, including criteria for non-drug therapists and the prescription of different drug treatments. The guidelines may include a limited list of drugs to ensure cost-effectiveness whilst taking into account special needs

- FHSAs and purchasing authorities should consider allocating resources to fund suitably qualified cognitive therapists to improve the range of effective treatment options

- guidelines should also consider strategies for compliance with treatments

- given the multifactorial causation of depression, FHSAs, purchasing authorities and local authorities should identify ways in which coordinated interventions in the health and social spheres can be developed to help depressed individuals, and populations with high rates of depression.

Source: Effective Health Care, 1993

More recently, a centre for the analysis of results from clinical trials has been established (Chalmers *et al.*, 1992), which will disseminate up-to-date reviews of randomised controlled trials in health care. The NHS is also emphasising the value of a common database on Research and Development activity and the importance of outcome measurement in health technology assessment (Department of Health, 1993d).

These approaches are examples of how the NHS is seeking to improve its intelligence in identifying which services are effective and which are ineffective.

Using the Information We Have

Though existing information systems are by no means ideal for monitoring patient outcome, there are data available that are of value. The type of outcome indicator that we can develop from existing data are biased towards mortality, clinical measures or proxies for outcome based on some process (Charlton *et al.*, 1984; Middleton, 1987). Table 8.2 gives some examples.

Information on mortality is widely collected and disseminated throughout the health service. Indeed the national health strategy has been driven to a large extent by information on mortality. As well as the use of crude or standardised mortality rates broken down by area, there are also a series of mortality rates specifically for conditions amenable to treatment (Charlton *et al.*, 1983). Such data are widely distributed throughout the NHS in the form of the Public Health Common Data Set (Department of Health, 1993c).

There are also a variety of surveys which address health and lifestyle and can be used to monitor health improvement targets. The most recent to be developed has been aimed at issues associated with the national health strategy (Office of Population, Censuses and Surveys, 1992).

Table 8.2   Examples of routinely available outcome indicators

Outcome indicator	Example sources
Mortality rates General "Avoidable deaths" Perinatal Maternal	Public Health Common Data Set OPCS Population Health Outcome Indicators
Immunisation and vaccination rates	Public Health Common Data Set Health Service Indicators OPCS
Abortion rates	OPCS
Indicators of adverse events e.g. hospital admission for diabetic ketoacidosis and coma	Population Health Outcome Indicators
Conceptions under 16	OPCS
Uptake of cancer screening Breast cancer Cervical cancer	Health Service Indicators
Notifications Infectious disease Congenital abnormalities	OPCS

In some circumstances, a process measure may be an appropriate description of how a service is delivered. Examples include data on abortion rates, immunisation uptake or cervical cytology screening. Alternatively, a process measure may be a proxy for outcome. For example, in the case of asthma, emergency attendance or in-patient admission for asthma may be indicative of health status in the community (Logan, 1991; Strachan and Anderson, 1992). It is important to stress that such values are only indirect indicators of health outcome and that very often we are unclear as to their validity. Though efforts are put into establishing validity and responsiveness for new health status or quality of life scales, such work also needs to be done for these proxy measures.

The Department of Health has recently published a series of population health outcome indicators (Department of Health, 1993b) which are based on existing data. These are specifically aimed at comparative analyses of indicators where health service performance is felt to be a key factor in the observed outcome.

Development of New Information Systems and Data Sources

Though some progress can be made in identifying outcome indicators from existing information, in many cases new information systems and innovative approaches to outcome measurement will be necessary.

Increasingly, there is emphasis on the development of patient-completed questionnaires dealing with either general health status or disease-specific aspects of well-being. The terminology used to describe such scales varies and includes health status, quality of life, functional status, well-being etc. (Bowling, 1991; Wilkin et al., 1992). The development of such instruments is discussed in detail in other chapters within this book. For the commissioning health authority, these instruments have the advantage that they might offer better descriptions of health than more limited clinical or technical measures. In the right context, they may generate some important questions over the value of services that are offered (Ellwood, 1988; Tarlov et al., 1989).

Such instruments clearly have great potential in improving the ways that we assess services. However, they are not without their problems. One of the biggest is the uncertainty over the validity of a particular measure in a particular context. To date, most effort has been devoted to developing the scales, with less attention being paid to their application to specific managerial issues.

There is also the case for developing information systems which exploit routine clinical assessments of patients. Very often the information needed to assess changes in health states over time is the information used by the clinician every time he/she sees the patient. Thus for example, Jones et al. (1992) have proposed a simple scale to assess the problems of people with asthma (Box 8.2) using questions that are part of any routine consultation. Exploiting such approaches can be tied in to work developing chronic disease registers for conditions such as diabetes (Donaldson, 1992).

Box 8.2   A simple assessment of asthma morbidity

Morbidity Index

Are you in a wheezy or asthmatic condition at least once a week?

Have you had time off work or school in the past year because of your asthma?

Do you suffer from attacks of wheezing during the night?

No to all questions	= low morbidity
One yes	= medium morbidity
Two or three yeses	= high morbidity

Source: Jones *et al.*, 1992

The key problem facing the development of clinical information systems is ensuring consistency and reliability. This involves the need to clarify the terms used to describe patients and the ways that these are encoded. It also means establishing consistent criteria for inclusion in the database and enlisting the support of a great many different actors in contributing to that database. Typically such schemes tend to be led by the enthusiast during the early stages of development, such as in the Royal College of General Practitioners' survey of morbidity (Fleming and Crombie, 1992). Alliances between interested practitioners are possible as a way to test outcome measurement in different settings. One example would be an audit of the outcome of knee replacement across one regional health authority (Cleary, 1993).

APPLYING THE KNOWLEDGE

The use of outcome measures in commissioning can cover both prospective planning of services as well as retrospective monitoring of quality. These two approaches appear in a variety of settings.

Formulation and Monitoring of Health Strategies

Within the NHS one of the most significant applications of outcome information is in the recently launched national health strategy (Department of Health, 1992b). *The Health of the Nation* has identified six priority areas for health services development and a series of explicit health targets to be met over the next ten to twenty years. These targets are primarily based on mortality indicators and have for the most part been driven by available data and a shared database, the Public Health Common Data Set, which can provide annual information on progress.

As a consequence of a national strategy, local health strategies are being increasingly used in assessing performance of RHAs, DHAs and FHSAs. In particular, corporate contracts between these organisations are aiming to make explicit the health benefits that are likely to emerge and the links to shorter-term plans or actions.

Other examples of health strategies exist. The Welsh Health Planning Forum, established in 1988, has been developing a series of documents called *Protocols for Investment in Health Gain* that aim to identify the health benefits for key disease areas (Welsh Health Planning Forum, 1991). A number of English RHAs are also active in this area.

Developing Local Purchasing Plans and Needs Assessment

Health authorities are required not only to purchase services in a way that is consistent with strategies developed at higher levels in the organisation, but also to develop local purchasing plans detailing the configuration of services for the next few years.

Whilst the nature of such purchasing plans can often be driven by historical relationships with providers, there is a need to consider the contribution to the health of the population. The process of assessment of needs is fundamental to the development of such plans (Stevens, 1991). Conceptually the exploration of need and outcome are the same process and can use the same measures (Wilkin, 1992).

For example, one health authority in East Anglia has approached the problems of high termination of pregnancy rates amongst young women. It has developed local plans for the provision of advice on contraception, concentrating on younger women by instituting special clinics and working with schools, youth clubs and local family doctors. Contracts for these services are being drawn up and a series of outcome indicators identified, ranging from the uptake of services to rates of unplanned/unwanted pregnancy.

Very often, the decisions about which service to buy include not only uncertainty about differences in outcome but also about differences in cost. Information on the relative costs and benefits of treatments is even rarer and almost always absent in terms of local services (Donaldson and Mooney, 1991).

In addition, service specifications can be developed which identify key elements that must be offered as part of a given service. The nature and detail of service specifications can vary. They offer an opportunity to look in some detail at how services for particular client groups can be configured and what the objectives of care may be. In this way they can help to foster the application of outcome assessment in the dialogue between purchaser and providers. As an example, Box 8.3 shows some detail from a service specification for diabetes drawn up jointly by a DHA and FHSA. The document clearly specifies the types of outcome that it hopes to achieve for people with diabetes.

Box 8.3   An example of outcomes in service specifications

Health outcomes for the district diabetes programme

An effective overall district diabetes programme should result in the following desired health outcomes:

- Increased proportion of patients diagnosed at an early stage of the disease, before the onset of complications, compared to the total number of patients diagnosed

- Decreased incidence of the short-term consequences of diabetes e.g. ketoacidotic coma

- Decreased incidence of the iatrogenic consequences of treating diabetes e.g. hypoglycaemia

- Decreased incidence of psychological problems attributable to diabetes

- etc.

Extract from Purchasing specification for diabetes. Suffolk FHSA, Suffolk DHA. September 1992

One innovative approach to linking specific outcomes to purchasing that is being pursued by some health authorities (for example, Wandsworth Health Authority, in the London area) is the idea of a health gain fund. A sum of money is reserved and bids for specific projects approved on the basis of agreed health objectives and the means to monitor progress towards those goals.

Making Specific Requirements of Providers

The previous sections have been concerned with the ways that health authorities or other purchasers of care can use outcomes to identify and monitor their own plans, albeit in discussion with providers. There are circumstances where outcomes may be an explicit part of agreements between the health authority and the providers. This is an area that is more sensitive as the potential for conflict between the wishes of health authorities and their providers may come to the surface.

Commissioning authorities can increase their knowledge of outcome by requiring providers to undertake more systematic evaluations, audits or data collection. This is one way of exploiting the experience and often enthusiasm within provider units for examining their own outcomes. As an initial approach to developing outcome standards for quality assurance, it is also appealing since it is relatively non-threatening and encourages sharing of purchaser and provider perspectives on appropriate indicators of outcome. There is also the potential to recognise some of the uncertainties in interpretation of outcome data.

In primary care, additional payments are made available for family doctors who undertake clinics specifically for the management of selected chronic diseases such as diabetes. In return, these doctors can be expected to collect basic information on patients who are attending, some of which may be related to outcome.

Promotion of Good Practice

In many cases certain processes can be assumed to be linked to better outcomes, and monitoring of the process of care will provide a more practical and satisfactory assessment of quality than attempts to measure outcome.

Box 8.4 Example of how a health authority can use requirements for information or specific process in purchasing intentions

---

Reducing mortality from accidents: priorities for 1993 and onwards

Targets

Accidents under age 15	- 33% reduction by the year 2005
Accidents age 15-24	- 25% reduction by the year 2005
Accidents age 65+	- 33% reduction by the year 2005

Policies

Contracts with providers must include a requirement for clinical audit of Accident and Emergency Departments
A policy is needed on osteoporosis in the older people and the possibility of hormone replacement therapy
The health services should give unreserved support to accident-reducing initiatives such as the use of smoke alarms or the loan of child car safety seats

Further research

Identify groups at special risk through A&E audit
Study of young people's attitude to risk-taking behaviour

Advice and support

Information to families on minimising accident risks for children

Collaboration

The County Advisory Group on Health has put accident prevention as one of the priorities for action in 1994/95. At present existing prevention programmes are being reviewed and better coordination considered

---

There is considerable scope for using contracts to promote the adoption of protocols or guidelines which make explicit the types of care that should be undertaken (Sheldon and Borowitz, 1993). Box 8.4 gives one example of how the purchasing intentions of one health authority (in collaboration with the local FHSA) addresses the problem of high mortality from accidents (a *Health of the Nation* priority area). These show a local outcome target (albeit based on a national aim) linked to specific processes, using examples of good practice and addressing the need for better information.

Specifying Desired Outcomes
The extent to which explicit outcome standards become part of the commissioning process will be limited. The exercise requires defining measurable outcomes that are sufficiently valid and accepted by purchaser and provider. Achieving a consensus seems more likely for some services or conditions than for others. In the first instance, it is more likely that outcome measures in contracts will look at the avoidance of negative outcomes rather than at positive health improvement. There are still relatively few examples of where providers are required to achieve certain health outcomes. One example from East Anglia is of a purchaser who has required all providers to attain a defined level of success in screening for congenital abnormalities.

In other areas of quality assurance, there are more examples of where explicit standards are being added as quality clauses in contracts. Nationally *The Patient's Charter* (Department of Health, 1991) specifies a number of specific rights or standards of service (for examples, see Box 8.5). At a more local level, many providers agree to adhere to standards concerning the environment of care. In some cases these can be quite exacting, with agreed monitoring mechanisms.

Box 8.5 Examples of explicit standards in The Patient's Charter

Examples
To be guaranteed admission for treatment by a specific date no later than two years from the day when your consultant places you on the waiting list.
Waiting time in out-patient clinics - the Charter standard is that you will be given a specific appointment time and be seen within thirty minutes of that time.

Given the uncertainties of measuring outcome, there are concerns about whether precisely defined outcome targets for providers is really the best place to start. The inevitable questions is: what happens when a provider fails to acheive its target? How much of the failure is due to a deficiency on the part of the provider and how much to circumstances beyond their control, perhaps, for example, a change in the case mix of patients? If a provider does not meet the defined target, should the purchaser automatically transfer the contract elsewhere? The answer is that, as with any other aspect of the purchaser-provider relationship, there must be a dialogue about how and why a particular failure in performance happened. The advantages of using outcome measures is the potential for illuminating that dialogue by concentrating on the things that really matter - the health and well-being of the patients.

CONCLUSION

There is clearly a large gap between where we would like to be and where we are currently in terms of using outcome measurement in commissioning health services. There are opportunites for developing the use of outcome measures and these are being taken.

The present situation suggests that development will happen in a number of different ways and will take some time. The ability to measure outcome directly may take second place to the application of proxy measures for which data are more easily available. Where direct outcome measures are used, they will tend to be for selected client groups in specific circumstances, rather than across the board. And the link between the outcome measures and the commissioning process will be established in a variety of ways, in the first instance by affecting the planning of services before application of specific outcome requirements in contracts.

The picture offered here is one of a patchwork of development and application of outcome measures. The specification of explicit requirements for certain outcomes in contracts will take time to develop. There are too many uncertainties concerning the validity of outcome measures to suggest it would be otherwise. Perhaps most important is the contribution that outcome measurement can make to clarifying the objectives of care. In many instances it may be that the process of identifying the criteria by which services will be judged will yield the greater benefit.

REFERENCES

Bardsley, M. and Coles, J. (1992) Practical experiences in auditing patient outcomes. *Quality in Health Care*, **1**, 124-130.

Bowling, A. (1991) *Measuring health: a review of quality of life measurement scales*. Buckingham: Open University Press.

Brazier, J.E., Harper, R., Jones; N.M.B., O'Cathain, A., Thomas, K.J., Usherwood, T. and Westlake, L. (1992) Validating the SF-36 Health Survey Questionnaire: a new outcome measure for primary care. *British Medical Journal*, **305**, 160-164.

Birch, S. and Maynard, A. (1986) Performance indicators and performance assessment in the UK National Health Service: implications for management and planning. *International Journal of Health Planning and Management*, **1**, 145-156.

Chalmers, I., Dickerson, K. and Chalmers, T.C. (1992) Getting to grips with Archie Cochrane's agenda. *British Medical Journal*, **305**, 786-788.

Charlton, J., Bauer, R. and Lakhani, A. (1984) Outcome measures for district and regional health care planners. *Community Medicine*, **6**, 306-315.

Charlton, J., Hartley, R., Silver, R. and Holland, W. (1983) Geographical variations in mortality from conditions amenable to medical intervention in England and Wales. *Lancet*, **1**, 691-696.

Cleary, R. (1993) Establishing inter-hospital comparisons of outcome. *Proceedings of the 10th International Society for Quality Assurance meeting, Maastricht.*

Coulter, A. and Bradlow, J. (1993) Effect of NHS reforms on general practitioners' referral patterns. *British Medical Journal*, **306**, 433-437.

Department of Health (1989) *Working for patients.* London: HMSO. (Cm. 555)

Department of Health (1991) *The patient's charter.* London: HMSO.

Department of Health (1992a) *Health and personal social services statistics for England.* London: HMSO.

Department of Health (1992b) *The health of the nation: a strategy for health in England.* London: HMSO. (Cm. 1986)

Department of Health (1992c) *Health service indicators handbook.* London: Department of Health.

Department of Health (1993a) *Managing the new NHS: a background document.* London: Department of Health.

Department of Health (1993b) *Population health outcome indicators for the NHS 1993: England. A consultation document.* Brighton: Institute of Public Health, University of Surrey.

Department of Health (1993c) *Public Health Common Data Set 1993.* Brighton: Institute of Public Health, University of Surrey.

Department of Health (1993d) *Research for health.* London: Department of Health.

Deyo, R.A and Inui, T.S. (1984) Towards clinical applications of health status measures: sensitivity of scales to clinically important changes. *Health Services Research*, **19**, 275-289.

Donaldson, C. and Mooney, G. (1991) *Needs assessment, priority setting, and contracts for health care: an economic view.* Aberdeen: Health Economic Research Unit, University of Aberdeen. (Discussion Paper No 05/91)

Donaldson, L. (1992) Registering a need. *British Medical Journal*, **305**, 597-598.

Donabedian, A. (1985) *Explorations in quality assessment and monitoring, (3 vols).* Ann Arbor, MI: Health Administration Press.

Donabedian, A. (1988) Unity of purpose, diversity of means. *Inquiry*, **25**, 173-192.

Effective Health Care (1993) *The treatment of depression in primary care.* Bulletin No.5. Leeds: School of Public Health, Leed University.

Ellwood, P.M. (1988) Outcomes management: a technology of patient experience. *New England Journal of Medicine*, **318**, 1549-1556.

Fleming, D.M. and Crombie, D.L. (1992) *Weekly returns service.* Birmingham: Royal College of General Practitioners.

Glennerster, H., Matsaganis, M. and Owens, P. (1992) *A foothold for fundholding: a preliminary report on the introduction of GP fundholding.* London: King's Fund Institute.

Ham, C. (1988) *Health care variations: assessing the evidence.* London: King's Fund Institute. (Research report No.2)

Ham, C. (1991). *The new National Health Service: organisation and management.* Oxford: Radcliffe Medical Press.

Hopkins, A. and Maxwell, R. (1990) Contracts and quality of care. *British Medical Journal*, **300**, 919-922.

Huntington, J. (1993) From FPC to FHSA to health commision? *British Medical Journal*, **306**, 33-36.

Jones, K.P., Bain, D.J.G., Middleton, M. and Mullee, M.A. (1992) Correlates of asthma morbidity in primary care. *British Medical Journal*, **304**, 361-364.

Jenkins, L., Bardsley, M., Coles, J. and Wickings, I. (1988) *Use and validity of performance indicators in the National Health Service.* London: CASPE Research.

Liddell, A. (1992) Health gain. In: *The Standing Conference on Health Gain '92.* Cambridge: East Anglian Regional Health Authority.

Logan, S. (1991) Outcome measures in child health. *Archives of Diseases in Childhood*, **66**, 745-748.

Lohr, K. (1989) Advances in health status assessment. *Medical Care*, **27**, S1-S11.

Long, A.F. and Sheldon, T.A. (1992) Enhancing effective and acceptable purchaser and provider decisions: overview and methods. *Quality in Health Care*, **1**, 74-76.

Mawhinney, B. (1993) The vision for purchasing. In: *Purchasing for health: a framework for action.* London: Department of Health.

Metcalfe, D.H.H. (1990) Measurement of outcomes in general practice. In: Hopkins A. and Costain D. (Eds.) *Measuring the outcomes of medical care.* London: Royal College of Physicians.

Middleton, J.D. (1987) A discussion paper on outcomes for a non-teaching district. *Community Medicine*, **9**, 343-349.

Office of Population, Censuses and Surveys. Social Survey Division (1993) *Health survey for England 1991.* London: HMSO.

Patrick, D.L. and Deyo, R.A. (1989) Generic and disease-specific measures in assessing health status and quality of life. *Medical Care*, **27**, S217-S232.

Pollitt, C. (1989) Performance indicators in the longer term. *Public Money and Management*, **9** (3), 51-55.

Roberts, H. (1990) *Outcome and performance in health care: a guide to developments in outcome and performance assessment in the NHS.* London: Public Finance Foundation. (Discussion Paper No.33)

Sheldon, T.A. and Borowitz, M. (1993) Changing the measure of quality in the NHS: from purchasing activity to purchasing protocols. *Quality in Health Care*, **2**, 149-150.

Starey, N., Bosanquet, N. and Griffths, J. (1993) General practitioners in partnership with management: an organisational model for debate. *British Medical Journal*, **306**, 308-310.

Stevens, A. (1991) Needs assessment needs assessment. *Health Trends*, **23**, 20-23.

Strachan, D.P. and Anderson, H.R. (1992) Trends in hospital admission rates for asthma in children. *British Medical Journal*, **304**, 819-820.

Tarlov, A.R., Ware, J.E, Jr., Greenfield, S., Nelson, E.C., Perrin, E. and Zubkoff, M. (1989) The Medical Outcomes Study: an application of methods for monitoring the results of medical care. *Journal of the American Medical Association*, **262**, 925-930.

Welsh Health Planning Forum (1991) *Protocols for investment in health gain.* Cardiff: Welsh Office.

Williams, R. (1992) *Epidemiologically based needs assessment. Report 1: diabetes mellitus.* London: NHS Management Executive.

Wilkin, D. (1991) Health outcomes and general practice. *Primary Health Care Management*, **10**, 2-4.

Wilkin, D., Hallam, L. and Doggett, M. (1992) *Measures of need and outcome for primary health care.* Oxford: Oxford University Press.

Chapter 9 _____

WHAT IMPACT CAN OUTCOME ASSESSMENT HAVE ON A NATION'S HEALTH: AN ILLUSTRATION FROM ENGLAND

AZIM LAKHANI

INTRODUCTION

"To secure continuing improvement in the health of the people of England through efficient and cost-effective use of resources."

This summarises the goals to which both the United Kingdom (UK) Government's Department of Health and the National Health Service (NHS) in England work (Department of Health, 1992; Department of Health, 1994b), while acknowledging that health is influenced by wider efforts of society as well as by health care. The Department of Health aims to improve the health of the population directly by its own efforts, and also by working with other governmental departments. The NHS aims to do this through the use of its allocated resources as well as by acting in alliance with other relevant organisations at national, regional and local level. The NHS reforms which came into effect in 1991 created a system whereby resources are allocated to health authorities mainly on a resident population basis, using a weighted capitation formula (Department of Health, 1989). Health authorities have a responsibility to assess the health needs of their resident populations and use available resources to meet these defined health needs, through the purchase of appropriate services from a variety of providers. Following a report on the state of public health in England (Department of Health and Social Security, 1988), a special role has been created for public health departments within health authority structures to support such work. In parts of the NHS, fundholding general practitioners are allocated some funds to purchase a limited range of services on the same basis as described for health authorities.

This context is important in demonstrating the potential for outcome assessment to have an impact on a national population's health. There are several considerations. Firstly, there is an explicit, published goal of improving health. Secondly, the Government has published a strategy for health in England, *The Health of the Nation* (Department of Health, 1992), which not only sets targets for improvements in health but also identifies areas for action and those involved in taking the action forward. Thirdly, the health care system is working towards equitable allocation of resources by resident geographical population. Explicit goals for efficient and cost-effective use of these resources to improve the health of the populations have been set. An implementation and accountability structure to assure these have been set in place. Outcome, in this context, must thus relate to the extent to which such improvement is achieved. Primary and out-patient care (ambulatory care) are two of many contributors to such achievement and can not be examined in isolation.

Assessment of Health Outcomes: National Initiatives

While there is a general belief that the resources being used for health intervention (health care or otherwise) must be improving health, it is not possible at present to quantify that improvement fully nor is it possible to attribute a link to the use of resources. It is thus difficult to demonstrate that available resources are leading to the maximum possible improvement.

In order to help overcome some of this constraint, the Department of Health has set up a Central Health Outcomes Unit (CHOU) to coordinate the development of health outcomes assessment and promote its use. One strand of this work is the coordination of a structured programme to develop the technical ability and systems within the NHS to undertake routine and comprehensive assessment of outcomes. The Central Health Outcomes Unit is also working with the NHS, health professionals and others to disseminate and apply some of the results of the programme. As part of this initiative, the Central Health Outcomes Unit has commissioned, jointly with other health departments in the UK, a Clearing House for Information on Health Outcomes, based at the Nuffield Institute for Health in Leeds (UK Clearing House, 1994). The Clearing House acts as a resource centre of outcomes assessment materials; a source of critical reviews of methods; a focal point for networking and exchange of information; an education and training centre; and a provider of an advisory and consultancy service.

This chapter aims to show current approaches to outcomes assessment in the above context, to provide a macro perspective of such assessment and its likely impact on health at a national level.

POPULATION HEALTH OUTCOME MODELS

The Central Health Outcomes Unit uses as its definition of health outcome, "attributable effect of intervention or its lack on a previous health state" (Department of Health, 1994a). Change in health is often a cumulative effect of a multitude of influences over a period of time. Any attempt at health outcome assessment at a national population level needs to reflect this. Figure 9.1 (Department of Health, 1994a) is a generic population health outcome model developed by Central Health Outcomes Unit, based on previous such approaches (Lakhani, 1989; Department of Health, 1990). The left-hand side shows a sequence of health events, from risk of ill health to manifestation of ill health, its

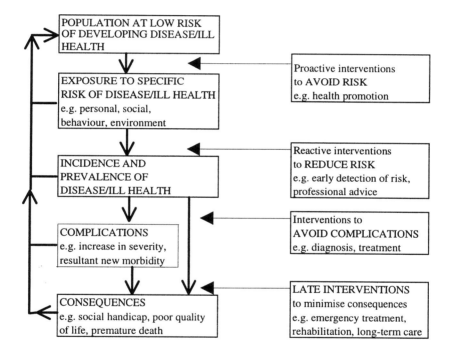

Figure 9.1 Population health outcome model

complications and consequences such as poor quality of life and early death. Health and ill health in this context cover the broader aspects of function, disability, handicap and well-being, not just signs, symptoms and disease. The right-hand side of Figure 9.1 shows how each part of the sequence may be influenced by targeted interventions. Using this model for asthma, for example, risks would include known allergens; ill health would include acute attacks; complications might include prolonged severe attacks; consequences would include misery caused by sleepless nights, days off school and work, loss of income, premature death. Interventions would include personal attempts at minimising contact with allergens; prophylactic drugs to prevent attacks, early detection and appropriate treatment of attacks; hospitalisation for very severe, prolonged attacks; to quote but a few examples. Potential uses of this approach for commissioning health care and working in alliance with other organisations to coordinate wider interventions have been described elsewhere (Lakhani, 1993). Figures 9.2 and 9.3 provide selected examples to illustrate outcomes assessment within such models at a national level, using currently available data from Department of Health Population Health Outcome Indicators (Department of Health, 1993c), national health surveys (Office of Population Censuses and Surveys, 1994) and Health Service Indicators (Department of Health, 1993d).

LIKELY IMPACT ON HEALTH

Outcome was defined earlier as "an attributable effect" of intervention or its lack. For the purpose of improving health, outcomes assessment thus requires the intervention or lack of a particular intervention to be specified as part of the assessment. Without this, a measure of health or any other kind of status on its own can not be called an outcome because it is not clear what, if anything, it is an "effect" of. This aspect is very important if outcomes assessment is to have any role in improving health. Unless the intervention or lack of it can be causally linked to health, it will not be possible to modify practice to improve health.

A proactive attempt to improve health, based on outcome assessment, requires two issues to be considered: what improvement can be expected; and how successful is the organisation in its endeavour to improve health. This is implicit in what many health professionals do in their clinical practice and also in what many health organisations do. Few, however, are able to demonstrate this at a macro level.

The Central Health Outcomes Unit has defined the following steps towards addressing these two aspects (Department of Health, 1994a):

a) Specify expectation of health outcome:
   i)   assess baseline level of health, ill health, disease severity and health determinants
   ii) access knowledge about effectiveness and cost-effectiveness of interventions
   iii) define health outcome objectives of interventions (plus targets if possible)
   iv) specify standards of intervention required to achieve desired outcomes.
b) Audit achievement of health outcome:
   i)   audit delivery of interventions to the standards specified (proxy)
   ii) audit end-point health, severity and determinants and attribute to interventions.

Figure 9.2 presents a model of how these steps may be used at national level to improve health. It shows firstly that individual interventions should not be considered in isolation. Change in health is often a cumulative effect of a number of influences over time. It may, however, be possible to assess baseline levels of risk, disease and ill health, and their complications and consequences. Based on assessments, it may be possible to set targets for change and audit achievement. The examples quoted are inevitably disease-based as they are dependent on current routine data. Aspects such as physical function, disability, mental health state, handicap, well-being could equally be placed within such models if data on these aspects were available. Similarly, health outcome objectives could be stated in terms of expected changes in some of these broader aspects of health. Assessment of this would then need objective measures as well as patient perceptions. There is a substantial effort underway in England currently to develop such broad data as part of routine data systems (National Health Service Management Group, 1992). When developing health outcome objectives, it is necessary to consider perspectives, values and cultures of individual patients, communities, carers, policy makers, managers, researchers and other interests, not just those of the health professionals.

Approaches such as Figure 9.2 present a macro perspective and need to be underpinned by a lot of detailed, supporting information. The example is illustrative only and based on different populations at different points in time. Therefore, no attempt should be made to infer associations, let alone causality from them. They are quoted essentially to illustrate an approach. They do, however, show how the working definition of health outcomes could be used, i.e relating health to intervention or its lack. What is immediately apparent is how patchy the coverage of the model is, highlighting inadequacies of current routine data systems to provide a full understanding of outcomes in a way that supports proactive action.

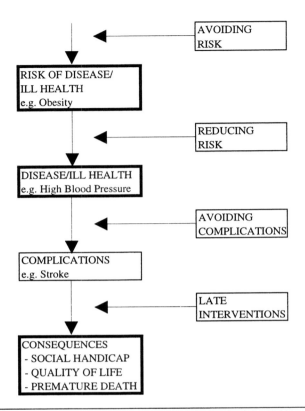

Comments: Stroke accounted for 12% of all deaths in England in 1991 and was a major cause of disability, particularly among older people. It accounts for 6% of total NHS expenditure and results in loss of about 7.7 million working days each year. Shown above are a few selected examples of how routine data may provide a macro perspective of ourcome. Obesity in England actually increased between 1986/7 and 1991. The target for mean systolic blood pressure is a reduction of 5mm by the year 2005 from the above 1991 baseline. There is considerable geographical variation in mortality between districts in England. It is not currently possible to assess key outcomes such as incidence of stroke, physical functional disability, social handicap and health-related quality of life using routine data. Completion of the model requires collection of data on interventions such as health promotion to avoid risk; professional advice to reduce risk; early detection and treatment of high blood pressure; and treatment, rehabilitation and care following a stroke, the majority of which are based in the ambulatory care sector. Any attempt at improving health needs to allow for complex interactions between all of these.

Figure 9.2 Action for health: stroke

Example: Risk of disease/ill health

Percentage distribution of adults by body mass index
(age 16-64 by sex; Great Britain/England; 1980, 1986/7 and 1991)

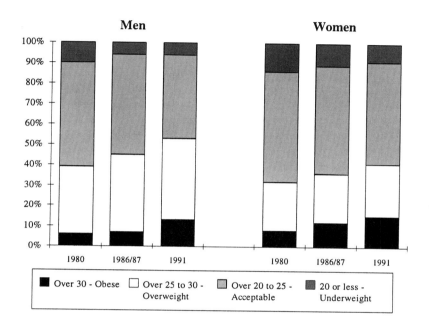

Example: Disease/ill health

	Mean systolic blood pressure	% hypertensive (Untreated)	% hypertensive (Treated)
Men 16 +	140mmHg	13%	4%
Women 16+	137mmHg	11%	6%

Source: Health Survey for England, 1991

Figure 9.2   Action for health: stroke (continued)

Example: Consequences

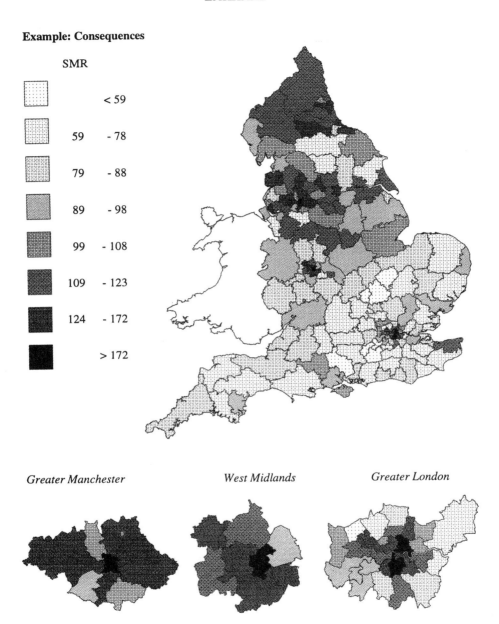

Figure 9.2   Action for health: stroke (continued)

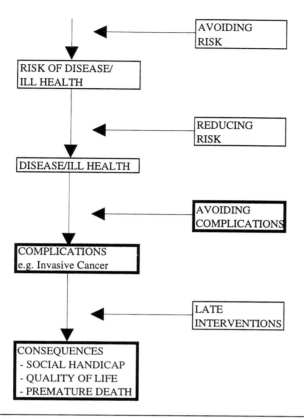

Comments: Although deaths from cervical cancer have fallen over the last 20 years, more than 1,500 women still die of the disease each year in England. In 1988 the Government introduced a national cervical cancer screening programme using computerised call and recall systems, building on earlier screening programmes. Health Authorities are required to invite women aged 20-64 for cervical screening, and to recall them at least every five years. A system of target payments was introduced in 1990 for general medical practitioners who screen women on their practice lists. As the objective is to detect abnormal cells before they become cancerous, key outcomes include the incidence of invasive cancer and death, both of which are potentially preventable. Coverage of the population by the screening programme acts as a proxy for outcome and although by 1991/2 it had increased to 80% of women being screened in the 5.5 years up to then, there is geographical variation in coverage between NHS Districts and Regions.

Figure 9.3 Action for health: cervical cancer

Example: Avoiding complications

Screening for cervical cancer
(Women aged 20-64 years by District, England, 1991/92)

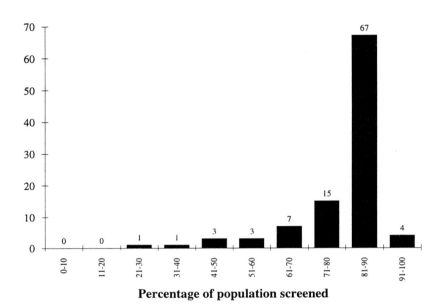

Percentage of population screened

Example: Complications

Health of the Nation Target - To reduce the incidence of invasive cervical cancer by at least 20% by the year 2000 from 15 per 100,000 population to no more than 12 per 100,000

Figure 9.3   Action for health: cervical cancer (continued)

Example: Premature death

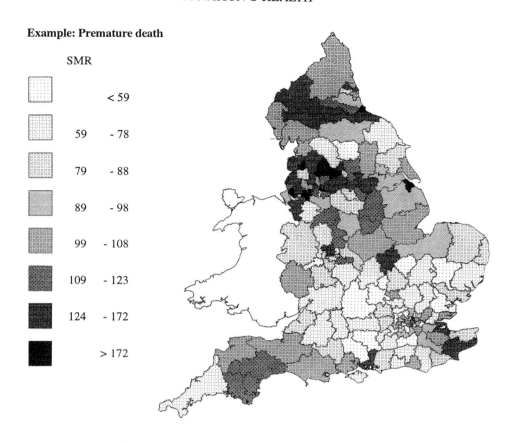

SMR

< 59

59   - 78

79   - 88

89   - 98

99   - 108

109   - 123

124   - 172

> 172

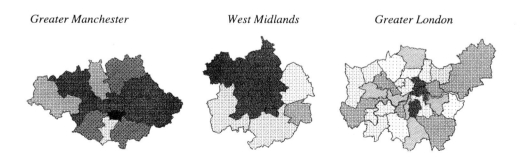

Greater Manchester   *West Midlands*   *Greater London*

Figure 9.3   Action for health: cervical cancer (continued)

A further consideration is the complex interactions and the differences in time lag between different parts of the model. The model should be seen as dynamic, not static. For example, in Figure 9.2, a population reduction in obesity may lead to a beneficial shift in the population distribution of systolic blood pressure which will impact on the need for treatment of high blood pressure, the incidence of strokes and their treatment, and premature death, each with its own time lag. An intervention at one level might thus have a multiple cascade effect. Any other intervention might then interact with every part of this cascade.

Such assessments could lead to changes in policy and management action. For example, with reference to Figure 9.3, early data on lower than expected population coverage of cervical cancer screening after implementation of the national screening programme led the national management tier of the National Health Service (Department of Health, 1994b) to issue guidance on improving coverage. By targeting areas with low coverage as well as making performance assessment part of the reporting and accountability process, there has been a cumulative national increase from 74% in 1990/1 to 80% in 1991/2. There is scope for further improvement and much of the remaining variation in coverage between regional and local health authorities is currently being addressed through specification of targets and action in corporate contracts between the NHS headquarters and districts.

Such contractual structures do not exist for those health problems that are only partially amenable to health care. For example, in considering morbidity, disability, handicap and premature death from road traffic accidents, much of the health care intervention comes at a fairly late stage, i.e ambulances, resuscitation, treatment at accident and emergency departments, hospital treatment, rehabilitation. A population health outcome model on health consequences of road traffic accidents shows that much of the action required to prevent accidents and severe injury is outside the direct control of the health care system (Lakhani, 1993). For such health issues, the Government, and in particular the Department of Health, is promoting working through common purpose alliances at national, regional and local level (Department of Health, 1993d). Health outcomes assessment, as described above, should help focus attention on key issues, hence policy and management action.

CONCLUSIONS

This chapter has sought to demonstrate the potential for outcomes assessment to lead to improvement in a population's health by: describing a structured framework for outcomes planning and assessment at a population level; showing how such assessment may relate to health policy and management action; describing an environment which is conducive to this, i.e a government policy to improve health, and a health care system with an explicit goal to improve health as well as structures, financial allocation and accountability systems to assure this.

It is still too early to demonstrate the effectiveness of this. Evaluation will require demonstration of appropriate change in the processes of health intervention as well as attributable improvement in health over time, a complex task. *The Health of the Nation* initiative already has, within it, proposals for monitoring and evaluating the strategy and a first anniversary publication describes activity to date as well as progress towards the targets (Department of Health, 1993b). Similarly, the national management tier of the National Health Service negotiates and monitors activity as well as health targets for the National Health Service, covering both *The Health of the Nation* and other health issues where the National Health Service has an important role. The foundations for an impact on health have been well laid.

Acknowledgements
The contents of this chapter are based on synthesis by the Central Health Outcomes Unit of contributions by numerous people over many years, as part of a national development programme.

REFERENCES

Department of Health and Social Security (1988) *Public health in England: the report of the committee of inquiry into the future development of the public health function.* London: HMSO. (Cm. 289)

Department of Health (1989) *Working for patients.* London: HMSO. (Cm. 555)

Department of Health (1990) *On the state of the public health : the annual report of the Chief Medical Officer of the Department of Health for the year 1989.* London: HMSO.

Department of Health (1992) *The health of the nation: a strategy for health in England.* London: HMSO. (Cm. 1986)

Department of Health (1993a) *Health service indicators handbook.* London: Department of Health.

Department of Health (1993b) *One year on: a report on the progress of the health of the nation.* London: Department of Health.

Department of Health (1993c). *Population Health Outcome Indicators for the NHS 1993: England. A consultation document.* Guildford: Institute of Public Health, University of Surrey.

Department of Health (1993d) *Working together for better health.* London: Department of Health.

Department of Health (1994a) *Central Health Outcomes Unit.* London: Department of Health.

National Health Service Management Executive Information Management Group (1992) *Information management and technology strategy for the NHS in England*. London : HMSO.

Lakhani, A. (1989) What do we need to measure? In: *Towards informed action for health: first annual report of the Director of Public Health*. London: West Lambeth Health Authority.

Lakhani, A. (1993) The role of health outcomes assessment in health care commissioning. In: *Best practice in health care commissioning*. Peel and Sheaff (Eds.) Harlow: Longman.

Office of Population Censuses and Surveys. Social Survey Division (1994) *Health survey for England 1992*. London: HMSO.

UK Clearing House for Information on the Assessment of Health Outcomes (1994) *Outcomes briefing, No. 4*. Leeds: Nuffield Institute for Health.

Chapter 10 _____

OUTCOME MEASURES IN OUT-PATIENT ASTHMA CARE

FIONA MOSS, PENNY FITZHARRIS, ALISON FRATER, DUNCAN KEELEY AND DUNCAN FATZ

INTRODUCTION

It is estimated in the United Kingdom (UK) that six per cent of the adult population suffer from asthma. Much attention has been focused on the problems associated with acute asthma. There are 2000 asthma deaths each year (Alderson, 1987), a figure that has not changed with the introduction of new therapies, and asthma is a frequent cause of hospital admission. The frequency of asthma attacks in the community has been estimated at 14.3/1000 patients per year (Neville *et al.*, 1993). However, for the majority of people with asthma, their symptoms represent a chronic and often intermittent problem which does not result in admission to hospital nor referral to a hospital-based respiratory physician.

This chapter will discuss the outcomes of asthma in the context of the aims and objectives of care in an ambulatory setting of patients with chronic persistent asthma (in line with the description given by the British Thoracic Society (BTS)). We chose this definition to distinguish between the care of this patient group, and those with acute asthma. Nevertheless, we recognise that for some patients asthma may be neither chronic nor persistent. We also recognise that the distinction between acute severe and chronic persistent asthma may not be clear cut, and that these two clinical descriptions only partly describe the complexity of the range of clinical presentation of asthma.

Chronic asthma remains a leading cause of morbidity in the developed world despite the introduction of effective interventions. Widespread asthma-related morbidity in the general population suggests that many people with this condition

139

are not getting therapy that would improve their symptoms and diminish lifestyle restrictions. A better understanding and use of patient outcomes in the care of individuals with asthma is essential if the morbidity from asthma is to improve. But outcome in ambulatory asthma care has several dimensions and may not be straight forward.

The Nature of Asthma

Asthma, now understood as a chronic inflammatory condition affecting the airways, is defined by variability in airflow. Variation of symptoms is a hallmark of clinical presentation. Symptoms often improve over time, may vary diurnally or seasonally or with exposure to specific allergens.

In addition to the variable natural history of asthma within one individual, the degree of morbidity between individuals also varies widely. Aside from acute episodes of asthma, morbidity from asthma ranges from minor exercise-, cold- or seasonally induced symptoms, to situations where asthma itself causes a profound limitation on daily activity, and to circumstances where the burden of therapy adds further to morbidity and cramping of lifestyle. The long-term implications and impact of asthma on lifestyle varies also. For many people with asthma, asthma affects their health and activity for only part of their lifetime and then recedes as a health problem. For others, asthma represents a life-long burden on their quality of life.

Treatment of Asthma

The intended mainstay of therapy is regular anti-inflammatory medication, usually in the form of inhaled steroids. The dose is, in theory at least, adjusted to response and outcome. Some patients may need occasional courses of oral steroids to counter exacerbations. Short-acting β_2-agonists, in general, are meant to be used for symptomatic relief on an "as needed" basis. Effective anti-inflammatory medication will minimise the need for such symptomatic relief. For people with more severe asthma, other medications may be required; some will need treatment with long-term oral steroids.

Aims of Asthma Care

The aims of asthma treatment and principles of management are set out at the beginning of the British Thoracic Society (BTS) guidelines on the management of asthma (1993) (see Box 10.1). Patient participation and the requirement of a partnership between patient, family and health professional are emphasised as important aspects of management. The general principle of adjusting treatment to minimise symptoms, while avoiding the use of unnecessary therapy, applies to all people with asthma, regardless of severity.

Box 10.1 Aims and principles of asthma management

Aims of asthma management
*   To recognise asthma
*   To abolish symptoms
*   To restore normal or best possible long-term airway function
*   To reduce the risk of severe attacks
*   To enable normal growth to occur in children
*   To minimise absence from work or school

Principles of management
*   Patient and family participation
*   Avoidance of identified causes where possible
*   Use of lowest effective doses of convenient medications minimising short- and long-term side-effects

---

OUTCOME MEASUREMENT IN ASTHMA

Understanding and acknowledging the variable nature of asthma is central to any discussion about outcome of chronic persistent asthma and highlights the importance of focusing on outcome for the individual patient. While prevention of death, or prevention or quick amelioration of acute episodes of asthma, or reduction in the need for admission to hospital with acute asthma, are important aims of asthma care at the population level, these outcome objectives are the immediate focus of care for only some individuals with asthma. For example, for a schoolboy with exercise-induced asthma, care may focus on the appropriate use of drugs to enable full participation in school sports. For a woman with chronic severe asthma the main objective of care may be to adjust oral steroid therapy to the minimum which enables her to carry out the routine tasks of daily living.

Linking Outcome with Care

The importance of outcome assessment in the context of the service arm of health care is based on assumptions regarding the relationship of health care interventions and outcome. The question of attributality of health care intervention is central to any discussion about outcome of care - and, for this, good research evidence is needed. Thus if the health care interventions (processes of care) are known to be effective and are used appropriately then the resulting outcomes for people with asthma should be positive; that is there will be a reduction in symptoms, a reduction in the effect of asthma on daily life and, assuming a minimal burden of therapy, an improvement in the health-related quality of life. However, for individuals with asthma in some instances improvement in symptoms may occur spontaneously without the use of an appropriate intervention - although an appropriate intervention may have hastened recovery.

Three levels of outcome have been described, each of which may apply to asthma (Shanks and Frater, 1993). A *health outcome* is an effect manifest as a change in health status without specified cause or effect. A *health care outcome* occurs when an outcome or result is attributable to health care but itself may not necessarily be a change in health status (for example, a change in social circumstances). A *health outcome of health care* is when a change is one of health status and is attributable and responsive to a health care intervention.

All three categories of outcome need to be recognised in the management of chronic persistent asthma. The first results from the natural variation in asthma symptoms. Failure to recognise asthma in the out-patient setting or to manage it correctly does not inevitably lead to further deterioration and most people with mild episodes will recover spontaneously, albeit after some time and at the expense of unnecessary morbidity and impaired quality of life. The natural variation of asthma partly explains the finding that it takes on average 16 visits to a general practitioner before a child is given a positive diagnosis of asthma and has the opportunity to start appropriate therapy (Ley and Bell, 1984). Some people with asthma become convinced that their asthma improves with two or three courses of antibiotics, not because the antibiotics are relevant to the asthma, but simply because the episode eventually subsides as part of the natural pattern of the asthma.

Asthma care may affect aspects of life other than health status and these should be considered important outcomes of asthma care by health professionals. For example, enabling a person with asthma to understand its nature may reduce anxiety; rationalising preventative treatment to a twice daily regime may enable a school pupil to manage more confidently at school.

Improving health outcome by health care intervention is clearly the key objective of asthma care. The use of outcome measures are central to self-management of asthma. There are several ways of assessing health outcome in asthma care; clinical outcome, patient-assessed outcome, physiological outcome and management outcome. There is clearly overlap between these categories. Each is important in asthma management but none can be used alone.

Clinical outcome includes symptoms such as cough, nocturnal disturbance, wheeze and shortness of breath; the frequency of untoward episodes, for example admissions to hospital, attendance at casualty departments or emergency attendances at general practitioner surgery; the use of a short course of oral steroids, and the number of extra doses of β_2-agonist needed each day. Although the latter categories are proxies for outcomes rather than health care outcomes in their own right, they are useful objective indicators of the effectiveness of care.

Patient-assessed outcomes are partly an extension of clinical outcomes. Their inclusion as a separate category emphasises the importance of understanding and using an individual's own perception of the effects of asthma on lifestyle, quality of life, and on general health in the management of chronic persistent asthma.

Limitation of activity, days off work or school and nights disturbed because of nocturnal asthma are three key features of chronic persistent asthma whose presence or frequency, as reported by the patient or parent, could form the basis of a simple morbidity index for recording and reporting the level of interference with everyday life experienced by individuals and groups. In addition there may be highly personalised outcome events - for example, the woman who reported that she knew when her asthma was beginning to become troublesome when she had difficulty in square dancing. Health professionals should aim to understand on an individual basis the limitations that asthma produces on normal activity.

Box 10.2   Outcomes expected from treatment of chronic persistent asthma

Outcome for mild to moderately severe asthma
(steps 1-3 on British Thoracic Society (BTS) stepwise approach to management)

* Minimal (ideally none) chronic symptoms
* Minimal (infrequent) exacerbations
* Minimal need for bronchodilators
* No limitations on activities
* Circadian variation in PEFR <20%
* PEFR >80% of best or predicted
* Minimal side-effects from medicine

Outcome for moderately severe to severe asthma
(steps 4-5 of BTS stepwise approach to management)

* Least possible symptoms
* Least possible need for relieving bronchodilators
* Least possible limitation of activity
* Least possible circadian variation in PEFR
* Best PEFR
* Least adverse effects from medicine

Asthma is described physiologically in terms of air flow resistance. Air flow may be monitored in terms of peak expiratory flow rate, measured using a portable peak flow meter, and forced expiratory volume in one second, and forced vital capacity, measured using a standard spirometer. Traditionally these physiological outcome measurements are recorded at each clinic, but the diurnal variation of asthma limits the usefulness of such "one-off" measurements for the assessment of asthma. The availability of relatively cheap, portable peak flow meters allows people with asthma to measure and to chart their own peak flows at home, usually on a twice daily basis, as part of ambulatory care management. This provides the important diurnal monitoring that will demonstrate the presence or absence of morning falls in air flow that for many people indicates relative instability of asthma. In addition to providing important physiological outcome information, ambulatory monitoring of peak flow measurement gives the responsibility and ownership of measurement to the asthma sufferer and allows patients to adjust therapy accordingly.

Such self-management by the patient is a central feature of asthma care. This is necessary as asthma is a variable condition. Treatment is varied in response to symptoms, using the lowest effective doses. There is a requirement for prompt treatment of acute episodes and worsening symptoms by adjusting medication accordingly, either by increasing inhaled steroids or, where indicated, by adding oral steroids. The ability of patients to self-manage asthma confidently and appropriately by assessing symptoms and peak flow measurement and taking appropriate action is itself an important management outcome of asthma care.

Self-managed care plans, such as the credit card plan (D'Souza *et al.*, 1994) place an emphasis on individualised skills rather than general knowledge acquisition. They require the patient's active participation and this may be more effective in facilitating long-term behavioural change than other approaches.

The BTS Guidelines outline outcomes expected in the treatment of chronic persistent asthma; these are a combination of the physiological, clinical and patient-assessed outcome (Box 10.2). The crucial issue, particulary for severe asthma, is the relationship between the level of morbidity and health care intervention. The aim of abolishing symptoms of asthma is not applicable to all people with asthma all of the time and thus a level of morbidity - even with good care - is inevitable.

Quality of Life Measurement in Asthma

To date, validated generic instruments measuring general health status, such as the Sickness Impact Profile and the Quality of Well-Being Scale, have been used more in chronic airways disease than in asthma. These well-validated questionnaires differentiate between severe and moderate airways disease but have little sensitivity for mild to moderate disease (Jones, 1991). More recently, disease-specific measures of quality of life for patients with airways disease have been developed. These are likely to have greater sensitivity than general health status measures. Again the emphasis has been more on assessment of patients with chronic airways disease than asthma.

The Living with Asthma questionnaire is an asthma-specific questionnaire designed to be used as an outcome measure in clinical trials and as a tool for helping in the management of individuals with asthma. Its 68 items and 11 domains were derived from focus group discussions with people with asthma (Hyland, 1991).

The St George's Respiratory Questionnaire, a self-completed questionnaire, provides a total "score" derived from three parts; symptoms, which quantify the distress from respiratory symptoms; activity, which measures the disturbance to physical activity; and a measure of the overall disturbance to daily life and well-being. This validated questionnaire demonstrates responses to improvements in health following therapy (Jones *et al.*, 1991). Another questionnaire, the Asthma Quality of Life Questionnaire, measures the component of asthma of immediate relevance to patients, and has been shown to discriminate between those who are stable, those who respond to treatment, and those who have natural fluctuations in severity (Juniper *et al.*, 1993).

Whilst the use of such questionnaires is being recognised as important for clinical research into asthma, the place of such instruments in ambulatory care has not been established. Their length makes them impracticable for use in routine practice.

Using Outcomes in Asthma Care

Part of the process of consultation is a discussion between health care professional and patient about expectation of outcome and deliberation over choices of health care intervention. Education about asthma and patient participation in management plans are part of modern asthma care. The need for self-management in asthma care - as distinct from a general desirability for all patients to take part in decision-making about health care intervention - arises from the variability and uncertainty that characterises asthma. It is often not possible to predict when and if asthma will deteriorate. Linking peak flow measurement with symptoms and patient-assessed limitations on lifestyle enables many people with asthma to self-manage their condition. While peak flow gives an objective measurement of airflow, teaching people with asthma the significance of symptoms and the linkage of symptoms to fluctuations in peak flow may also be important in highlighting when to take appropriate action if their asthma worsens (Charlton *et al.*, 1990; D'Souza *et al.*, 1994). Thus, setting outcome goals must become part of individual patient management plans. For this to be a useful approach to care, asthma and its positive and negative outcomes must be discussed in terms that clearly relate to an individual's daily life and usual activity, but this varies enormously between people. Each person with asthma needs to be able to assess clinical outcome, to relate changes to variation in physiological outcome e.g. peak flow, and alter therapy in response to these changes. Thus a central tenet of modern asthma care - self-management - requires people with asthma to have an understanding of outcomes both positive and negative. All types of outcome, patient-assessed outcomes with clinical, physiological and management outcomes, need to come together for each individual.

TARGETING CARE

Current Status of Morbidity from Asthma

Several studies in the UK have surveyed the incidence of symptoms amongst populations of patients identified as having asthma in primary care settings and in the general population. Whilst these studies do not provide direct information about the link between morbidity and health care they outline the extent of the current burden of morbidity and the challenge to those who work in asthma care.

Asthma morbidity in the primary care setting has been measured using an index of reported morbidity, based on three questions asked of patients receiving repeat prescription for asthma (Horn and Cochrane, 1989). Such an approach using a simple questionnaire might help identify and target those people with worst outcomes from asthma but has yet to be validated.

Nocturnal waking is a problem reported by between one third and half of patients identified as having asthma from primary care records (Horn and Cochrane, 1989; Turner Warwick, 1989; Jones *et al.*, 1992). Furthermore, asthma restricts to some extent the daily activity of between one quarter and a half of all asthma sufferers (Charlton *et al.*, 1990; Hilton *et al.*, 1986; Juniper *et al.*, 1993). Data from 140 patients with asthma attending three chest clinics in North West London shows a similar pattern of morbidity (Figures 10.1 and 10.2). The data from these and from other studies suggests that for many patients outcome for asthma was not meeting the aims set out in the British Thoracic Society guidelines.

There is marked variation in the care of people with asthma. Unnecessary morbidity is thought to equate with under-use of inhaled anti-inflammatory medication possibly accompanied by overuse of β_2 agonists. The use of general practice Prescribing Analyses and Cost (PACT) data has been suggested as an approach determining good prescribing for asthma (Jones, 1992). General practitioners with a known interest in asthma care have higher than average prescribing costs for respiratory drugs. The link between prescribing data - and in particular the use of prophylactic anti-inflammatory medication for asthma - and morbidity and outcome has yet to be established. Nevertheless PACT data may be an approach to targeting initiatives for improving asthma care.

Assessing the Quality of Care

Outcome is one measure on a spectrum of quality of care measures. No simple outcome measure for assessing the quality of care in out-patient asthma exists. Whether a particular outcome represents good care of chronic persistent asthma will vary between patients. The importance of balancing the burden of morbidity with the burden of therapy adds an important dimension to the assessment of outcome in chronic persistent asthma. For some people with asthma most of the time and probably for all people with asthma some of the time, there is a trade-off between the effect of asthma on daily life and the amount of therapy taken. In particular, for some people with asthma, fear of steroids in any form conditions acceptance of symptoms and reluctance to increase inhaled steroid therapy. In the best circumstances these trade-offs are made through discussion between the asthma specialist and the patient.

There is also such a range of severity that outcome goals are difficult to apply to a population of patients - for example to use clinical outcome to assess the care of patients on a general practice asthma register. Waking one night a week and having a morning cough most mornings with a limitation on sporting activity might be a good outcome for a person with moderately severe asthma currently taking a high dose of inhaled steroid therapy, whose symptoms were much more prominent and disruptive. On the other hand such symptoms for another patient with mild asthma may represent asthma at its most bothersome and failure to increase therapy to deal with these could be judged a poor health outcome of health care.

ASTHMA OUTCOMES

Short- and medium-term health outcomes of health care in asthma vary over time. So the current status of a person attending for a routine appointment at an asthma clinic might not give a true reflection of the outcome of asthma care. For example a person with asthma might be well now but over the past month may have had eight days away from work because of asthma and experienced nocturnal disturbance for 15 out of 30 nights.

There is, as yet, little firm evidence that maximising lung function in the short term affects lung health in the future. Unlike diabetes care where there is a link between aspects of the process of care and long-term outcome, the imperatives for asthma care relate to current symptoms and quality of life. The only exception to this is care of asthma in childhood when failure to treat asthma may result in growth retardation. A major challenge for research is to design and carry out studies to determine the implications for respiratory health in later life of asthma and asthma management and to quantify any risks which may attach to the long-term use of commonly used therapeutic agents.

CONCLUSION

Understanding a range of outcome measures is central to the management of asthma. Outcome of asthma care should include patient-assessed outcome as well as clinical and management outcomes and physiological measures. The outcome of asthma care varies between patients and varies over time. There is no simple outcome measure that can be used to assess the quality of care of chronic persistent asthma. But the need to develop effective measures remains important, for the level of morbidity from asthma in the general population suggests that many people with asthma are receiving less than adequate treatment. Outcome measures are one means of identifying those inadequacies.

REFERENCES

Alderson, M. (1987) *Trends in mortality and morbidity form asthma.* London: HMSO.

British Thoracic Society (1993) Guidelines on the management of asthma. *Thorax,* **48**, S1 - S24.

Charlton, I., Charlton, G., Broomfield, J. and Mullee, M.A. (1990) Evaluation of peakflow and symptoms only self management plans for control of asthma in general practice. *British Medical Journal,* **301**, 1355-1359.

D'Souza, W., Crane, J., Burgess, C., Te Karu, H., Fox, C., Harper, M. and Robson, B. (1994) Community based asthma care: trial of a "credit card" asthma self management plan. *European Respiratory Journal,* **7**, 1260-1265.

Hilton, S., Sibbald, S., Anderson, H. R. and Freeling, P. (1986) Controlled evaluation of the effects of patient education on asthma morbidity in general practice. *Lancet,* i, 26-29.

Horn, C.R. and Cochrane, G.M. (1989) An audit of morbidity associated with chronic asthma in general practice. *Respiratory Medicine,* **83**, 71-75.

Hyland, M.E. (1991) The living with asthma questionniare. *Respiratory Medicine,* **85 (Suppl B)**, 1306.

Jones, K. (1992) Impact of an interest in asthma on prescribing costs in general practice. *Quality in Health Care,* **1**, 110-113.

Jones, K.P., Bain, D.J.G., Middleton, M. and Mullee, M. (1992) Correlates of asthma morbidity in primary care. *British Medical Journal,* **304**:361-364.

Jones, P.W. (1991) Quality of life measurement for patients with airways disease. *Thorax,* **46**, 676-682.

Jones, P.W., Quirk, F.H. and Baveystock, C.M. (1991) The St George's Respiratory Questionnaire. *Respiratory Medicine,* **85, (Suppl B)**, 25-31.

Juniper, E.F., Guyatt, G.H., Ferrie, P.J. and Griffith, L.E. (1993) Measuring quality of life in asthma. *American Review of Respiratory Disease,* **147**, 832-838.

Levy, M.L. and Bell, L.C. (1984) General practice audit of asthma in childhood. *British Medical Journal,* **289**, 1115-1116.

Neville, R.G., Clark, R.C., Hoskins, G. and Smith, B. (1993) National asthma attack audit 1991-92. *British Medical Journal,* **306**, 559-562.

Shanks, J. and Frater, A. (1993) Health status, outcome and attributality: is a red rose red in the dark? *Quality in Health Care,* **2**, 259-262.

Turner Warwick, M. (1989) Nocturnal asthma: a study in general practice. *Journal of the Royal College of General Practice,* **39**, 239-243.

Chapter 11 _____

WHICH OUTCOME MEASURE?
A METHODOLOGICAL REVIEW

MAX JACOBS AND JOS A G DESSENS

_____

INTRODUCTION

Doctors within Western societies have been confronted with important changes in levels of morbidity because of developments such as a higher standard of living, better housing, better hygiene, and growing life expectancies. Nowadays, health care is increasingly concerned with clinical care in people with chronic illness and patients with common, non-invasive disorders (Tarlov, 1983).

The central objective of a doctor's involvement with most of these patients is no longer exclusively restricted to the cure of a patient's disease but increasingly focuses on the improvement of a patient's functioning in daily life (Cluff, 1981). This has led to a view that the effects of medical care on a patient's health can no longer be efficaciously assessed merely by ascertaining absence or presence of signs or symptoms of a disease. Changes, not only in a patient's physical but also mental and social (dys)functioning, have become important standards in judging the management of care by physicians and the success of health care programmes (Ellwood, 1988).

Since the early fifties numerous instruments have been designed for measuring these non-biomedical aspects of a patient's health. These health status measures clearly differ from the traditional biomedical process or outcome parameters such as results of blood and urine tests, or an X-ray finding. Most of these measures are questionnaires in which patients, by self-assessment, report on one or more domains of their health status such as presence of pain, feelings of anxiety or physical immobility.

Feinstein (1983) coined the name "clinimetrics" for the science of applying these measures in health care assessments. By doing so he not only aimed at highlighting a difference in the psychometrical background of clinimetric instruments compared to biomedical instruments, but he also wanted to stress the importance of carefully considering the specific methodological implications when applying these instruments in health care assessments.

Clinimetric measures have proved useful in various applications within health care, such as in answering research questions, for the purpose of assessing group needs, for resource allocation, and for screening, assessing, monitoring and maintaining a patient's functioning in routine practice. The application of these clinimetric measures in clinical practice and research has thus become widely accepted (Feinstein, 1987). Lately, however, critical remarks about the clinical relevance of these instruments have been made when used to measure health outcomes. In particular, are these clinimetric instruments responsive in measuring effects of clinical treatment over time? Additionally, do these measures point to the same quantitative outcomes as the diagnostic tests physicians are familiar with?

Part of this scepticism stems from a lack of knowledge of the diversity in contents and applications of these instruments (Walker and Rosser, 1988). Selection of a measure often seems to be made on an arbitrary basis, without due attention to whether it is appropriate in addressing the research question of interest. Moreover, the psychometric properties of the rival instruments are often given scant regard.

Another reason for scepticism stems from the fact that in many situations doctors (as well as researchers) are confronted with health status outcomes which in their opinion do not relate to the medical treatment or observed changes on clinical outcome parameters (Shanks and Frater, 1993). However, as Feinstein (1987) pointed out, it is necessary to pay attention to methodological fallacies which must be taken into account in order to attain unbiased results. Most health professionals are unaware of this consideration.

The aim of this chapter is to clarify some basic issues one encounters in the process of adequately selecting and applying a clinimetric outcome measure. First, we describe how the choice of an instrument should be based on the objectives for which it will be used, the situation for which it was designed, and the situation in which it will be applied. Second, some basic methodological considerations that should be examined before applying a measure will be presented. Third, several of the pitfalls that one can come across in relating clinimetric outcomes to clinical outcomes and to treatment will be described. This will be illustrated by examples of applications of three outcome measures which have been widely used in ambulatory and primary care, and which cover diverse health status domains and have different psychometric characteristics (Table 11.1).

PURPOSE AND CONTENT OF AN INSTRUMENT

In the introduction we pointed out that the choice of a specific clinimetric instrument depends, among other things, on the application and the particular goals of the health status assessment. Consequently, an important consideration in choosing an appropriate outcome measure concerns the correspondence between the content of the measure and the goals of the assessment, in other words will the data provided by the outcome measure address the questions asked? This can be illustrated more clearly by comparing the differences in purpose and content of the three instruments described in Table 11.1: the Sickness Impact Profile (SIP) (Bergner *et al.*, 1981), the Barthel Index (Mahoney and Barthel, 1965) and the Dartmouth COOP Charts (Nelson *et al.*, 1987; Rogers, 1990).

For instance, when a researcher or clinician is especially interested in measuring the degree of independence of a group of older patients in performing self-care activities, this requires an instrument which focuses solely on activities of daily living (ADL) functioning, such as the Barthel Index. In such a situation an instrument like the Dartmouth COOP Charts would be less appropriate, because it does not address self-care activities.

On the other hand, if the objective was to explore the health status of a general population, inclusion of as many dimensions as possible would seem to be indicated. A multidimensional measure such as the Dartmouth COOP Charts seems less adequate in this situation, because it only yields global information on its dimensions. While the Sickness Impact Profile (SIP) gives detailed information on behavioural dysfunctioning in various areas of daily life, the Dartmouth COOP Charts only give a general measure of the degree of dysfunctioning (physical, emotional, social etc.).

In general, clinimetric instruments can be used for producing clinically valuable information for doctors in their patient care or for health care policy makers utilising research findings. For both of these applications, different objectives can be pursued. The goal(s) of applying clinimetrics in daily patient care includes a wide variety of possible objectives. Initially, a main objective was screening for functional problems, findings which might contribute to the discovery of previously undiagnosed conditions or facilitate a clinical decision. A second important objective concerned the monitoring of disease progress and therapeutic response by evaluating changes in functioning of individual patients or groups of patients.

Nowadays, clinimetric data are often gathered in daily patient care for improving the doctor-patient communication about the effects of health problems and their treatments. Furthermore, assessing quality of care and providing case mix adjustment for comparing other outcomes between groups of patients has become another common objective.

Table 11.1 *Purpose and content of three broadly used clinimetric outcome measures*

Outcome Measure	Sickness Impact Profile	Barthel Index	Dartmouth COOP Charts
Conceptualisation	A general purpose measure for the impact of disease expressed in sickness-related behavioural dysfunction in usual daily activities.	A measure of functioning with a conceptual focus on a patient's dependence on others for actual physical assistance.	A multidimensional general health profile which focuses on global physical, mental, social function and overall health.
Purpose	Developed to fulfil a variety of different needs for a measure of perceived health including outcomes of care, health surveys, programme planning, policy formulation and monitoring patient progress.	Developed as a means of assessing the degree of independence in patients with neuromuscular or musculoskeletal disorders in clinical practice.	Especially developed to provide doctors in primary care with an efficient system for screening, assessing, monitoring and maintaining patient function in routine practice.
Health status dimensions	Sleep and rest, eating, work, home management, emotional behaviour, recreation and pastimes, ambulation, mobility, alertness behaviour, body care and movement, social interaction, communication.	Basic ADL functioning such as independence in toilet use, bathing, transfers, dressing, stairs, mobility, feeding, grooming, and continence of bowels, bladder.	Feelings, physical fitness, daily activities, social activities, overall health, change in health.

Applying clinimetrics in research contributes to building up and extending existing databases of information on health status which can be linked in turn with treatment and diagnostic information. The aim is to determine which treatments are most effective, and to ascertain the effects of medical intervention under various conditions. The Medical Outcomes Study, undertaken in the United States, is an excellent illustration of the importance of building up this kind of database (Tarlov et al., 1989).

The purpose and content which a candidate instrument should possess depend on the type of application. One type of application is discriminating between individual patients or groups at a single point in time to determine the impact of a disease at that point in time. In this context, the sensitivity of the instrument, in other words, its ability to correctly measure the "between patients or patient groups" variability at a certain point in time, will be of prime importance.

A second type of application relates to evaluating patients' outcome over time, or to predicting patients' likely future "health gain" from treatment. In this situation the responsiveness of the instrument, that is its ability to correctly measure the variability within patients over time, will be the main focus. Here, too, attention must be given to whether the instrument yields separate scores for each of the different aspects of health that it taps. Many multidimensional clinimetric instruments only provide separate scores for each domain of health, resulting in a health profile of the studied patients. However, for some of these instruments, an overall or index score can also be calculated. The importance of this distinction lies in the fact that evaluating changes over time is easier when indices exist, because only the aggregated scores need to be taken into account. By contrast, aggregated scores are of less interest when screening is the primary goal (Bullinger, 1993).

The third type of application relates to the setting in which the clinimetric data must be gathered. When measurements will be carried out in a busy clinical practice, issues concerning the mode of administration and the practicality of the measurements must be taken into account. For example, a short self-completion questionnaire may be preferred to a longer, more complex instrument requiring a trained interviewer.

Sometimes two or more of these types of application will need to be considered simultaneously in selecting an instrument, because clinimetrics are often used for more than one purpose. For instance, studying the effectiveness of a health intervention in a clinical trial means not only that the power to measure meaningful change over time in a reliable manner is an important feature but also that the instrument must be capable of discriminating between groups of patients who differ in severity of illness.

WHAT HEALTH OUTCOME ARE WE INTERESTED IN?

As we have seen in the last paragraph, the process of clarifying which goal(s) should be satisfied by an outcome measure restricts the number of possible candidates. A further restriction occurs in considering the question: to what extent is the instrument capable of assessing what the constructors intended to measure? This question relates to the aspects of health which are of interest to the investigator and to the properties of the candidate health status instruments. Methodological concepts involved here are the "validity", "reliability" and "clinical utility" of a clinimetric measure.

Validity addresses the extent to which the instrument actually records what it purports to measure and for which purposes it has already been proven suitable (Anastasi, 1986). Three basic types of validity can be distinguished: content, criterion-related and construct validity. These types of validity can be used to judge the overall validity of an instrument. Content validity refers to how well the actual health domain one is interested in is indeed covered by a specific instrument. In choosing a measure, the clinician or researcher should first decide what domains of a patient's health status are relevant to the patient's illness, to the outcomes of health and to the intervention under investigation. In general, an instrument should tap dimensions of health that are likely to be affected by the intervention or that have been troublesome to the patient's health status in the past, those that may be affected in the future, and perhaps outcomes that are very unlikely to occur but are possible. It is, however, no easy task to delimit the health domain under study.

In deciding whether the content validity of a specific instrument is satisfactory, one should take into account the measurement precision that is required. When only broad distinctions in patient outcomes are necessary, high content validity is far less important than when fine distinctions are wanted. For instance, in looking at health-related quality of life in end-stage cancer patients, a crude measure will do in assessing the quality of basic ADL activities. But such a crude measure would be unsatisfactory if in such patient groups effects of different management on change in mental health were to be assessed, since only relatively small differences would be expected.

Content validity also concerns the extent to which the full continuum of a health domain is represented within the instrument. Some instruments are designed to assess only major functional impairment. For example, most measurements of functional disability in daily activities focus on strong dysfunctional impairments. This also applies to the Barthel Index (Table 11.2). Other instruments are designed to assess the impact of illness at varying levels of impairment. For instance, the SIP has proven to be a generic index that has a high degree of validity for measuring cross-sectional differences in a variety of different populations (Patrick and Deyo, 1989). It has been shown to be a valuable instrument, not only in patients with severe physical impairment, but also in patients with combined medical and psychiatric problems, and in patients with minor functional impairment.

The criterion validity of an instrument is typically assessed by comparing the scores on the instrument with one or more external criteria, known or believed to measure the domain under study. The interest is not so much in what the instrument measures (content validity), rather it is in the predictive ability of the instrument. However, identifying relevant criteria will in general be difficult. A "gold standard" which can be used as a criterion for measuring health does not exist. For this reason, the choice of an instrument may be based primarily on judgements regarding relevance or content validity, with the need for evidence of criterion validity accorded less importance.

The third type of validity, construct validity, is of primary importance because it links the measurement to theoretical notions. In fact, construct validity is concerned with an indirect test of content validity. Assuming content validity, one can - on theoretical grounds - make predictions with respect to the behaviour of the instrument in specific conditions. For example, if a certain type of functional impairment is known to go with certain individual characteristics, the instrument for measuring that type of functional impairment should give distinctive mean scores for individuals who differ on those characteristics. The judgement of the content validity of a subjective measure progresses by empirically testing well-constructed hypotheses.

Several strategies can be used in obtaining an insight into the construct validity of a clinimetric instrument. First, empirical information on the construct validity of the instrument may have been gathered. Perhaps descriptive statistical analyses have been performed, such as factor analysis of item clusters or sub-sets of a health status measure. These analyses present descriptive information on how well the dimension structure of an instrument suits the intended health concepts.

Second, an instrument may have been tested by a "multitrait-multimethod" approach (Campbell and Fiske, 1959). This is a testing strategy in which the instrument's conceptual content is evaluated against a test battery of comparable indices and alternative methods known to address the same health concepts and partly known to address different concepts. Two kinds of validity can be distinguished in such studies: convergent and discriminant validity. Convergent validity relates to the correlation with indices that address the same health dimension, while discriminant validity concerns the correlation between clinimetric indices measuring health concepts from which the instrument is supposed to deviate. Researchers and clinicians can inform themselves about whether the clinical measure actually distinguishes between different health status dimensions.

Third, the construct validity of the instrument may have been tested by evaluating hypotheses about the correlations between measurements in patients with a clear clinical picture. This known-group validity involves comparing mean scores on a certain health measure across groups known to differ in the concept being validated. For example, long-term functional impairment in patients with

Table 11.2 *Psychometric aspects of three broadly used clinimetric outcome measures*

Outcome Measures	Sickness Impact Profile	Barthel Index	Dartmouth COOP Charts
Evidence of construct validity	A comprehensive behaviourally based measure with clearly distinct psychosocial and physical dimensions.	A good measure of needs for care, potential for rehabilitation in moderately to severely disabled populations.	Can discriminate between physical and emotional components of general function.
Content validity of the health dimensions	For the psychosocial dimension only moderate correlations exists with traditional depression and anxiety scales. The SIP may not possess adequate sensitivity if subjective states are of interest in evaluating patients' outcome.	Not suitable for less disabled populations and where assessment of a broader range of function is required.	The physical fitness measure is too restricted in scope to be sensitive to disability in older individuals.
Multitrait-multimethod approach	Satisfactory convergent and discriminant validity.	Factor analyses of results have confirmed that the instrument is measuring a single dimension.	All charts have convergent validity but the charts for daily and social activities have no discriminant validity.
Known-group validity	The instrument performs well in detecting different impacts to patients' physical and psychosocial functioning caused by many types of illnesses.	The index has been shown to predict survival, length of stay and progress, but mainly among stroke patients.	The instrument has the ability to detect moderate effects in physical and emotional functioning due to medical illness or health status.
Cross-cultural applications	Several international versions exist. Evidence of conceptual agreement was found between international versions and the original version.	The instrument has been used in different countries, but no documentation exists addressing cross-cultural equivalence.	Recently, the instrument has been applied in many countries. Equivalence of the verbal response choices and pictures in the various language versions has not been fully assessed.
Response categories	Yes/No statements.	Three response choices: dependent, with help, independent.	Five Likert-scaled response choices. Each response choice is translated by a picture.
Scaling characteristics - *dimensionality* - *items per dimension* - *index v profile*	Twelve dimensions. Multi-item scales, 136 items. Index and profile.	One dimension. Multi-item scale, 10 items. Index, no profile.	Five dimensions. Single-item scales, 6 items. Profile, no index.

severe abdominal disorders, such as cancer, should be poorer than in patients with chronic non-serious abdominal complaints, as has been demonstrated with the Dutch version of the SIP (Jacobs, 1993).

Careful consideration of the construct validity of the instrument is particularly needed when considering the application of a clinimetric instrument in groups of patients in which an instrument has not been used before. An instrument that is valid and reliable in one situation does not necessarily have these properties when used in another situation.

Finally, and perhaps most importantly, it is necessary to recognise that an instrument that has been proved valuable for use in patient care may be of no value for research, and vice versa. The Dartmouth COOP Charts have been extensively studied for their use in family medicine research as an evaluative instrument on the effectiveness of individual patient care. Preliminary test results show that their improved conceptual structure make them more valuable for monitoring patient care, but that their single-item structure and their restricted multidimensional structure limit their use in research (McHorney *et al.*, 1992).

ERROR VARIABILITY AND HEALTH CHANGES OVER TIME

If an instrument is invalid, the observed scores are systematically biased. That means that the measurement instrument misses the mark. In the stage of designing the instrument, this kind of systematic bias or error must be identified and as far as possible corrected. A typical source of systematic bias relates to anxiety-arousing questions. For example, questions referring to maintaining a diet or taking medicines regularly might be better asked as an indirect question, i.e. how the respondent thinks people in general will behave with respect to maintaining a diet or taking medicines regularly.

Observed scores may also be affected by random error. For example, if a patient is asked how he or she feels today the answer may be biased because the patient feels very well or very bad at that very moment. To eliminate this sort of random "noise" it may be more appropriate to ask how a patient felt last week or last month. The extent to which an instrument is free of this type of random error is called the reliability or precision of the instrument. If a measure is reliable, a respondent's score would be expected to be roughly the same on repeated administrations, the observed score on average being equal to that patient's "true score" (assuming no systematic bias). Of course, it is not generally possible to establish a patient's score on successive trials of the same instrument and to average the obtained scores. Nevertheless, the reliability of an instrument can be estimated by assuming the patients are replicates of each other, or by posing a number of different questions designed to tap the same dimension of interest. The issue of reliability can be summarised by stating that an observed score can be considered to have three components: observed score = *true score + systematic error + random error*. The *true score* refers to the actual underlying value of the health status attribute being measured.

In analysing the reliability of an outcome measure, three approaches can be distinguished (Bravo and Potvin, 1991). The first approach is to examine the extent to which all scale items measure the same underlying concept. This yields a reliability coefficient with regard to the internal consistency of the health status measure. The second approach concentrates on the stability of measurements by studying the extent to which, in case of repeated administration, test findings are consistent over time. In the literature this is denoted by reproducibility or test-retest reliability. Finally, and most importantly, the magnitude of the different error sources can be estimated within the context of analysis of variance. Analysis of variance enables the calculation of intra-class reliability and generalisability coefficients, taking into account the influence of the error components under various measurement conditions.

When considering the reliability of an instrument, it is again necessary to consider the aim and context of the measurement. If, for instance, the attention is focused upon the individual patient, the random error in individual changes in the outcome scores is important. Most clinical research, however, is aimed at the possible effects of different treatments. In that case, the average change in health status in a group of patients is important. Nunnally (1978) recommends that the level of random error must be low when measurements are used to evaluate effects of treatment on an individual level. By contrast, a substantial higher level of random error in individual patients' scores is acceptable for group measurements, because the random error tends to average out across people. Although this tendency already appears even in small samples, the corrective effect improves when the number of individual patients in a sample grows. For instance, in small groups of less than 20 patients, a lower level of random error in individual patients' scores is important in order to obtain unbiased conclusions.

When a researcher or clinician wants to compare the reliability of indices, care should be exercised in interpreting and using the internal consistency of an instrument. For single-item scales, such as the Dartmouth COOP Charts, it is not possible to calculate a measure of internal consistency (Table 11.3).

Another source of random error involves the use of proxy scores. Most clinimetric instruments are self-report measures. However, in cases of serious illness, patients are not always able to complete the form and proxy scores are needed. These can be achieved, for instance, by asking their physician or a close relative. However, the accuracy of physicians in estimating a patient's health has been shown to be not very high (Epstein *et al.*, 1989) and, in close relatives, psychological proxy-generated SIP scores appeared to be strongly influenced by the proxy's own psychological distress and perceived burden of care-giving (Rothman *et al.*, 1991). Furthermore, the issue of inter-rater reliability needs to be

Table 11.3   Accuracy and ease of administration of three broadly applied clinimetric outcome measures

Outcome Measures	Sickness Impact Profile	Barthel Index	Dartmouth COOP Charts
Administration/ acceptability	Interviewer and self-administered (explicit instruction required). Self-assessment or by proxy. Administration takes between 20 to 30 mins. Patient acceptance is high, but especially in follow-up administration its length asks for extra attention to avoid response-set bias. Length of administration restricts application, field work must be well organised in clinical practice.	Only interviewer administered. Self-assessment or by proxy. Administration takes between 2 to 5 minutes. High reported response rates. No problems in administration.	Interviewer and self-administered. Self-assessment or by proxy. Administration takes between 2 to 3 minutes Both patients' and doctors' acceptance is high. No problems in administration There are a number of versions of the original Dartmouth COOP Charts and care is needed in ensuring the updated version is selected.
Reliability: - reproducibility, test/retest	High reproducibility for the total, psychosocial and physical index scores, low reproducibility for the individual item scores. Lower reported reproducibility in case of self-administration.	Reported test-retest in reliability is high but in general there has been little attention to this aspect.	High test-retest reliability.
- internal consistency	Internal consistency of category scores is moderate to high, but low for eating.	Reported internal consistency is high, but in general there has been little attention to this aspect.	Analyses of internal consistency of scales are not applicable because the instrument encloses only single-item scales.
Responsiveness	Responsiveness is not fully established.	The crude categories employed in the instrument may be insufficient to detect important changes. Substantial change can occur within the broad categories without altering index scores.	The responsiveness to change of the charts in various patient samples is under study.

considered since two different proxies may give quite different reports of the same patient. Consequently, if proxy-generated scores are used, careful consideration of possible sources of error is important in order to avoid erroneous interpretation of the results.

When a researcher or clinician wants to use clinimetrics for assessing outcome changes over time or for predictive purposes, reliability interpreted as reproducibility of test results seems problematic. In those situations, one is not interested in an instrument which produces stable results over time, but one which responsively measures the effects of therapeutic interventions over time. To address responsiveness properly, the issue of the clinical significance of changes over time must be separated from the statistical significance of change. Responsiveness coefficients should express to what extent changes over time are due to statistical coincidence or to random error in scores of a clinimetric index. Other statistical coefficients, such as relative effect sizes, can provide a standardisation of the magnitude of the changes (Kazis et al., 1989). In addition, clinical criteria are needed to judge the clinical relevance of the established responsiveness. Thus, analysing the responsiveness of an outcome measure correctly also means choosing clinical indicators, which are appropriate to measure clinical changes over time, and stating the kind of health status change that can be expected to occur during the assessment period.

For instance, Sullivan et al. (1990) found the Swedish SIP version to be responsive to pre- and post-treatment changes in 96 female patients with rheumatoid arthritis over a one year period, showing both improvement and deterioration. Their suggestion that these results partly depended on the selection of better clinical indicators of change (which were able to detect small changes better than in the analyses of the SIP responsiveness in patients with rheumatoid arthritis by Deyo and Inui (1984)), is in line with our argument.

One should also be aware of the possibility of spurious change when assessing change over time in an outcome study of health status. Several possible sources of misleading or spurious change can be identified. First, changes over time can be masked by statistical effects such as the regression to the mean effect, especially in non-randomised observational or correlational studies. Central to the effect of regression to the mean is the concept of selection. This can be demonstrated in the following way. Suppose a group of patients is being selected on the criteria of blood pressure being below a specific value. On a subsequent occasion the mean blood pressure of this selected group will be higher irrespective of any treatment given. This is because blood pressure within a person varies around a true value. By selecting patients with low values, patients with values below their true value are over-represented.

A second source of spurious change is the existence of highly skewed distributions of the scores. Especially in general populations with low levels of functional impairment, which is characteristic for the morbidity in populations encountered in family medicine, inadequate attention to the congruence of the level of the health status assessed by the clinimetric outcome measure and that of the intended research sample will result in a skewed distribution of health status scores. Many statistical techniques are based on the assumption that variables are more or less normally distributed. This means that, starting from an average level of health, scores are symmetrically spread over the continuum. Where this is not the case, non-parametric statistical methods of analysis must be used or outcome scores must be transformed to obtain a more symmetrical distribution of health status scores.

In recording change over time in populations, one should also take into account the possible differences in the restricted range of candidate instruments. The candidate instrument should be sensitive in that part of the health continuum that applies to the majority of the study population. Ignoring this can lead to so-called floor and/or ceiling effects. For instance, applying the SIP or the Barthel Index in a primary care population with asthma to evaluate positive effects of a care programme seems less appropriate because of the minimal impairment in general function and basic ADL present in most of these patients at the baseline. This is an instance of a so-called floor effect (Bindman *et al.*, 1990). In such a situation the Dartmouth COOP Charts with their global focus on physical fitness, on general health, on perceived change in health and on feelings may be more suitable.

For those outcome instruments which provide the possibility of calculating an index, one should be alert to cancelling out opposite changes within the individual health domains. In those cases, scores of the separate health aspects should be analysed, or health profiles should be used. A study with the Dutch SIP by Mulders *et al.* (1989) illustrates the importance of conducting analyses of change in separate health dimensions instead of looking at total SIP scores over time, depending on the clinical expectations about changes over time during a follow-up period. The SIP confirmed the functional improvement in only the two health dimensions in which patients were expected to change over time.

The influence of heterogeneity between patients' groups can also have a confounding influence on change itself, besides causing differences at the baseline measure. This "patient mix" can be defined as the differences between patients' characteristics which may help to explain the patients' outcome, such as difference in socio-demographic characteristics, baseline functional status, disease-specific severity of the studied condition, and comorbidity. Usefully, several statistical methods can be used to adjust the outcome measurements for the influence of patient mix. For instance, these factors can be included as covariates when analysing the relation between management and outcome.

The timing of the measurement may be another masking factor in assessing change over time. This necessitates answering questions about the hypothesised relationships between the processes and the outcomes of care that can be expected to occur within the time interval in which the health status assessments take place.

The right timing of the data collection is a critical, but often neglected, factor. For each outcome and for each episode of care an optimum time window exists that is maximally sensitive and specific to the care delivered. To approach this timing issue appropriately, a number of criteria have to be defined: the episode of care, the content and process of care delivered, the patient's outcome expected from those processes, and the course of time in which the outcome can be expected.

The final source of spurious change is the presence of response bias. This also is an often neglected factor for systematic error in self-reported health status scores over time. Response bias refers to systematic errors which might arise when collecting the clinimetric data. Before drawing conclusions from the observed clinimetric outcomes, a researcher or clinician must examine his data for the presence of response bias. Did the instrument or the assessment situation comprise aspects that invited patients to represent themselves favourably? This may lead to an under-reporting of socially undesirable characteristics or behaviour and to over-reporting of desirable behaviour. If behavioural aspects of a personal nature (e.g. sexual behaviour or being suicidal) are part of an index, these might be under-reported because respondents may feel uneasy talking about those subjects in the presence of an interviewer. If an index consists of complicated questions which are difficult to understand, this may cause the tendency to agree or disagree with any question regardless of the behaviour which was addressed. A second source of response bias may exist because of "response shift" effects, which are caused by changes in the patient's standards over time or by a shift in the perception of the response scaling. In using self-report instruments, researchers assume that subjects have an internalised perception of their level of functioning with regard to a given dimension and that this internalised standard will not change from one test to the next. However, sometimes treatments alter subjects' perceptions. This contaminates self-report assessments of a treatment if such a shift happens between successive measurements. This kind of systematic error may occur particularly in the case of self-measurements of perceived changes in health (Howard *et al.*, 1979). For instance, due to the absence of real change, patients might become more pessimistic during their illness episode about the possibilities of positive change. The possible effect then is that a patient rates himself higher on the post-test response scale although no true gain on the variable of interest occurred. This type of response bias does not only occur in non-randomised observational studies, but also occurs in true experimental designs. Since treatment subjects have different experiences from control subjects, the possibility of confusion with the experimental treatment exists.

THE FEASIBILITY AND ACCEPTABILITY OF OUTCOME MEASUREMENTS

Once the goals for the use of the instrument and the test features are agreed upon, then it is essential to carefully analyse the population and setting in which the candidate instrument will be used. Two main facets should be focused upon.

First, it is important to explore the expected utility to clinicians and patients of knowing these clinimetric patient outcomes. The content of the measurement must appeal to the physicians as eliciting important information to benefit the understanding of a patient's impairment or the effects of their care. This understanding is often self-evident when applying clinimetrics in patient care, but an initial understanding influences the doctor's willingness to collaborate in clinical research. This means examining such characteristics as whether the instrument is easy to understand and simple to score (Greenfield and Nelson, 1992).

Apart from the issue of the utility of the outcome measure to the doctor, the patient's recognition of the relevance of the measurement to his/her health needs some thought. For instance, if an index is intended to demonstrate a patient's improvement in health, it is important to consider whether the content of the index from the patient's perspective actually addresses specific entities whose improvement would be most gratifying for him/her. Otherwise not only will the willingness to collaborate be low, but the observed change in scores will be of minor relevance to a patient's health-related quality of life.

Second, one must address the practical implications of the measurement process. If, for instance, a clinician wants to use a clinimetric measure in his/her patient care, the first consideration will be how to fit the measurement in with a patient encounter of limited duration. An instrument that is used routinely in the physician's office will not be tolerated if it takes too much time and therefore interferes with daily practice. Several factors related to the office ecosystem complicate the execution of clinimetrics in patient care: "integrating functional assessment into a busy clinical practice is difficult because the necessary steps require time, thought, recording and follow-up" (Greenfield and Nelson, 1992). For instance, if a clinician wants to apply a clinimetric instrument for use in daily patient care, application of a long instrument such as the SIP does not seem feasible. One assessment takes about twenty minutes and few clinicians are either willing or able to schedule this in their regular practice hours. Short-form instruments which have been developed specifically for use in clinical care should be considered first, such as the Barthel Index and the Dartmouth COOP Charts (Applegate, 1987).

The understanding of possible differences in the level of clinimetric outcome should also be looked at. Adequate interpretation of the health status scores should be given prior thought: which health outcomes can be considered normal? Sometimes data of the health status in an open population are present, which can serve as a point of reference, or the scores can be compared with other samples of patients with the same clinical characteristics. Analysing subsets with varying patient characteristics such as age and gender can give an insight into deviations in outcome if no reference scores are known.

CONCLUSION

We have given a global guideline in answering the question of how to approach the selection of an outcome measure in an appropriate manner. It was not our intention to present an overview of all currently available generic and disease-specific outcome measures that can be applied in ambulatory or primary care. Several texts give excellent comprehensive summaries of the most important outcome instruments (Scrivens *et al.,* 1985; Wilkin *et al.,* 1992). Most of these texts clearly describe the theoretical concept of each instrument, the purposes for which the instrument can be used, the strategy that was followed to address the content and construct validity, and whether a valid international version has been developed (Anderson *et al.,* 1993).

Rather, we have set out the conditions a researcher or clinician should consider before selecting an outcome measure, a process described by Stewart *et al.* (1989) who formulated criteria for selecting an outcome instrument to be used by clinicians in patients with chronic conditions in daily patient care.

There are many pitfalls when using health status indicators. These can be avoided by keeping in mind the key aspects of applying an outcome measurement: the goal of the study, the validity and appropriateness of the instrument, the clinical utility and feasibility of the measurements. Only such a strategy will result in actually reaching the right selections of outcome measures in research or patient care.

REFERENCES

Anastasi, A. (1986) Evolving concepts of test validation. *Annual Review of Psychology,* **37**, 1-15.

Anderson, R.T., Aaronson, N.K. and Wilkin, D. (1993) Critical review of the international assessments of health related quality of life. *Quality of Life Research,* **2**, 369-395.

Applegate, W.B. (1987) Uses of assessment instruments in clinical settings. *Journal of the American Geriatrics Society,* **35**, 45-50.

Bergner, M., Bobbitt, R.A., Carter, W.B. and Gilson, B.S. (1981) The Sickness Impact Profile: development and final revision of a health status measure. *Medical Care,* **19**, 787-805.

Bindman, A.B., Keane, D. and Luri, N. (1990) Measuring health changes among severely ill patients: the floor phenomenon. *Medical Care*, **28**, 1143-1152.

Bravo, G. and Potvin, L. (1991) Estimating the reliability of continuous measures with Cronbach's Alpha or the intra-class correlation coefficient: toward the integration of two traditions. *Journal of Clinical Epidemiology*, **44**, 381-390.

Bullinger, M. (1993) Indices versus profiles: advantages and disadvantages. In: Walker, R. and Rosser, R.M. (Eds.), *Quality of life assessment: key issues in the 1990s*. Dordrecht: Kluwer Academic Publishers.

Campbell, D.T. and Fiske, D.W. (1959) Convergent and discriminant validation by the multitrait-multimethod matrix. *Psychology Bulletin*, **56**, 81-105.

Cluff, L.E. (1981) Chronic disease, function and the quality of care. *Journal of Chronic Diseases*, **34**, 299-304.

Deyo, R.A. and Inui, T.S. (1984) Towards clinical applications of health status measures: sensitivity of scale to clinically important changes. *Health Services Research*, **19**, 275-289.

Ellwood, P.M. (1988) Outcomes management: a technology of patient experience. *New England Journal of Medicine*, **318**, 1549-1555.

Epstein, A.M., Hall, J.A., Tognetti, J., Son, L.H and Conant, L. (1989) Using proxies to evaluate quality of life. *Medical Care*, **27**, S91-S98.

Feinstein, A.R. (1983) An additional basis science for clinical medicine. IV: The development of clinimetrics. *Annals of Internal Medicine*, **99**, 843-848.

Feinstein, A.R. (1987) *Clinimetrics*. New Haven: Yale University Press.

Greenfield, S. and Nelson, E.C. (1992) Recent developments and future issues in the use of health status measures in clinical settings. *Medical Care*, **30**, MS23-MS41.

Howard, G.S., Ralph, K.M., Gulanick, N.A., Maxwell, S.E, Nance, D.W. and Gerber, S.K. (1979) Internal invalidity in pretest-posttest self report evaluations and a re-evaluation of retrospective pretests. *Applied Psychological Measurement*, **3**, 1-23.

Jacobs, H.M. (1993) *Health status measurement in family medicine research: the Sickness Impact Profile and its application in a follow-up study in patients with non-specific abdominal complaints*. Utrecht: University of Utrecht Press. (OMI-offset)

Kazis, L.E., Anderson, J.J. and Meenan, R.F. (1989) Effect sizes for interpreting changes in health status. *Medical Care*, **27**, S178-S189.

Mahoney, F.I. and Barthel, D.W. (1965) Functional evaluation: the Barthel Index. *Maryland State Medical Journal*, **14**, 61-65.

McHorney, C.A., Ware, J.E., Rogers, W., Raczek, A.E. and Lu, J.F.R. (1992) The validity and relative precision of MOS Short- and Long-Form Health Status Scales and Dartmouth COOP Charts. *Medical Care*, **30**, MS253-MS265.

Mulders, A.H.M., de Witte, L.P. and Diederiks, J.P.M. (1989) Evaluation of a rehabilitation after care programme for stroke patients. *Journal of Rehabilitation Science*, **2**, 97-102.

Nelson, E.C., Wasson, J. and Kirk, J. (1987) Assessment of function in routine clinical practice: description of the Dartmouth COOP Chart method and preliminary findings. *Journal of Chronic Diseases*, **40**, S55-S63.

Nunnally, J.C. (1978) *Psychometric theory*. New York: McGraw-Hill.

Patrick, D.L. and Deyo, R.A. (1989) Generic and disease specific measures in assessing health status and quality of life. *Medical Care*, **27**, S217-S232.

Rogers, T.B. (1990) The development of a new measuring instrument. In: *Functional status measurement in primary care: report from the Classification Committee of WONCA*. New York: Springer Verlag.

Rothman, M.L., Hedrick, S.C., Bulcroft, K.A., Hickam, D.H. and Rubenstein, L.Z. (1991) The validity of proxy generated scores as measures of patient health status. *Medical Care*, **29**, 115-124.

Scrivens, E., Cunningham, D., Charlton, J. and Holland, W. (1985) Measuring the impact of health interventions: a review of available instruments. *Effective Health Care*, **2**, 247-261.

Shanks, J. and Frater, A. (1993) Health status, outcome, and attributability: is a red rose red in the dark? *Quality in Health Care*, **2**, 259-262.

Stewart, A.L., Greenfield, S., Hays, R.D., Wells, K.B., Rogers, W.H., Berry, S.D., McGlynn, E.N. and Ware, J.E. (1989) Functional status and well-being of patients with chronic conditions: results from the Medical Outcomes Study. *Journal of the Americal Medical Association*, **262**, 907-913.

Sullivan, M., Ahlmen, M. and Bjelle, A. (1990) Health status assessment in rheumatoid arthritis: further work on the validity of the Sickness Impact Profile. *Journal of Rheumatology*, **17**, 439-447.

Tarlov, A.R., Ware, J.E., Greenfield, S., Nelson, E.C., Perrin, E. and Zubkoff, M. (1989) The Medical Outcomes Study: an application of methods for monitoring the results of medical care. *Journal of the American Medical Association*, **262**, 925-930.

Tarlov, A.R. (1983) The increasing supply of physicians, the changing structure of the health services, and the future practice of medicine. *New England Journal of Medicine*, **308**, 1235-1244.

Walker, S.R. and Rosser, R.M. (Eds.) (1988) *Quality of life: assessment and application*. Lancaster: MTP Press Limited.

Wilkin, D., Hallam, L. and Doggett, M.A. (1992) *Measures of need and outcome for primary health care*. Oxford: Oxford University Press.

HEALTH OUTCOME MEASURES FOR OLDER PEOPLE

JAN HEYRMAN AND KATELIJNE VAN HOECK

INTRODUCTION

The Importance of Health Outcome

It can be argued that health outcome measurement can prove of greatest value in relation to older people. The need to introduce notions of outcome assessment in the care of the older person was felt a number of years ago. Katz *et al.* published an "Index of Independence in Activities of Daily Living" (ADL) in 1963 in response to the growing interest in this area.

Generally speaking, the interest of the medical world in the health outcome of its interventions has traditionally been linked to the belief that it is possible to make people healthy again simply by eliminating their diseases. For a long time this was the great illusion of medicine. The profession grew in stature when it succeeded in eliminating acute infectious diseases and epidemics. But chronic diseases, for which there is no ultimate cure, took their place. Medicine then became increasingly concerned with changing unhealthy lifestyles, in an effort to prevent these chronic diseases. The problems resulting from bad habits such as smoking, unhealthy eating or stressful behaviour tend to present themselves at a later stage in life, but changes in lifestyle need to be made earlier before the symptoms have manifested themselves. Convincing people to adopt new lifestyles in order to reap later benefits can not be done in the traditional way of prescribing pills and therapies. Medicine has become confronted with a need for new strategies and fresh questions regarding the effectiveness and efficiency of interventions have been raised. How much health gain can medical care produce and at what cost?

In the clinical care of older people, chronic diseases with a limited possibility of healing have always been recognised. It is clear to everybody that it is impossible to treat all the diseases that older people suffer from. People over 75 on average have seven important disease conditions. Most of them are chronic conditions without any prospect of a cure. Autopsy studies have shown that older people have three to four cancer localisations on average! From the beginning of geriatrics as a medical speciality, it has been recognised that realistic and attainable goals have to be the guideline as to whether or not diagnostic or therapeutic interventions are necessary or desirable. Functional status is promoted as the main yardstick to measure the outcome of medical intervention. This involves looking at the range of function of the patient, defining what is the functional problem, and then trying to discover if medically treatable conditions are the cause of this loss of function. It is necessary to ensure that side-effects from intervention do not neutralise or even counteract the positive influence of treatment. The clinical focus on functional status as an appropriate health outcome has become central to geriatric care. Health outcome measures are used as clinimetric instruments: to guide clinical decision-making.

The older population group will become more dominant in the future as their numbers increase and the social impact of an ageing population will become increasingly apparent. In Europe, there has been a social tradition that places a high value on caring for the older person, but at the same time society is increasingly being asked to take over the care which individual families are no longer prepared to guarantee themselves.

A concerned society tries to get a grip on its older population via population surveys; what are their special needs, perspectives and expectations, and how is this related to isolation, handicap, housing condition, physical possibilities, support systems etc. Health status measurement forms an important part of this assessment. A society feeling responsible for the care of its older people will have to allocate larger budgets to meet demand. Health policy makers are interested in foreseeing the necessary resource allocations. They want to plan the needs for health care, especially for the older population. Institutional care must be made available for those who need it most. Health outcome measures have also been used on an individual basis to describe functional loss and link it to the access to better organised care, special home care or more intensive institutional care. This need for better and more intensive care for older people created a positive climate for the development and acceptance of the Activities of Daily Living (ADL) scales of Katz. Linking changes in functional loss or dependency to costs and resources has made health outcome measurement a central issue in health technology assessment and human resource management, especially for older people.

Lessons learned from the care of older people can have important consequences for medicine as a whole. Mold *et al.* (1991) recently introduced the notion of goal-orientation as the new focus of medicine. They argue that the traditional problem-oriented medical model, with its focus on the identification and resolution of problems and diseases, is less suited to the management of a number of modern health care problems, including chronic incurable illnesses, health promotion and disease prevention, and normal life events such as pregnancy, well-child care, death and dying. Instead, Mold and his colleagues advocate goal-orientation as the basis of medical involvement. The aim of goal-oriented medicine is the maximum desirable and achievable quality and/or quantity of life, defined at the level of the individual. The definition of health goals, and the assessment of whether or not these goals have been attained, becomes a central issue in the individual patient's care. Health outcome measures will have an important role in this new goal-orientation of medicine.

An Overview
What is "good health" and which are the most important health-related goals for an older population? In goal-oriented medicine this should be answered by the older people themselves. Doctors easily confound better health with a higher life expectancy. Others define health as "life expectancy free of disability". Rowe and Kahn (1987) refer to the concept of "successful ageing", and they conclude from a literature overview that older patients judge successful ageing by the degree of autonomy they can preserve. A recent qualitative Belgian study showed that health is very much related to autonomy in opinions and thoughts, vitality and self-consciousness, diversity in activities and social contributions (Tilkin-Franssens, 1992).

Meyboom and Lamberts (1993) reported on one of the largest European compilations to date on the functional status of all patients, aged 65 and older, registered with 25 family physicians. There were 5502 people involved, with 26,000 doctor-patient encounters. A personal study done on a 75 and older population in ten practices represents 3370 encounters (Heyrman *et al.*, 1993). The ten most common problems listed in rank order were: hypertension, respiratory tract infections, osteoarthritis, diabetes, heart failure, cystitis, adverse effects of medication, death of the partner, depressive disorders and problems with neighbours. The overall limitation of function according to the Dartmouth COOP Charts showed that in 35% of the encounters, serious physical limitations were found to exist (although in 10% there were no physical limitations at all) and in 18% there was serious limitations in activities of daily living (27% had no ADL limitations at all). In 11% there were psychological and social contact problems (whereas in 25% no psychological and in 39% no social problems were reported). Doctors do not always express the same opinions on functional status as their patients. Meyboom and Lamberts as well as Nelson *et al.* (1983) reported discrepancies between doctors' and patients' assessments in one third of all encounters.

HEALTH OUTCOME MEASURES FOR OLDER PEOPLE

"At least 43 different indexes have been developed for classifying a patient's functional disability in the self-care and mobility area which we usually call ... 'activities of daily living'. At least 230 rating scales have been proposed for describing the condition of patients with arthritis and other impairments in locomotion. What the process lacks however is a name, a set of well-defined principles and strategies, and an intellectual home." (Feinstein, 1987)

Over the last 20 years, a wide variety of health outcome measures have been developed. A considerable number of the instruments have been designed specifically for use with older people. Besides the dimensions traditionally included in health outcome measures, they give more attention to cognitive impairment, memory function, social network and often they give a focus on the degree of (in)dependency. Not all instruments are completely unique; many include parts of other scales. Some examples of health status measures for use in geriatric care are listed in Box 12.1.

Box 12.1   Examples of health status measures for use in geriatric care

---

The Older American's Resources and Services Schedule (OARS): multidimensional functional assessment questionnaire (developed by Fillenbaum for use in adults over 55).

The Index of Activities of Daily Living (ADL): description of states of older patients (Katz; Barthel Index).

Townsend's Disability Scale: *idem.*

The Crichton Royal Behaviour Rating Scale (CRBRS): residents in homes for older people, geriatric and psychiatric wards.

The Clifton Assessment Procedures for the Elderly (CAPE): most extensively tested measure of dependency in UK, particularly in relation to psychological assessment in older people.

Geriatric Mental Status questionnaires (GMS) (AGECAT = computer version): diagnose dementia and depression.

The Mental Status Questionnaire (MSQ).

Life Satisfaction Index A (checklist version) and B (open-ended questionnaire).

The Philadelphia Geriatric Center Morale Scale: multidimensional scale for well-being.

Source: Bowling, A. (1991)

Instruments used in clinical situations often lack extensive validation, but have proved their usefulness. Instruments for psychometric use tend to be multidimensional, sometimes with differential weighting of the constituted sub-scales. Instruments for cost-benefit analysis or resource allocation or health policy making are often very extensive and time-consuming to apply.

DEVELOPING A HEALTH STATUS OUTCOME INSTRUMENT (HSOI) FOR OLDER PEOPLE

Ongoing research at the University of Leuven is aimed at the development of a generic instrument for health outcome evaluation of older people. Below, we present an overview of the steps, considerations, options and difficulties encountered in an area where instruments are needed but where appropriate tools do not yet exist.

In 1987, work started within the Department of General Practice to develop a clinimetric instrument to measure and quantify the health outcome of older patients (Heyrman et al., 1993). This instrument was intended for routine use in general practice care, as part of medical record-keeping. Eventually, it was hoped the instrument would become an integrated part of the general practitioner's computerised record. Software would guarantee that a health outcome assessment would be made at least once every year. The instrument is designed for use by the doctor, to support medical interventions, and to foster a goal-oriented approach to care in place of a disease orientation.

The instrument reflects some important conceptual dimensions which must be considered by the physician in assessing the health outcome of older patients. The conceptualisation of these aspects of health, relevant for decision-making by the general practitioner, are an important aspect of ensuring the content validity of the instrument.

The four individual instruments which make up the global outcome instrument refer to the four main goals in the management of chronic illness: reducing the severity of diseases, symptom relief and minimising side-effects of therapeutic interventions, and maintaining optimal functions concerned with maximum autonomy. Another basic option for the instrument was to represent a clinical and a functional status.

Clinical Status
Reducing the severity of the diseases
It is a clinician's job to monitor physio-biological and clinical parameters for patients. One development option was to include key biological parameters which could be measured easily and are generally considered to be markers for the most common diseases in older people (blood pressure, blood sugar, peak expiratory

flow, etc.). After deliberation however we realised that including a simple checklist of such biological parameters would be an over-simplification and might even be misleading in representing the clinical status of a patient. Determining the most appropriate indicators for inclusion in a generic measure and deciding how scores should be allocated would not be straightforward. Moreover, follow-up of these parameters on a regular basis would be both time- and cost-consuming. Dealing with comorbidity would also be a problem. One alternative solution identified was the active problem list (Weed, 1971) which is a feature of many computerised record files. However, a problem list cannot be quantified, and this option was also ruled out.

Finally, we chose to use the Duke Severity of Illness Score (DUSOI), as developed by Parkerson *et al.* (1993). The DUSOI represents a physician's opinion on a patient's clinical status, considering the symptoms, complications, prognosis and treatability of every problem or disease listed in the patient's record, taking an overall view of the impact of illness rather than disease.

Symptom relief and minimising side-effects of therapeutic interventions
The symptom status of a patient is an important aspect of clinical outcome. Symptoms may be an early manifestation of altered health or treatment side-effects. Although symptoms can be vague and non-specific, their number and severity may provide an indicator of general health status (Meyboom *et al.*, 1993). Interventions and treatment should not provoke too many side-effects, but as noted earlier, adverse effects of treatment are frequent problems in an older patient population (due to metabolic and physiologic changes with age). Early results of the Leuven Outcome Study show that it is almost impossible to distinguish symptoms due to drug side-effects from those due to illness. Indeed, it is likely that this will never be possible unless drug-specific questionnaires are used, an approach that does not coincide with the "generic" character of the outcome instrument. In the development phase, we combined the Bulpitt Symptom Questionnaire (SQ) (Bulpitt *et al.*, 1990) and the symptom questions of the Duke UNC Health Profile (Parkerson *et al.*, 1981). The Bulpitt SQ was chosen for the simple reason that an outcome study on hypertensives was planned in combination with the generic outcome study. Associating the Bulpitt questions with questions from the Duke UNC Health Profile resulted in a questionnaire covering all the body systems. In total there are 42 questions that most probably will be submitted to item reduction during the course of the project.

Functional Status
Maintaining optimal functioning
The Dartmouth COOP Charts have proven their usefulness and feasibility in scoring functional status in older people (Nelson *et al.*, 1983). In the Leuven outcome instrument, these charts are used to assess patients' views of their day-to-

day functional health status. The pain chart from older versions of the COOP Charts have also been included.

To be concerned with maximum autonomy

Autonomy is important when caring for older people: the maintenance or restoration of optimal function is fundamental. For this reason we deemed it important to include an autonomy/dependency scale in the Leuven outcome instrument. We chose the AMP-dependency scale (Heyrman *et al.*, 1990), a nine-item instrument, scoring the presence or absence of dependency in different areas of need (the physical, cognitive and psychosocial areas) and to a certain extent the degree of dependency. Dependency has been defined by Wilkin as a state in which an individual is reliant upon others for assistance in meeting recognised needs (1987). These needs might be recognised by society or significant others, but not by the individual him/herself. The author presents a matrix for dependency-classification according to the area of need (orientation, ADL, mobility, occupation etc) and a classification according to the aetiology (normal life cycle dependency, by crisis or resulting from disablement, as a personality trait or socially and culturally defined). A third dimension is the severity, which can be seen differently from the point of view of care givers and care receivers. In the AMP instrument the presence or absence of needs in the above mentioned areas is scored, according to the presence and quality of offered help. Aetiology notions are not included. We chose an instrument which covers any type of dependency. The AMP is designed to be scored by doctors. AMP scores are in accord with an ordinal scale pattern, with higher scores reflecting a higher demand on the general practitioner and the support network.

The Sense of Sum Scores

Each of the scores on the different sub-scales represent a quantification of an aspect of outcome. We considered the possibility of making a global sum score as a general interpretation of the health status. The advantage is to have one global number, like the APGAR score or the ADL index. This would give the general practitioner an overall idea as to the patient's health status at any given time. When the actual measured status differs in a negative way from the previous one, the physician can consult the contributing scales in more detail and compare this with the clinical findings to localise the problem.

Traditional researchers can have problems with adding up sub-scale scores. "A unique feature that differentiates clinimetric from laboratory (or research) measurement is the frequent use of global indexes and scales. The main advantage of global indexes is their simplicity and their direct focus on the selected phenomenon; their main disadvantage is the absence of the stipulations needed for scientific reproducibility" (Feinstein, 1987). The biological plausibility, the statistical isonometry and the scientific transparency are considered as main attributes for a combined index by Feinstein. Often the investigator will have to choose which of the competing goals should be given priority.

CONCLUSION

There is an increasing desire to incorporate functional status assessments into routine clinical practice. The American College of Physicians recommends that primary care practitioners should incorporate into their routine medical management of older adults procedures for measuring functional deficits and identifying dependency needs (Health and Public Policy Committee, 1988). The purposes served by these procedures in clinical practice would include: detecting, quantifying and identifying the sources of decreased functional capacity; providing information by comparing changes in function over time; guiding management decisions; guiding the efficient use of community resources; and improving the prediction of the course of chronic disease in the older population. Functional assessment instruments complement but are not a substitute for clinical judgement derived from questioning and observing the patient. Through continuing medical education, practising physicians should be prepared to perform and to utilise such examinations. It will certainly contribute to the aforementioned goal-orientation which needs to be introduced into daily clinical care. The proposed implementation within the computerised medical records can support daily routines, once clinical personnel are introduced to the practice and trained in its use.

REFERENCES

Bowling, A. (1991) *Measuring health: a review of quality of life measurement scales.* Buckingham: Open University Press.

Bulpitt, C.J. (1990) The measurement of quality of life in hypertensive patients: a practical approach. *British Journal of Clinical Pharmacology*, **30**, 353-364.

Feinstein, A.R. (1987) *Clinimetrics.* Yale: Yale University.

Health and Public Policy Committee (1988) Comprehensive functional assessment for elderly patients. *Annals of Internal Medicine*, **109**, 70-72.

Heyrman, J., Dessers, L. and van Hoeck, K. (1993) Problems elderly people present to their general practitioners in Belgium. In: Lamberts, H., Wood, M. and Hofmans-Okkes, I. (Eds.), *The international classification of primary care in the European Community*. Oxford: Oxford Medical Publications.

Heyrman, J., Dessers, M. and de Munter, B. (1990) Functional status assessment in the elderly. In: *Functional status measurement in primary care:report from the Classification Committee of WONCA*. New York: Springer Verlag.

Katz, S., Ford, A.B. and Moskowitz, R.W. (1963) Studies of illness in the aged: the index of ADL - a standardised measure of biological and psychosocial function. *Journal of the American Medical Association*, **185**, 914-919.

Metcalfe, D. (1992) *The measurement of outcomes in general practice: doing qualitative research.* Newbury Park: Sage.

Meyboom-de Jong, B. and Lamberts, H. (1993) The autonomy project: practical experiences with functional status indicators within the framework of ICPC. In: Lamberts, H., Wood, M. and Hofmans-Okkes, I. (Eds.), *The international classification of primary care in the European Community.* Oxford: Oxford Medical Publications.

Mold, J.W., Blake, G.H. and Becker, L.A. (1991) Goal-oriented medical care. *Family Medicine*, **23**, 46-51.

Nelson, E., Conges, B., Douglass, R., Gephart, D., Kirk, J., Page, R., Clark, A., Johnson, K., Stone, K., Wasson, J. and Zubkoff, M. (1983) Functional health status levels of primary care patients. *Journal of the American Medical Association*, **249**, 3331-3337.

Parkerson, G.R. Jr., Gehlbach, S.H., Wagner, E.H., James, S.A. and Clapp, N.E. (1981) The DUKE UNC Health Profile: an adult health status instrument for primary care. *Medical Care*, **19**, 806-828.

Parkerson, G.R. Jr., Broadhead, W.E. and Tse, C.K. (1993) The Duke Severity of Illness Checklist for measurement of severity and comorbidity. *Journal of Clinical Epidemiology*, **46**, 379-393.

Rowe, J.W. and Kahn, R.L. (1987) Human aging: usual and successful. *Science*, **237**, 143-149.

Tilkin-Franssens, D. (1992) *Vitàal oud worden.* Antwerpen.

Weed, L.L. (1971) *Medical records, medical education and patient care.* Chicago: Yearbook Medical Publishers.

Wilkin, D. (1987) Conceptual problems in dependency research. *Social Science and Medicine*, **24**, 867-873.

Chapter 13 _____

ANTENATAL CARE: AN ASSESSMENT OF OUTCOME

PEDRO L FERREIRA

INTRODUCTION

In the last few years there has been a paradigm shift in health-related perspectives from disease to health, and also a shift from a problem-oriented to a goal-oriented approach. We are moving from a focus solely on disease and traditional epidemiological measures to a more encompassing vision which includes such concepts as functioning, well-being and quality of life. Until at least the middle of this century, health care had been guided by the rationale of correct diagnosis and resolution of health problems, and providers were mainly concerned with physiological dysfunction. Now, clinicians are dealing with a significant portion of patients with chronic diseases and little hope of a full cure. There is a shift in emphasis towards more proactive areas such as health promotion and prevention of diseases (Mold *et al.*, 1991; Greenfield and Nelson, 1992). Sometimes, in degenerative or debilitating diseases, health providers' goals are limited to the reduction or the elimination of the dysfunction, improving the ability of the patients to live with chronic diseases rather than attempting cure.

The introduction of health status measurement has its foundations in the sociological approach to defining the concept of health; in this approach, health is seen as the physical and mental fitness necessary for daily social activities. This is a broader focus than the traditional focus on biophysical indicators such as blood pressure, cholesterol level, liver and lung function, and mortality. The assumption behind the use of such traditional measures is that if we treat these biological problems, the patients will improve physically and, eventually, will be able to perform their daily and social activities better.

In fact some authors consider that the biophysical measures do not reflect other important health dimensions and are not enough for a complete understanding of what happens in the patient's body. As mentioned by Greenfield and Nelson (1992), for instance, not all patients with coronary artery disease have angina. The defenders of this new vision argue that we need to measure, as a minimum, physical function, mental function, and social function. Physical function corresponds to the individual's mobility and how easily the various types of motion are performed; mental function includes the ability to think (cognitive function) and the emotions (mental health); role and social functions are concerned with activities in the family, in school, in work and in the community.

The concept of quality of life, another layer of this new paradigm, includes dimensions of physical well-being and the cognitive skills as well as satisfactory relationships, adequate living conditions, and sufficient income to enjoy life beyond the basic level required to ensure biological survival (Hopkins, 1992). It encompasses such dimensions as pain, sleep, energy, and sexual function.

However, some factors contributing to quality of life are beyond the physician's control and therefore beyond the scope of health outcomes research. Therefore, in our work, we concentrate on the health-related quality of life, sometimes called health functional status, which has also become a standard to evaluate clinical practice (Ware *et al.*, 1980). This may be defined as the ability of a person to perform and participate in daily social activities and to cope with environmental constraints, measured subjectively and objectively over time (Scholten and Weel, 1992). Ellwood (1988) supports this focus, stating that one of the most agreed upon goals of health care is to restore and maintain patients' functional status and well-being. This is particularly true in the context of pregnancy and maternity care. The reduction of infant mortality has been observed with great enthusiasm all over the world. One of the reasons for this reduction has to do with the improvement of the quality of the health care provided during the pregnancy, the delivery and post-partum periods (Mahler, 1987).

The World Health Organisation, in *Health for All by the Year 2000,* stressed the need for the creation of health systems based on primary health care, and recognised the importance of this type of health care in the global context of health policies (WHO, 1981). General practitioners play a vital role in health promotion and the detection of early risk situations (Ryan *et al.*, 1980). In countries like Portugal, where the family doctor is usually the first point of contact with the health care system, general practitioners have major responsibilities in terms of monitoring and supporting special groups of individuals such as children, pregnant women and older people. The World Organisation of National Colleges, Academies and Academic Associations of General Practitioners/Family Physicians (WONCA) has created a task force which aims to develop a health outcomes classification system for clinical practice. The United Kingdom's Department of Health has also recognised the need for outcome measurement to go alongside evaluation of the process of care (Department of Health, 1988; Hutchinson and Fowler, 1992). More recently, the United States Department of Health and Human Services (1991), in its document *Healthy People 2000,* defended the importance of increasing the proportion of people who live long and healthy lives, including a "full range of functional capacity at each life stage, from infancy through old age, allowing one the ability to enter into satisfying relationships with others, to work, and to play."

Pregnant women are usually not sick people; instead, they constitute a cluster of individuals characterised physiologically and psychologically. They experience physical symptoms related to hormonal changes at the endocrine level and in physical terms with the increase of the uterus as well as emotional states such as happiness, depression and anxiety (Bricker *et al.,* 1977). There are a large number of factors, not completely understood, which influence the physical, psychological and social equilibria of the pregnant woman. The short time of pregnancy may sometimes prevent a woman from being able to cope with these changes (Raphael-Leff, 1991). The future mother-child relationship is dependent upon the way the mother experiences the pregnancy and the recognition of this is important because it allows a better follow-up and psychological support during the pregnancy. On the other hand, the large majority of post-partum depressions (more than 95%) can be seen as a consequence of a status not diagnosed during the pregnancy (Gotlib *et al.,* 1989).

In summary, as John Ware Jr (1991) stated, it is important to have a comprehensive model for understanding health status in pregnancy, "one that includes traditional clinical measures of disease status measured in parallel, in the same data base, and in the same analysis, as with generic concepts that represent the patient view of disease and treatment."

MEASURING FUNCTIONING OF PREGNANT WOMEN

The corpus of research in this field suggests that it makes sense to focus our attention on the measurement of health status in pregnant women and on maternal health, with "positive or negative outcomes - physical, social or mental - in a woman from any cause related to childbearing or its management" (Graham and Campbell, 1992). The reasons for measuring maternal health include the definition and identification of levels and trends in specific health outcomes, their characteristics and determinants, and the monitoring and controlling of the effectiveness of the processes that influence them. This includes being able to look at the natural history of health in pregnant women and to study the impact of pregnancy on a woman's health in terms of physical function, emotional and mental functions, role and social functions, and quality of life.

Currently very little is known about physical and mental well-being as a woman goes through the process of having a baby, delivery and recovering from that delivery. At the Maternity Department of the Coimbra University Hospital we are looking at the overall health effect of being pregnant on a woman. This work is based mainly on the self-health perceptions of the women. This project has been supported in part by the European Communities' BIOMED Programme, including the activities of the European Research Group on Health Outcomes (ERGHO), and in part by the Coimbra University Hospital Quality Committee. The study aims at gaining a better knowledge regarding the natural history of pregnancy from the first time a woman goes to the primary care health centre or presents herself at the hospital maternity department through delivery, discharge and any possible follow-up for complications. We adopted the sociological/humanistic view of health where optimal autonomy, personal strength, happiness and the positive meaning of life are placed in a central position. While a pregnant woman's physical needs are taken care of by the providers, her psychosocial needs require much more intense attention. The following objectives are being pursued in this project:

1) to gain knowledge about the natural history of pregnancy
2) to initiate a study about the impact of pregnancy on a woman
3) to show evidence of the utility of functional health measures to support decisions regarding the care provided to a pregnant woman, to improve clinical decision-making
4) to enhance the communications and information flow between the Hospital Maternity Department and the health centres of the region.

A coordination team was formed to carry out this project, including the author, a hospital administrator, two obstetricians and an administrator from the Maternity Department, and one general practitioner from each of the three health centres participating in this project.

To measure functional health status we decided to use the Portuguese version of the COOP Pregnancy Charts and the Portuguese version of the Medical Outcomes Study SF-36. Both are self-administered measurement instruments. The instruments, originally written in English and designed for the US population, needed to be validated for cross-cultural use, to ensure that Portuguese versions were as correct as possible; that is, there was semantic, content, technical and conceptual equivalence. Two translations from English to Portuguese and two back-translations were performed by different bilingual translators. For a more in-depth explanation of the cross-cultural validation procedure please refer to Chapter 15.

COOP Pregnancy Charts (Friedrichs *et al.*, 1992) were initially developed at the Dartmouth Medical School by the Primary Care Cooperative Program with the aim of producing a valid and reliable measurement instrument which was quick to administer. They comprise scales to measure various dimensions of maternal health: impact of the pregnancy on the woman's physical well-being; mental health;

availability of someone to help, if needed; readiness to deal with the new-born's needs; and quality of life. The SF-36 is an instrument derived from the Medical Outcomes Study (Stewart and Ware, 1992), and comprises the following scales: general health now and compared to one year ago; health and daily activities; physical health; emotional health; pain; feelings; and health in general. The main dimensions from both health status instruments have been empirically and statistically confirmed by us through principal component analyses with varimax rotations. Other studies performed by us included reliability tests and how feasible and understandable the instruments were for the subjects. Figures 13.1 and 13.2 represent the Portuguese versions of the COOP readiness scale for pregnancy and the SF-36 physical functioning scale respectively.

Socio-demographic data and data related to the pregnancy (context variables) have also been collected. Among those selected were age, number of previous pregnancies and deliveries, and gestational age. In the cases where the woman was admitted and stayed on a ward, we also collected information regarding the admission and discharge dates, the reasons for the admission, diagnoses and procedures performed, and the corresponding Diagnostic Related Groups.

The research project can be split into two main parts. In the first part we tested and validated the health status measures and initiated a discussion with the participants in the project. In the second part, we intend to gain knowledge about the natural history of pregnancy, comparing the outcome measurements to other information taken from the medical records (e.g. diagnoses, complications, socio-demographics).

For the first phase, already concluded, three health centres (Arganil, Cantanhede and Lousa) agreed to participate. All women attending for antenatal care at each site during one month were included, yielding a sample of 930 women. Six hundred and seventy women were seen in out-patient antenatal clinics, 158 were admitted to hospital wards and 102 were seen in the three primary care health centres. Their ages were normally distributed, with an average age of 26.9 years of age (standard deviation = 5.3 years). Seventy-six percent of them had not experienced any complication during the pregnancy, 14% were in the first trimester of pregnancy, 27% in the second trimester, 35% were at the end of their pregnancy, and 24% were in the post-partum period.

By stratifying the sample on the period of pregnancy, we found some results that were also used as validation of the instruments. As an example, using non-parametric statistics, we found evidence of a significant difference between the second and third trimesters, especially in the questions related to the physical well-being of the woman and to her mental health.

Preparação
[Readiness]

Sente-se preparada para cuidar do seu bebé quando ele estiver barulhento, comer mal, chorar frequentemente ou acordar muitas vezes durante a noite?
[How ready do you feel you are to care for a baby that: acts fussy, or eats irregularly, or cries frequently, or awakens often at night?]

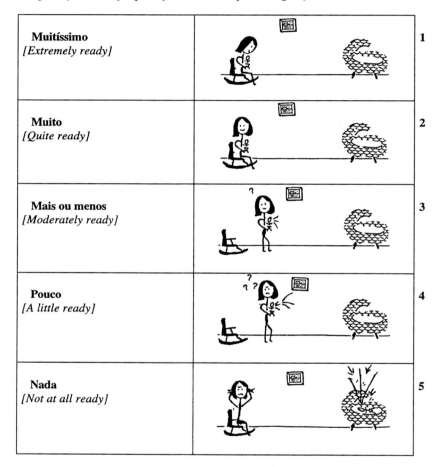

Muitíssimo *[Extremely ready]*		1
Muito *[Quite ready]*		2
Mais ou menos *[Moderately ready]*		3
Pouco *[A little ready]*		4
Nada *[Not at all ready]*		5

Figure 13.1   COOP readiness for pregnancy scales

- As perguntas que se seguem são relativas às actividades do seu dia-a-dia. Será que a **sua saúde** a limita nestas actividades? Por favor **assinale com um círculo um número em cada linha**.
  [The following questions are about activities you might do in a typical day. Does your health limit you in these activities? If so, how much? Please circle one number on each line.]

	Sim, muito limitada *[Yes, limited a lot]*	Sim, um pouco limitada *[Yes, limited a little]*	Não, nada limitada *[No, not limited at all]*
a. **Actividades violentas**, tais como correr, levantar pesos, participar em desportos violentos *[Vigorous activities, such as running, lifting heavy objects, participating in strenuous sports]*	1	2	3
b. **Actividades moderadas**, tais como deslocar uma mesa ou aspirar a casa. *[Moderate activities, such as moving a table, pushing a vacuum cleaner, bowling or playing golf]*	1	2	3
c. Levantar e carregar as compras de mercearia *[Lifting or carrying groceries]*	1	2	3
d. Subir **vários** lances de escada *[Climbing several fights of stairs]*	1	2	3
e. Subir **um** lance de escadas *[Climbing one fight of stairs]*	1	2	3
f. Inclinar-se, ajoelhar-se or baixar-se *[Bending, kneeling or stooping]*	1	2	3
g. Andar **1500 metros** *[Walking more than a mile]*	1	2	3
h. Andar **500 metros** *[Walking several blocks]*	1	2	3
i. Andar **100 metros** *[Walking one block]*	1	2	3
j. Tomar banho ou vestir-se sozinha *[Bathing or dressing yourself]*	1	2	3

Figure 13.2 SF-36 Portuguese version - health and daily activities

Confident with the validity of our instruments, and following discussion of the results with the providers involved in this study, we were able to enter into the second phase of this project. In this phase, aimed at acquiring an even better knowledge about the perceptions pregnant women have at different stages of their pregnancy about their own functional health status, we chose a longitudinal study design. Five hundred women (all those attending for a first antenatal consultation in the hospital out-patient clinics and in the primary care health centres over a period of one month) are being followed through their pregnancies.

After explicit consent and the completion of an enrolment form, each of these women is subject to measurements at four time points: before 18 weeks gestation; between 26 and 30 weeks gestation; between 35 and 40 weeks gestation; and after the delivery. Should the woman be seen for any subsequent complication of pregnancy or delivery she will be asked to provide data on a fifth occasion. A special label will be placed in the subjects' medical records to make it easier to follow them over time.

CONCLUSION

We are finding a wide consensus regarding the concepts that should be included in the term "health status" including: physical function, mental and emotional well-being, social and role activities, general health perceptions, pain, energy and vitality (Lohr, 1992). To this list of dimensions we usually add physiological and biological indicators. Generic and disease-specific or condition-specific outcome measures already exist that have been validated and accepted as good measures of the health states (Nelson and Berwick, 1989; Spilker et al., 1992). Furthermore, we are facing an enormous evolution regarding the understanding and the solving of some methodological issues. Health services researchers are working hard to go beyond their current knowledge.

On the other hand, some forces are still limiting our ability to measure the health status of an individual or a population (Thier, 1992). We deal with extremely complex health systems subject to enormous pressures, the costs are high and, at the same time, the health coverage of the population is not complete. The solution for this situation lies in an improvement of the quality of the care provided and the measurement of its effectiveness by process and outcome indicators, including the measurement of its impact on the individual's health and on satisfaction.

Other challenges to the science of health status and health outcome measurement include the shift of the most prevalent diseases from acute to chronic, the ageing of the population, some migration phenomena changing the disease patterns of various populations, and finally, the enormous movement led by patients and patient-interest groups in fighting for their rights to be informed and to be involved in the medical decision-making process.

The utility of the project being carried out at Coimbra is threefold. Firstly, it will allow us to gain knowledge about the expected changes in health status and to initiate actions to prevent some unwanted outcomes of pregnancy; secondly, it will start giving us an idea of the impact caused by complications on physical functioning, role and psychological status. Thirdly, it has a structural utility in linking more closely the care provided by the health centres and by the maternity units.

The health of the women in developing countries is a matter of fundamental importance to human rights and dignity (Graham and Campbell, 1992) and all efforts to better understand and dignify the pregnant condition are vital for all of us as human beings. Enormous challenges are waiting for us in the difficult field of outcomes measurement. However, it seems that we are in the right place, at the right time.

REFERENCES

Bricker, M.C., Gmanion, L., Beadnell, B., Yaple, K. and Moires, K.A. (1977) Anxiety, depression and stress in pregnancy: a multivariate model of intra-partum risks and pregnancy outcomes. *Journal of Psychosomatic Obstetrics and Gynecology*, **7**, 77-92.

Department of Health (1988) *On the state of the public health for the year 1988.* London: HMSO.

Ellwood, P.M. (1988) Outcomes management. *New England Journal of Medicine*, **318**, 1549-1556.

Friedrichs, P. Hamilton, N. and Jette A. (1992) The Dartmouth COOP Pregnancy Charts. *Interactive Newsletter Annual Meeting Edition*, **April**, 4.

Gotlib, I.H., Whiffen,V.E., Mount, J.H., Milne, K. and Cordy, N.I. (1989) Prevalence rates and demographic characteristics associated with depression in pregnancy and the postpartum. *Journal of Consulting and Clinical Psychology*, **57**, 269-274.

Graham, W.J. and Campbell, O.M. (1992) Maternal health and the measurement trap. *Social Science and Medicine*, **35**, 967-977.

Greenfield, S. and Nelson, E. (1992) Recent developments and future issues in the use of health status measures in clinical settings. *Medical Care*, **30**, MS23-MS41.

Hopkins, A. (1992) How might measures of quality of life be useful to me as a clinician? In: Hopkins, A. (Ed.), *Measures of the quality of life.* London: Royal College of Physicians of London.

Hutchinson, A. and Fowler, P. (1992) Outcome measurement for primary health care: what are the research priorities? *British Journal of General Practice*, **42**, 227-231.

Lohr, K.N. (1992) Applications of health status assessment measures in clinical practice. *Medical Care*, **30**, MS1-MS14.

Mahler, H. (1987) The safe motherhood initiative: a call to action. *Lancet*, **i**, 668-670.

Mold, J.W, Blake, G.B. and Becker, L.A. (1991) Goal-oriented medicine care. *Family Medicine*, **23**, 46-51.

Nelson, E. and Berwick, D.M. (1989) The measurement of health status in clinical practice. *Medical Care*, **27**, S77-S90.

Raphael-Leff, J. (1991) *Psychological processes of childbearing*. London: Chapman and Hall.

Ryan, G.M., Sweeney, P.J. and Solola, A.S. (1980) Prenatal care and pregnancy outcome. *American Journal of Obstetrics and Gynecology*, **137**, 876-881.

Scholten, J.H.G. and van Weel, C. (1992) Report of an international workshop of the WONCA Research and Classification Committee. In: Scholten, J.H.G. and van Weel, C. (Eds.), *Functional status assessment in family practice*. Lelystad: MediTekst.

Spilker, B. Simpson, R.L. and Tilson, H.H. (1992) Quality of life bibliography and indexes. *Journal of Clinical Research and Pharmacoepidemiology*, **6**, 205-266.

Stewart, A.L. and Ware, J.E. (Eds.) (1992) *Measuring functioning and well-being: the Medical Outcomes Study approach*. Durham, NC: Duke University Press.

Thier, S.O. (1992) Forces motivating the use of health status measurement. *Medical Care*, **30**, MS15-MS22.

US Department of Health and Human Services (1991) *Healthy people 2000*. Washington, DC: US Government Printing Office. (No (PHS) 91-50213)

Ware, J.E, Brook, R.H, Davies-Avery. A. (1980) *Conceptualization and measurement of health for adults in the Health Insurance Study. Volume I: Model of health and methodology*. Santa Monica, CA: The Rand Corporation. (publication no. R-1987/1-HEW)

Ware, J.E. (1991) Conceptualizing and measuring generic health outcomes. *Cancer*, **67**, 774-779.

World Health Organization (1981) *Health for all by the year 2000*. Geneva: WHO.

Chapter 14 _____

WHOSE LIFE IS IT ANYWAY?

BERIT ROKNE HANESTAD

INTRODUCTION

Interest in the concept and measurement of quality of life in relation to health care, especially in the area of chronic diseases, is shown by the increase in publications which include "quality of life" as a keyword. Baker and Meadows (1992) found in their Medline search, which covered the period from 1982 to 1991, a growing interest in applying quality of life assessment to conditions such as coronary heart disease, diabetes, arthritis, cancer, renal disease and epilepsy.

Quality of life research has a number of different objectives. Fitzpatrick *et al.* (1992) discuss alternative applications: screening and monitoring for psychosocial problems in individual patient care, population surveys of perceived health problems, medical audit, outcome measures in health services or evaluation research, clinical trials, and cost-utility analysis. Irrespective of the objectives for using the quality of life concept within the health care context, issues such as the definition and operationalisation of the concept are of importance. Yet, despite extensive applications, no formal and consistent definition of the concept exists. Instead the concept is defined and operationalised differently in different settings. Additionally, there have been discussions as to whether health personnel, other individuals, such as relatives who have an impact on a patient's well-being and.are in turn affected by that well-being, or the patients themselves, should determine and judge that patient's quality of life. To explore these issues, the intention of this chapter is first to provide a review of the different ways the concept has been, and continues to be, defined and operationalised. Second, it sets out to discuss who should assess quality of life. Finally, the usefulness of the quality of life concept and its measurement within a health care context is discussed.

THE ORIGIN AND EXPANSION OF THE QUALITY OF LIFE CONCEPT

Although the concept of quality of life has gained increasing popularity within the context of health care in the 1980s and 1990s, it first appeared in other research fields, particularly in the social sciences. Over time a range of different disciplines have had an impact on the conceptual issues of quality of life: philosophy; social sciences, economics, sociology, psychology; medicine; and nursing science.

Discussions as to what constitutes "the good life" has been the topic for philosophers for years (Lindstrom, 1992), but "quality of life" is a relatively new concept emerging from social and political discussions in America in the 1960s. Initially the concept was associated with measurable, objective conditions of living including income, education, health and housing; this emphasis stemmed from a belief that improved material welfare resulted in a better quality of life. However, as it became apparent that higher levels of material and social standards did not necessarily lead to increased subjective well-being, it was claimed that what mattered was not the objective working and housing conditions, but rather satisfaction with these conditions (Naess, 1989). As a consequence, quality of life became associated with perceived satisfaction and/or happiness with life rather than objective conditions. This resulted in researchers endeavouring to identify what constitutes a good life (Cantril, 1967; Bradburn, 1969; Andrews and Withey, 1976; Campell *et al.,* 1976).

Application of the concept within the social sciences has influenced research within the health care context and in the last decade interest has increased in quality of life measurement, focusing on different levels of health, symptoms, illnesses and treatments. Within medicine, patients' subjective feelings regarding the quality of their lives have increasingly become recognised as important outcomes in clinical research, which need to be considered alongside the more traditional biomedical outcomes. This change in focus from the use of traditional biomedical outcomes, such as survival or cure, to a more humanistic, holistic and democratic view of the patient, encompassing physical, psychological and social aspects of life, may be attributed to a number of factors. One reason is the recognition of the limitations of traditional outcomes of treatment effects, such as survival, in deciding the effect of treatment. Patients may have improved quality of life despite low survival rates, or treatment effects may improve survival rates but reduce quality of life. Second, in the treatment of various diseases, a range of different treatments may be available, all of which may be satisfactory in meeting medical criteria of what constitutes a "good outcome". The choice of treatment, however, should be based both on optimising the reduction or elimination of symptoms, as well as maintaining or increasing the patient's quality of life. Third, the increase in the prevalence of chronic diseases with life-long treatments has also resulted in the recognition of quality of life as an important outcome variable. It is not sufficient to find a suitable treatment alone, but also to enable the patient to cope with the disease over time (Spilker, 1990).

In nursing research, as well as in more general medical and health services research, quality of life has received increasing attention in recent years. Padilla *et al.* (1992) enumerate five areas of quality of life research as relevant to nursing research:

1) to describe patients' psychosocial and physical responses to specific diseases
2) to examine symptom management responses to disease and treatment
3) to compare patient and/or family responses to treatment
4) to demonstrate the effect of specific rehabilitation approaches
5) to identify vulnerable periods in the health-illness continuum.

This preoccupation with quality of life in nursing science is due to the fact that the concept reflects the essentials of nursing, which include helping patients to be comfortable, delivering appropriate treatment and enhancing well-being. Quality of life encompasses the biological, psychological and sociocultural aspects of life, all of which are within the domains of nursing.

The focus on the relationship between quality of life and different degrees of health, symptoms, illnesses and treatments has resulted in studies measuring the quality of life of different disease populations, assessing the benefit of alternative use of resources, comparing the effectiveness of interventions in clinical trials and evaluating decision-making on treatment for individual patients (Cox *et al.*, 1992). Yet, despite the recognition of the importance of the concept of quality of life and its assessment within different disciplines, there remains no clear agreement on its definition.

THE DEFINITION OF QUALITY OF LIFE

Because of the subjective nature of the concept, quality of life has been variously expressed in terms of self-fulfilment, usefulness, satisfaction, functional ability, realisation of life plans, happiness, pleasure, management and personal control (Fowlie and Berkely, 1987; Goodinson and Singleton, 1989). However, a number of ways of describing the concept can be outlined. Maeland (1993) states that the definitions of quality of life can be categorised as:

1) *happiness*, reflecting the affective component of the individual's experience and involving emotional aspects
2) *satisfaction*, reflecting the cognitive component of the individual's experience and referring to the rational or intellectual aspects
3) *need fulfilment*, relating to the different needs which have to be satisfied before the individual may experience a "good life"
4) *self-realisation*, emphasising personal growth and development

5) *functional ability*, in relation to physical, social and psychological aspects of life.

Furthermore, quality of life is frequently referred to as a sense of *well-being* (Padilla *et al.*, 1992).

From a philosophical point of view quality of life as "happiness" has been described by Nordenfelt (1991) and Tatarkiewicz (1976). Nordenfelt perceives happiness as related to the degree to which the individual experiences attainment of aspirations or wishes. This indicates that one experience might for one person increase happiness because it is in accordance with that individual's wishes or aspirations, while for another the same experience will have no significance. Tatarkiewicz defines happiness as a kind of satisfaction which includes both affective and cognitive components. Happiness is then defined as:

1) *complete*: to be considered complete it must pervade the whole of the consciousness and not just flow over its surface

2) *lasting*: in the sense that the satisfaction is not transitory but endures throughout the whole of an individual's life; when people contemplate their lives, their reaction and judgement should be favourable and whenever they ask themselves if they are satisfied with life the answer should be in the affirmative

3) *satisfying*: the person who is satisfied is not only emotionally gratified but also regards that satisfaction as justified, indicating the intellectual element in happiness

4) *touching the life as a whole*: even though only a fragment of an individual's life is focused in the mind, satisfaction with parts of life can be emotionally equivalent to satisfaction with the whole of it.

Tatarkiewicz's description represents an ideal happiness and the happy person is one who at least approaches this ideal or maxim.

Within social sciences also, quality of life defined as happiness, satisfaction or both has been widely used. The distinction between quality of life as happiness (reflecting positive and negative affect) and satisfaction (reflecting the cognitive aspect) has been the subject of some debate (Naess, 1989). Campell *et al.* (1976) suggest that the use of satisfaction is a better indicator of quality of life because it implies the cognitive judgement of a situation in which external standards may be used for comparison. Surveys of global quality of life have found that older adults report lower levels of happiness than do younger adults, but higher levels of satisfaction, suggesting that cognitive evaluations of life as a whole may rise with age, while positive affect may decline.

Within the areas of psychology and psychiatry, quality of life has been defined as "need fulfilment". Different authors have suggested different needs. Hornquist (1982, 1989) defines quality of life as the degree of need fulfilment within the physical, social, psychological, structural, activity/behavioural and material life domain including well-being. Aggernaes (1988), strongly influenced by Maslow's needs hierarchy, defines the following needs which have to be satisfied to obtain an adequate quality of life: biological needs; need for close relationships; need for meaningful occupation; and need for change. A further psychological view of quality of life is that of Naess (1989) in which she emphasises self-realisation and defines quality of life as the degree to which the person is active, relates well to others, has positive self-esteem and a basic mood of happiness.

Quality of life as functional ability has been described especially in the health care context. De Haes and van Knippenberg (1985) claim that, within the clinical field, quality of life has to be approached as a multidimensional construct comprising at least four domains: physical and functional status; disease- and treatment-related physical symptoms; psychological functioning; and social functioning. Padilla *et al.* (1992) describe quality of life as well-being comprising:

1) *psychological well-being* i.e. satisfaction with life, usefulness, body image, adjustment, emotions such as anxiety, personal control, recreational/vocational concerns, developing/learning concerns, goal achievement, fulfilment, meaning in life, normality of life, and happiness

2) *physical well-being* i.e. functional ability, activities of daily living, eating, appetite, sex, sleep, strength, fatigue, perceived health-illness, and sequelae of diagnosis and treatment

3) *social and interpersonal well-being* i.e. interpersonal function, social activities, support from significant others, privacy, rejection, role function

4) *financial or material well-being* i.e. sense of present/future security, housing/shelter concerns, health insurance, job security, mobility/transportation ability.

Each of these aspects of quality of life can be characterised in relation to the level of intensity, degree of satisfaction or distress experienced, and the importance of the attribute to perceived well-being and extent of congruence between present experience and expected outcome.

Some authors combine different concepts in their description of quality of life. Sullivan (1992) lists six core dimensions of quality of life in clinical research: physical complaints/well-being; psychological distress/well-being; functional status; role functioning; social functioning/well-being; and health/quality of life perceptions.

Bergner (1989) suggested ten domains of quality of life: symptoms; functional status, encompassing self-care, mobility and physical activity; role activities, including work and household management; social functioning, including personal interactions, intimacy and community interactions; emotional status, comprising anxiety, stress, depression, locus of control and spiritual well-being; cognition; sleep and rest; energy and vitality; health perceptions; and general life satisfaction.

Although these definitions have much in common, they vary in their complexity, with some expressing a more global approach to the phenomenon, while others express a more focused and specific view. Nonetheless, the majority of definitions indicate a multidimensional concept by focusing on the individual's total situation. Because quality of life is an abstract phenomenon it seems to be inevitable that more than one definition exists and it is a fact that both clinicians and researchers have to accept and take account of. As a consequence the concept has been operationalised in a number of ways and many instruments to measure quality of life have been developed to reflect these different perspectives (Bowling, 1991). In choosing a measure, therefore, careful consideration needs to be given not only to its practical and psychometric properties but also to the conceptual definitions on which it is based; researchers and practitioners alike should try to choose a measure which best fits their own aims and concepts of quality of life.

WHO SHOULD ASSESS QUALITY OF LIFE ?

Consideration also needs to be given as to the most appropriate source of quality of life data, since different sources can provide assessments of the patient's quality of life: health personnel; patients themselves; and proxies. Traditionally, health professionals have provided assessments of the patient's situation; for example, in relation to functional status, the Karnofsky (Karnofsky and Burchenal, 1949) and Spitzer (Spitzer et al., 1981) scales are physician-based rating systems addressing quality of life dimensions including psychological and social well-being. If quality of life is conceptualised and defined in purely objective terms, observation based on the perception of health personnel would appear to be practical and suitable. If, however, quality of life is defined as a subjective phenomenon (which it usually is) then observation by others is problematic, because subjective phenomena such as feelings and thoughts which are representative of quality of life are, by definition, unobservable by others. Research has shown there to be low levels of agreement between ratings by health personnel and patients, with a tendency for health personnel to rate the patient's quality of life lower than the patient herself (Pearlman and Uhlmann, 1988; Slevin et al., 1988). The differences, not surprisingly, are greater for more subjective aspects of quality of life than for dimensions that are more observable, such as functional status (Uhlmann and Pearlman, 1991; Sprangers and Aaronson, 1992). However, findings suggest that nurses and other ancillary health care personnel may provide more reliable ratings than physicians (Yates et al., 1980). There is also reported low concordance between subjects and proxy responses when assessing emotional health and satisfaction, with the tendency for relatives to underestimate the patient's quality of life (Epstein et al., 1989). Therefore, it would appear necessary to ask patients themselves questions regarding the impact of disease, treatment and symptoms such as pain, fatigue or distress on quality of life. Even in the case of more observable symptoms, patient feedback may provide important insights into their meaning and impact on daily living (Aaronson, 1989).

The tendency for health personnel and relatives to underestimate the quality of life in patients may be due to the coping and adaptation mechanisms which may be developed by people with a chronic disease. Actually having a disease appears to be perceived differently to the theoretical notion of what it means. This mismatch may also explain the small differences in perceived quality of life in people with different diseases and between different disease and non-disease groups compared to the larger differences in health measured by more objective indicators (Cassileth *et al.*, 1984). Patients with significant illnesses differ from healthy individuals only modestly in overall psychological well-being; they vary less with regard to psychological and social dimensions of quality of life than they do in terms of physical function. Similarly, patients with different illnesses differ from each other less in relation to psychological and social dimensions of quality of life than they do in terms of physical function. Furthermore, patients with significant illnesses emphasise more psychological and social dimensions of quality of life rather than assessing quality of life mainly in terms of physical function (Fitzpatrick, 1993).

As a consequence, patients' self-reports should be regarded as the "gold standard" for quality of life assessments. However, in cases where self-reports are difficult to obtain, such as with children and patients with senile dementia, it is better to use the assessment of health personnel or proxies than to ignore quality of life completely.

ISSUES IN THE USE OF QUALITY OF LIFE AS A CONCEPT IN A HEALTH CARE CONTEXT

The ultimate aim of using quality of life as a concept, and of carrying out quality of life research, is that patients should experience a higher level of quality of life. Success in realising this aim will depend on the extent to which health personnel find the concept meaningful and the research relevant and applicable. Although there is increasing interest in and willingness to include quality of life assessments in clinical research and practice, there are still some issues which merit further consideration including: conceptual; ethical; cultural; and methodological.

Above all, there is still a need for conceptual clarification. Although the different definitions of quality of life outlined above reflect some common underlying themes, some have been developed from a theoretical standpoint while others have their basis in clinical practice and research. Within philosophy, where the concepts of happiness and satisfaction are used to describe the good life, definitions tend to be theoretical and less pragmatic than those used in the health care context. Fitzpatrick (1993) states that health care research is highly pragmatic and formal conceptual definition of quality of life has not been a major preoccupation. This has resulted in the conceptualising of the concept in terms of anything from severity of angina to frequency of bowel movements. In clinical research and practice, dimensions are often chosen from an empirical rather than a theoretical standpoint. This can lead to problems in distinguishing between the different concepts used to describe quality of life and between different related concepts such as health and quality of life. That the "health" and "quality of life" concepts can and do overlap is shown in the framework of the Medical Outcomes Study (MOS), which presents as indicators of "health" such domains as physical, role and social functioning, and psychological distress/well-being which in other studies are referred to as "quality of life" indicators (Stewart and Ware, 1992).

HEALTH   **QUALITY OF LIFE**

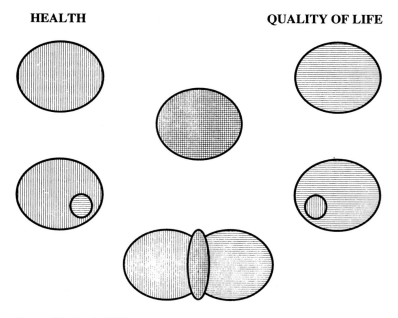

Source: Maeland, 1993

Figure 14.1 Possible relationships between the health and quality of life concept

Figure 14.1 gives an illustration of four possible and alternative relationships between the concepts of health and quality of life (Maeland, 1993). The first pair of circles indicate that health is something quite different from quality of life. The second single circle indicates that quality of life and health are synonymous. The third possibility, represented by the nested circles, is that health is only one aspect of quality of life, or conversely, that quality of life is but one dimension of health; in other words that either quality of life or health is superior to the other. Finally, the interlocking circles represent the fourth alternative, namely that both the quality of life and health concepts represent something unique, but have overlaps. Which alternative to choose depends on the way both the health and quality of life concepts are conceptualised and operationalised. Therefore, when using the concepts and terms, they should be clearly defined and their relationship should be stated. If health is defined as absence of disease, alternative one is the most appropriate. However, if health is defined according to the WHO definition "as a state of complete physical, mental and social well-being, and not merely the absence of disease and infirmity", then alternative two might be the most useful. How the concepts are defined in a specific setting will influence which of the alternatives need to be used.

This conceptual framework might profitably be used in research where the linking of measurement to a body of theory may enable the researcher to use the method analytically, rather than simply employing it descriptively. For instance, this would make it possible to explain the patient's condition in term of the underlying theory, rather than simply describing it.

In much research and practice, the value judgements underpinning the choice of the concepts remain implicit and are not clearly expressed. However, it should be recognised that the selection of dimensions of quality of life may both be influenced by, and have influence on, the aspects of life which are considered to be important and for which improvement is sought. The dimensions do not only serve as a passive marker of quality of life, but may provide the basis for specific health care reforms such as greater emphasis on home care compared to residential nursing. Health care reforms are based on the information available so the choice of quality of life dimensions reflect and in turn come to influence political goals. In the end, the choices of dimensions tends to affect the quality of life of the population.

Therefore, it is very important to consider to what extent the dimensions included in measurement of quality of life intuitively reflect a generally accepted definition of quality of life. For example, even if there is no clear and consistent pattern regarding what patients regard as most important dimensions of quality of life, family relations seems to be a strong contributor to patients' quality of life (Fitzpatrick, 1993).

It must also be recognised that quality of life is a culture-related concept. Definitions of the concept can differ between different countries. Within developing countries, a quality of life definition emphasising personal growth and development might be meaningless when the population is starving. Interventions to improve quality of life in these areas would focus on nutrition, while in the developed countries interventions will focus on the effect of different advanced medical treatments. Different disciplines also define quality of life differently. In the social sciences, quality of life might be referred to as satisfaction with life as a whole, while in the health care context quality of life tends to be referred to as "health-related quality of life" focusing on those aspects of life and well-being specifically related to health such as physical functioning and emotional status. The emphasis on health-related quality of life indicates that health care is not generally concerned with those aspects of quality of life such as satisfaction with the environment, housing or income (Fitzpatrick, 1993), but concentrates on aspects of personal experience that might be related to health care.

Even in the health care context, quality of life may defined in different ways because it is of importance to identify a definition which is related to the actual context and condition of interest. For example, the concept and definition used in the context of diabetes care should cover areas of life that are important in the daily management of the disease and other disease-related aspects. This does not imply that quality of life needs to be or indeed could defined as "everything", but that patient reports on important aspects of their lives should be used as a basis for clinical practice and research.

The aims, objectives and potential for change of health care interventions need to be taken into account. Thus, the choice as to what dimensions be included must be influenced by the nature of the disease and the expected benefits and adverse effects of treatments as well as the more practical considerations such as length of study and available instruments (Fletcher *et al.*, 1992). For example, most patients with arthritis have functional restrictions and pain, and the benefits of different medical and rehabilitation treatments should be measured within these areas, while in hypertensive patients dimensions need to be chosen that reflect sexual function and mood. This demands active involvement in conceptual development and clarification and instrument development.

CONCLUSION

Quality of life is a subjective phenomenon leading to difficulties in defining and measuring the concept. Do these problems outweigh the usefulness of quality of life as a concept and preclude research activities within the area? We would argue that the use of quality of life in clinical practice and research has broadened the focus of patient care and is therefore a valuable concept within the health care context. By focusing on quality of life, patients have the opportunity to influence their own health care. Therefore, it can be concluded that applied quality of life research is valuable because it can improve our general understanding of experienced quality of life as an empirical phenomenon and in this way provide information that might improve the life situation and well-being of the individual concerned.

REFERENCES

Aaronson, N.K. (1989) Quality of life assessment in clinical trials: methodological issues. *Controlled Clinical Trials*, **10**, 195S-208S.

Aggernaes, A.E. (1988) *Livskvalitet*. Copenhagen: FADL.

Andrews, F.M. and Withey, S.B. (1976) *Social indicators of well-being*. New York: Plenum.

Baker, G.A. and Meadows, K. (1992) A review of quality of life assessment: diabetes mellitus. *Practical Diabetes*, **10**, 18-20.

Bergner, M. (1989) Quality of life, health status and clinical research. *Medical Care*, **27**, S148-S156.

Bowling, A. (1991) *Measuring health: a review of quality of life measurement scales*. Buckingham: Open University Press.

Bradburn, N.M. (1969) *The structure of psychological well-being*. Chicago: Aldine.

Cantril, H. (1967) *The pattern of human concerns*. New Brunswick: Rutgers University Press.

Campell, A., Converse, P.E. and Rodgers, W.L. (1976) *The quality of American life: perceptions, evaluations and satisfactions*. New York: Russell Sage.

Cassileth, B.R., Lusk, E.J., Strouse T.B., Miller, D.S., Brown, L.L., Cross, P.A. and Tengalia, A.N. (1984) Psychosocial status in chronic illness: a comparative analysis of six diagnostic groups. *New England Journal of Medicine*, **311**, 506-511.

Cox, D.R., Fitzpatrick, R., Fletcher, A.E., Gore, S.M., Spiegelhalter, D.J. and Jones, D.R. (1992) Quality of life assessment: can we keep it simple? *Journal of the Royal Statistical Society*, **155**, 353-393.

de Haes, J.C.J.M. and van Knippenberg, F.C.E. (1985) The quality of life of cancer patients: a review of literature. *Social Science and Medicine*, **20**, 809-817.

Epstein, A.M., Hall, J.A., Tognetti, J., Sou, L.H. and Conant, L. (1989) Using proxies to evaluate quality of life: can they provide valid information about patients' health status and satisfaction with medical care? *Medical Care*, **27**, S91-S98.

Fitzpatrick, R. (1993) *Contrasting approaches to quality of life in health*. Manuscript.

Fitzpatrick, R., Fletcher, A., Gore, S., Jones, D., Spiegelhalter, D. and Cox, D. (1992) Quality of life measures in health care. I: Applications and issues in assessment. *British Medical Journal*, **305**, 1074-1077.

Fletcher, A., Gore, S., Jones, D., Fitzpatrick, R., Spiegelhalter, D. and Cox, D. (1992) Quality of life measures in health care. II: Design, analysis, and interpretation. *British Medical Journal*, **305**, 1145-1148.

Fowlie, M. and Berkely, J. (1987) Quality of life: a review of the literature. *Family Practitioner*, **4**, 226-234.

Goodinson, S.M. and Singleton J. (1989) Quality of life: a critical review of current concepts, measures and their clinical implications. *International Journal of Nursing Studies*, **4**, 327-341.

Hornquist, J.O. (1982) The concept of quality of life. *Scandinavian Journal of Social Medicine*, **10**, 57-61.

Hornquist, J.O. (1989) Quality of life: concept and assessment. *Scandinavian Journal of Social Medicine*, **18**, 69-79.

Karnofsky, D.A. and Burchenal, J.H. (1949) The clinical evaluation of chemotherapeutic agents in cancer. In: MacLeod, C.M. (Ed.), *Evaluation of chemotherapeutic agents*, New York: Columbia University Press.

Lindstrom, B. (1992) Quality of life: a model for evaluating health for all. Conceptual considerations and policy implications. *Sozial-und Praventivmedizin*, **37**, 301-306.

Maeland, J.G. (1993) *Helse og livskvalitet - to sider av samme sak?* Medicinsk Arbok. Copenhagen: Munksgaard.

Nordenfelt, L. (1991) *Livskvalitet och halsa: teori and kritik.* Falköbing: Almqvist and Wiksell.

Naess, S. (1989) The concept of quality of life. In: Bjork, S. and Vang, J. (Eds.), *Assessing quality of life*. Linkobing: Samhall Klintland.

Padilla, G.V., Grant, M.M. and Ferell, B. (1992) Nursing research into quality of life. *Quality of Life Research*, **1**, 341-348.

Pearlman, R.A. and Uhlmann, R.F. (1988) Quality of life in chronic diseases: perceptions of elderly patients. *Journal of Gerontology*, **43**, M25-M30.

Spilker, B. (1990) Introduction. In: Spilker, B. (Ed.), *Quality of life assessments in clinical trials*. New York: Raven Press.

Slevin, M.L., Plant, H., Lynch, D., Drinkwater, J. and Gregory, W.M. (1988) Who should measure quality of life, the doctor or the patient? *British Journal of Cancer*, **57**, 109-112.

Spitzer, W.O., Dobson, A.J., Hall, J., Chesterman, E., Levi, J., Shepherd, R., Battista, R.N. and Catchlove, B.R. (1981) Measuring the quality of life of cancer patients: a concise QL-index for use by physicians. *Journal of Chronic Diseases*, **34**, 585-597.

Sprangers, M. and Aaronson, N. (1992) The role of health care providers and significant others in evaluating the quality of life of patients with chronic disease: a review. *Journal of Clinical Epidemiology*, **45**, 743-760.

Stewart, A.L. and Ware, J.E. (1992) *Measuring functioning and well-being: the Medical Outcomes Study approach*. Durham, NC: Duke University Press.

Sullivan, M. (1992) Quality of life assessment in medicine: concepts, definitions, purposes and basic tools. *Nordic Journal of Psychiatry*, **46**, 79-83.

Tatarkiewicz, W. (1976) *Analysis of happiness.* Warsaw: PWN-Polish Scientific Publishers.

Uhlmann, R. and Pearlman, R. (1991) Perceived quality of life and preferences for life sustaining treatment in older adults. *Archives of Internal Medicine*, **151**, 495-497.

Yates, J.W., Chalmer, B. and McKegney, F.B. (1980) Evaluation of patients with advanced cancer using the Karnofsky performance status. *Cancer*, **45**, 2220-2224.

Chapter 15 _____

CROSS-CULTURAL ISSUES IN OUTCOME MEASUREMENT

FRANSJE TOUW-OTTEN AND KEITH MEADOWS

INTRODUCTION

In many European countries there is currently a vastly expanding interest in health outcome assessment, particularly in the areas of chronic diseases; not only in terms of biological parameters but also in quality of life and health status. Against a background of increasing international collaboration there is also need for cross-cultural comparison on these parameters to enable the identification of the differences and similarities resulting from the various health care systems, differing attitudes of physicians and patient health care behaviour. Not only is health status assessment relevant for physicians in the evaluation of intervention procedures but also for health policy makers with regard to evaluating the effectiveness of health care programmes, health economics, epidemiological studies and clinical trials. There already exists equivalent measures to meet these objectives within the domain of biological parameters. However, within the domain of quality of life and health status, there still remains the need for reliable and valid cultural equivalent measures. An important issue here is the expression and conceptualising of health, both between cultures and nations, and the diversity which exists must be taken into account. For this to be achieved measures of quality of life and health status which have been developed within a specific culture are required to undergo adaptation for use in other cultures. In order that instruments are appropriate for cross-cultural use in terms of their content and other methodological criteria a number of specific criteria must be fulfilled .

Within the European Research Group on Health Outcomes (ERHGO) we have been developing a number of specific criteria for the adaptation of instruments for the evaluation of health status and quality of life in different European countries and which can provide both a conceptual and objective framework for other researchers and health care professionals in evaluating and selecting appropriate cultural equivalent instruments. The aim of this chapter is to provide a description of this framework, as well as to illustrate its practical application in the evaluation of specific health status instruments. In doing so we have taken as examples two commonly used multidimensional instruments which have undergone cross-cultural adaptation. These comprise the Sickness Impact Profile (SIP) (Bergner *et al.*, 1981), originally developed in the United States of America, and the Nottingham Health Profile (NHP) developed in the United Kingdom (Hunt *et al.*, 1985).

The following sections will focus first on the description of the specific criteria for the adaptation of health outcome measures for cross-cultural use, and second, as an illustrative example of the selection and application of one of these criteria in the evaluation of the selected measures. The chapter will conclude with an outline of the minimum criteria which we consider is required for the evaluation of instruments used for cross-cultural comparisons.

CRITERIA FOR THE ADAPTATION OF HEALTH OUTCOME MEASURES FOR CROSS-CULTURAL USE

In order to cross-validate health status measures for cross-cultural use a number of criteria are required (Flaherty *et al.*, 1988 and Bullinger *et al.*, 1993). These are: content equivalence; semantic equivalence; technical equivalence; criterion equivalence; and conceptual equivalence.

Content Equivalence
For cross-cultural research each item in the instrument must be examined to establish whether the concept it measures is relevant to the cultural setting in which it is to be used. It would be, for example, inappropriate to include items which are considered taboo in certain cultures, for instance certain aspects of sexual behaviour.

Semantic Equivalence
In the translation of each item or statement, its meaning must remain the same as the original version. Therefore in the translation process emphasis must be placed on retaining the essence of what is being asked or stated rather than obtaining a direct (literal) translation of the words.

Technical Equivalence
Technical equivalence of an instrument which has been cross-culturally adapted can be assessed in a number of different ways. One approach is to establish the concurrent validity of the measure, which involves obtaining data using a

multi-method approach (e.g. interview and self-report) or from different instruments (including the translated instrument) which measure the same phenomena. If there is agreement between the findings obtained from the translated instrument and the other measures of the same phenomena then concurrent validity of the translated measure is supported.

It is important to note that results obtained in the assessment of technical equivalence can also be influenced by the use of different measuring conditions. For example, different methods of assessment (e.g. self-report, interview, postal) as well as differing time intervals in their administration can influence the results. Therefore, comparable measuring conditions need to be taken into account in the measurement of concurrent validity.

Criterion Equivalence
Criterion validity of an instrument refers to its relationship to previously established and independent criteria which does not necessarily mean another instrument. For example criterion validity would be established if our translated instrument behaved in a predicted way with respect to the use of health services in the following year. However, criterion validity of our instrument would also be supported if we found satisfactory levels of agreement between our translated instrument and other measures of the same phenomenon (concurrent validity).

Conceptual Equivalence
Evidence relating to the conceptual equivalence of an instrument is when the instrument is found to be measuring the same construct/concept (e.g. physical, emotional functioning) in the different cultures. Methods of examining conceptual equivalence include assessing the known relationship between constructs measured by the instrument and responses to other variables in each of the study populations. For instance, if symptomatology is associated with the construct physical dysfunction in the original culture, then findings of significant predicted relationships between these variables and the construct in other cultures would be evidence of conceptual equivalence for the translated instrument. Another indicator of construct validity is discriminating between patient groups differing in severity of illness (known-group validity).

METHODS IN THE TRANSLATION OF CROSS-CULTURAL INSTRUMENTS

To obtain an appropriate cross-cultural outcome measure several steps have to be taken before satisfactory equivalence with the original language version is established. The first is the translation process and field-testing of the translated version. Secondly, when a final translated version is available this should be authorised by the authors of the original version in terms of its conceptual basis. Thirdly, the translated instrument should then be evaluated for its equivalence in terms of reliability and validity with the original version following the procedures outlined above.

Translation Process and Field-Testing

In order to establish the semantic equivalence of a translated instrument the most common procedure is forward and back translation. The first step in the procedure is to obtain an initial forward translated version which involves translating the original version into the chosen language. It is important to stress the importance of obtaining a good forward translation as any subsequent back translation is dependent on this. This process is generally carried out by the translators independently of one another. Any differences identified following this should be addressed and when necessary consultation with the original developer should be carried out, resulting in a first draft. This procedure should then be followed by back translation by one or more bilinguists whose native language is that of the original version. Both forward and back translation should be carried out until a suitable translated version is obtained for field-testing. It is worth noting that during this process many of the problems encountered are generally concerned with statements indicative of an emotional or psychosomatic nature (Hunt *et al.*, 1987).

Following forward and back translation of the instrument, the next step in the process is to get it completed by the target group of respondents in the presence of interviewers in order to identify problems in the interpretation of the content experienced by the respondent.

A number of multidimensional outcome measures, for instance the Sickness Impact Profile, comprise items which have been weighted according to their perceived importance (e.g. within the category social interaction comprising 20 items, each item is rated on an equal interval scale relating to the severity of dysfunction) (Bergner *et al.*, 1981). However, because the perceived importance of a particular dysfunction (e.g dysfunction in daily activities) may vary from one culture to another it is important that the evaluation of the weighting of such items in the different cultures is carried out. This procedure should involve similar groups of people (on which the original weightings were derived), for instance health professionals, patients and lay people (Patrick *et al.*, 1985 and Jacobs *et al.*, 1990).

Throughout the process of translation and field-testing the authors of the original version should be informed of the findings in order to obtain a final and authorised translated version of the instrument. Having achieved this, the final translated version needs to be evaluated for technical, criterion and conceptual equivalence in several populations comparable with the study populations on which the original instrument was developed and validated and/or the target population.

MEASURES CURRENTLY DEVELOPED FOR CROSS-CULTURAL USE

In this section of the chapter we will illustrate the application of the conceptual framework developed by ERGHO by reference to two existing health status instruments. These measures, the SIP and the NHP, have been developed to measure the psychosocial and functional domains of health status and have been translated into a number of different languages. Table 15.1 provides an overview of the different languages in which these instruments are available. To illustrate which aspects of our recommended criteria have been met, we reviewed the Dutch versions of the SIP and NHP as examples. For a more detailed critical review of the international assessments of these and other instruments, see Anderson *et al.*, 1993.

Table 15.1   Availability of translated versions of the SIP and NHP

Language	SIP	NHP
Danish	+	+
Dutch/Flemish	+	+
English	+[a]	origin
Finnish	?	+
French	+	+
German	+	+
Italian	+	+
Norwegian	+	+
Portuguese	-	?
Spanish	+	+
Swedish	+	+

+ = present;   - = not present;   ? = unknown

[a] The English version is known as the Functional Limitations Profile (FLP); the original version is from the USA.

In terms of the Dutch versions of the SIP and NHP both have been extensively validated (Jacobs *et al.*, 1990; Jacobs *et al.*, 1993 and Erdman *et al.*, 1993) which includes semantic and content equivalence (Table 15.2). Problems with the translations were the items indicative of emotional or psychosocial distress in the SIP and the use of double negatives in the NHP.

In the case of the NHP conceptual equivalence was established by comparing the results of general practice patients categorised as either healthy or ill. (Table 15.3) Healthy patients were defined on the basis of non-consultation with the general practitioner in the previous six months and ill patients on having consulted the general practitioner within the past month. Differences in the scores between these two groups of patients supported the construct validity of the instrument (Erdman *et al.*, 1993).

Table 15.2 Results of content and semantic equivalence of the Dutch versions of the SIP (Jacobs et al., 1990) and NHP (Erdman et al., 1993)

	SIP	NHP
Translation procedure	Forward independently by two health care staff members Backward by linguist experienced in native language	Six health care staff members bilingual
Feasibility testing	Yes	Yes
Field-testing	Yes	Yes
Problems in translation	Items indicative of emotional or psychosocial distress	Use of double negatives
Comparability of item weights	Same procedure as in original version .80 < r < .97	Not relevant
Cooperation with authors of original version	Yes	Yes
Authorised by original authors	Yes	Yes

For the SIP known-group validity was assessed by comparing scores in three samples differing in illness type and severity (Table 15.3). The three samples were respectively: non-specific abdominal complaints; rheumatoid arthritis; and spinal cord lesions. The health status of the three samples was reflected in the increasing SIP scores in relation to morbidity (de Witte *et al.*, 1987).

For the SIP, comparisons were made between a Dutch general population with an equivalent American population (Jacobs *et al.*, 1990). The score profiles in both populations were very similar. Correlations of SIP categories and NHP sub-scales with other scales existed as hypothesised (Essink-Bot *et al.*, 1992). Furthermore the psychosocial dimension of the SIP discriminated psychosocial from physical illnesses in accordance with the original instrument (Jacobs *et al.*, 1993).

Table 15.3   Validity of the Dutch versions of the SIP and NHP

	SIP	NHP
Known-group validity	Predicted differences to severity of illness in patients with abdominal complaints, rheumatoid arthritis and spinal cord lesions (de Witte *et al.*, 1987)	Predicted differences in scores between healthy and ill and between young and older persons (Erdman *et al.*, 1993)
Construct validity	SIP scores resembled strongly between Dutch open population and comparable American population (Jacobs *et al.*, 1990) Strong correlations with patients' medical characteristics and SIP scores in the same way as in original version (Jacobs *et al.*, 1993)	
Convergent/discriminant validity	Correlations SIP categories with STAI, SDS, ADL and Karnofsky as hypothesised, except Eating with ADL (Essink-Bot *et al.*, 1992)	Correlations with NHP subscales and STAI, SDS, ADL and Karnofsky as hypothesised (Essink-Bot *et al.*, 1992)
Technical equivalence	Lower SIP scores (10.2) by self-administered compared to interviewer administration (16.3) (Hulsebos *et al.*, 1991)	Not applicable

STAI: State-Trait Anxiety Inventory
SDS: Zung Self-Rating Depression Scale
ADL: Activities of Daily Living

Table 15.4   Reliability of the Dutch versions of the SIP and NHP

	SIP	*NHP*
Test-retest reliability	.86 to .91 total SIP score and dimensions tested in several different patient categories	.69 to .92 for the 6 subscales .42 to .85 for part II; home life; .13 tested in patients awaiting for coronary artery graft surgery (Erdman *et al.*, 1993).
Internal consistency of sub-scales	.58 to .84 within 10 categories; sleep and rest (.39) and eating (.23) total SIP score .9 tested in patients with end-stage renal disease (12) .86 physical subdimension .80 psychosocial subdimension .86 total SIP score tested in older primary care patients with COPD (Jacobs *et al.*, 1993)	.70 to .85 within the 6 sub-scales ((Essink-Bot *et al.*, 1992)
Intercorrelations between sub-scales	Not applicable	Relatively independent constructs except the associations between energy and emotional reactions, social isolation Similarly between the Dutch study group and the original English study group
Reproducibility	High: total SIP score and dimensions; low for individual item scores. Same results as in original version	

The translated versions also need equivalence with the original version with regard to reliability. Results of reliability studies of the Dutch versions of the SIP and NHP showed comparable results as found in the original versions (Table 15.4).

CONCLUSIONS

In this chapter we have discussed and applied a number of recommended criteria for the cross-cultural adaptation of health status measures, based on existing methodologies (Flaherty *et al.*, 1988 and Bullinger *et al.*, 1993). The criteria which have been outlined clearly represent the ideal in achieving adaptation and as a result will not always be met. Adaptation of health status measures will not result from a single methodological procedure or piece of supportive evidence, but requires a continuing process lasting possibly for a number of years before all of the recommended criteria are met. Therefore, because of pragmatic reasons, often only one or two of the criteria can be met prior to the use of the instrument. As a result the ERGHO group has suggested that, both in the adaptation and selection of instruments for cross-cultural use, a minimum or intermediate set of criteria must be met before any confidence can be placed either in the choice of an instrument developed for cross-cultural use or findings obtained. Therefore the minimum criteria considered acceptable by ERGHO is content equivalence, together with semantic and conceptual equivalence. For an instrument to meet the intermediate criteria, this should also additionally include criterion equivalence.

In the measurement of outcome an instrument needs the property of responsiveness to clinically significant change in individuals over time and is a major consideration in any study concerned with evaluating the impact of treatment. In many cases though, responsiveness is not always evaluated as it may not be part of the conceptual base in the development of the original instrument. However, since such instruments are also used in evaluative research responsiveness to change is an important property. There are indeed a number of instruments where the property has been evaluated both in the original version as well as in translated versions (Anderson *et al.*, 1993).

An aid to researchers in the use of culturally developed instruments would be some form of national and international data bank. From this bank, information could be obtained relating to the nature and extent of the studies as well as results relating to specific patient groups etc. Such a coordinating centre could be in the position to disseminate findings relating to specific patient groups as well as the applied methodological framework.

In this chapter we have focused on the NHP and SIP as examples in illustrating the methodological framework, although a number of generic and disease- or condition-specific instruments have been evaluated for cross-cultural use (Anderson *et al.*, 1993). In the near future more results of cross-cultural use of instruments will become available. We hope that the methodological framework presented contributes to an appropriate use of health outcome measures in cross-cultural settings.

REFERENCES

Anderson, R.T., Aaronson, N.K. and Wilkin, D. (1993) Critical review of the international assessments of health-related quality of life. *Quality of Life Research*, 2, 369-395.

Bergner, M., Bobbitt, R.A., Carter, W.B. and Gilson, B.S. (1981) The Sickness Impact Profile: development and final revision of a health status measure. *Medical Care*, 19, 787-805.

Bullinger, M., Anderson, R., Cella, D. and Aaronson, N. (1993) Developing and evaluating cross-cultural instruments from minimum requirements to optimal models. *Quality of Life Research*, 2, 451-459.

de Witte, L., Jacobs, H.M., van der Horst, F., Luttik, A., Joosten, J. and Philipsen, H. (1987) De waarde van de Sickness Impact Profile als maat voor het functioneren voor patienten. *Gezondheid en Samenlving*, 8(2), 120-127.

Erdman, R.M., Passchier, J., Kooijman, M. and Stronks, D. (1993) The Dutch version of the Nottingham Health Profile: investigations of psychometric aspects. *Psychological Reports*, 72, 1027-1035.

Essink-Bot, M., van Agt, H.M.E. and Bonsel, C.J. (1992) NHP of SIP: een vergelijkend onderzoek onder chronisch zieken. *T soc Gezondheidsz*, 70: 152-159.

Flaherty, J.A., Gaviria, F.M., Pathak, D. *et al.* (1988) Developing instruments for cross-cultural psychiatric research. *J Nerv Ment Dis*, 176, 257-263.

Hulsebos, R.G., Beltman, F.W., Reis Miranda D dos. and Spangenberg, J.F.A. (1991) Measuring quality of life with the Sickness Impact Profile: a pilot study. *Intensive Care Medicine*, 17, 285-288.

Hunt, S.M., McEwen, J. and McKenna, S.P. (1985) Measuring health status: a new tool for clinicians and epidemiologists. *Journal of the Royal College of General Practitioners*, 185-188.

Hunt, S.M. and Wiklund, I. (1987) Cross-cultural variation in the weighting of health statements: a comparison of English and Swedish valuations. *Health Policy*, 8, 227-235.

Jacobs, H.M., Luttik, A., Touw-Otten, F.W.M.M. and de Melker, R.A. (1990) The Sickness Impact Profile: results of a validation study of the Dutch version. *Nederlands Tijdschrift voor Geneeskunde*, 134, 1950-1954.

Jacobs, H.M. (1993) *Health status measurement in family medicine research: the Sickness Impact Profile and its application in a follow-up study in patients with non-specific abdominal complaints*. Utrecht: University of Utrecht Press. (OMI-offset)

Patrick, D.L., Sittampalam, Y., Somerville, S.M., Carter, W.B. and Bergner, M. (1985) A cross-cultural comparison of health status values. *American Journal of Public Health*, 75, 1402-1407.

INDEX

abdominal disorders   157, 204-205

acceptability   20, 25, 28, 51, 78, 82, 159, 163, 181

accuracy   27, 34, 48-49, 59- 60, 159

activities of daily living   39, 48, 50, 52, 54-55, 78, 84, 88, 111, 140-146, 149, 151-152, 154, 156, 161, 168- 170, 173, 177, 178, 181, 183, 191-192, 202
see also lifestyle

acute care   14, 93, 106-107

acute illness   110-111, 139, 141, 144, 167, 184

administration - diary techniques   *see* diaries

administration - interviewer   *see* interviewer-administered measures

administration - observer   *see* observer-administered measures

administration - self-report   *see* self-report measures

adults   23-24, 51-52, 119, 131, 133-134, 139, 141, 174, 190

ambulatory care   9-21, 46, 126, 130, 139, 143, 145, 150, 164
see also primary care; out-patient care

AMP Dependency Scale   173

antenatal care   95, 177-185

anxiety   15, 52, 60- 62, 96, 111, 142, 149, 156, 179, 191

arthritis   12, 160, 169-170, 187, 196, 204-205

asthma   11-12, 15-18, 20, 23-43, 45-62, 115-116, 128, 139-148, 161

Asthma Quality of Life Questionnaire   145

attributability   10-11, 13, 25, 30, 91, 94, 97-100, 109-110, 126, 128-129, 137, 141-142, 147

audit   9, 14, 19, 43, 92-95, 100, 116, 118-119, 129, 187

autonomy   169, 171, 173, 180, 189, 191
see also dependency

back pain   15, 78-79, 82-88

Barthel Index   70, 151-152, 154, 156, 159, 161, 163, 170
see also Barthel Rating Scale

Barthel Rating Scale   65, 67-68, 70-74
see also Barthel Index

bias   27, 41, 71, 150, 157, 162

biological measures   184, 199

biomedical measures   11, 15, 23, 42, 66, 149-150, 171-172, 177-178, 188

Bulpitt Symptom Questionnaire   172

cancer   67, 114, 133-136, 154, 157, 168, 187

cardiovascular disorders   13, 15, 80-82, 96, 130-132, 136, 156, 169, 172, 178, 187, 193, 196, 206

case mix   108, 121, 151

ceiling effect   161
see also floor effect

childbirth   98, 110, 180

respiratory disorders   11-12, 15-18, 20, 23-43, 45-62, 78, 97, 115-116, 128, 139-148, 161, 169, 206

responsiveness to change   11-12, 16, 23, 36, 40-42, 72, 78, 82, 86-88, 97, 110, 115, 145, 150, 153, 159-160, 207

rheumatoid arthritis   *see* arthritis

role function   77, 84-85, 178-179, 184-185, 191, 194

St George's Respiratory Questionnaire   144

satisfaction   *see* life satisfaction; patient satisfaction

screening   150-153, 187

secondary care   108

see also acute care; hospital care

self-management   45-47, 61- 62, 111, 142, 144-145

see also patient management

self-report measures   19, 29, 47-49, 59-61, 71, 79, 115, 144, 149, 153, 158-159, 162, 180, 193, 201, 205

semantic equivelence   *see* equivalence - semantic

sensitivity   11, 16, 60-61, 66, 72, 97, 100, 144, 153, 156

severity   24, 26-28, 48, 54-61, 82, 84, 86, 127, 129, 139-141, 143-145, 147, 153, 156-157, 161, 171-172, 193, 201, 204-205

SF-36   17-18, 39-40, 42, 65, 70-74, 84-85, 88, 180-181, 183

Sickness Impact Profile   144, 151, 154, 156-161, 163, 200, 202-207

side-effects   15, 68, 118, 141, 143, 168-169, 171-172, 191

single-item scales   156-157, 159

social health status   19, 26, 71, 85, 111, 127, 130, 133, 149, 151-152, 156, 169, 178-179, 184, 188, 190-195, 202

Spitzer Index   192

Standardised Response Mean   86-87

State-Trait Anxiety Inventory   205

structure of care   12, 92-94, 110

survival   66, 69, 156, 188

see also life expectancy

symptom measures 16-18, 23-43

symptoms   17, 23-43, 47-49, 54-60, 66, 68, 77, 82, 84, 87, 96-98, 111, 128, 139-147, 149, 167, 171-172, 179, 188-189, 191-192, 201

technical equivalence   *see* equivalence - technical

terminal illness   15, 69, 96, 111, 154, 169, 206

test-retest reliability   *see* reliability - test-retest

Townsend Disability Scale   170

translation of instruments   180, 200-202, 204, 207

see also cross-cultural measures

unidimensional measures   31, 49

utility - clinical   19, 27, 37-38, 43, 154, 163-164, 172, 180

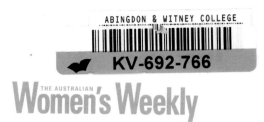

THE

EASY AUSTRALIAN DIET

By Pamela Clark

with nutritionist Catherine Saxelby

Test Kitchen

Food director Pamela Clark
Assistant food editor Amira Georgy

ACP Books

Published by ACP Publishing Pty Limited,
54 Park Street, Sydney; G.P.O. Box 4088,
Sydney NSW 2001.
Ph: (02) 9282 8618 Fax: (02) 9267 9438
acpbooks@acp.com.au
www.acpbooks.com.au
Printed by
Editorial director Susan Tomnay
Creative·director Hieu Chi Nguyen
Senior editor Lynda Wilton
Designer Mary Keep
Studio manager Caryl Wiggins
Editorial/sales coordinator Caroline Lowry
Editorial assistant Karen Lai
Publishing manager (sales) Brian Cearnes
Publishing manager (rights & new projects)
  Jane Hazell
Marketing manager Sarah Cave
Pre-press Harry Palmer
Production manager Carol Currie
Business manager Seymour Cohen
Business analyst Martin Howes
Chief executive officer John Alexander
Group publisher Pat Ingram
Publisher Sue Wannan
Editor-in-chief Deborah Thomas

UK Division
Director Laura Bamford
Managing Director Jean Gardiner
Sales Director Lynda Ayres
Office Manager Anna Pisani
Office Assistant Charlotte Brown

Production services by Book Production Consultants plc, UK
Printed and bound by Burlington Press, UK

To order books, phone 01604 497 531

Send recipe enquiries to: recipeenquiries@acp.com.au

UNITED KINGDOM: Distributed by Australian Consolidated Press (UK), Moulton Park Business Centre, Red House Rd, Moulton Park, Northampton, NN3 6AQ.
Ph: (01604) 497531 Fax: (01604) 497533
acpukltd@aol.com

AUSTRALIA: Distributed by Network Services,
GPO Box 4088, Sydney, NSW 2001.
Ph: (02) 9282 8777 Fax: (02) 9264 3278.

Clark, Pamela.
The magazine editors' diet: a revolutionary low-carb, low-fat diet from The Australian Women's Weekly test kitchen

Includes index.
ISBN 1-90377703-8
1. Clark, Pamela. 2. Women food writers – Australia – Biography. 3. Women cooks – Australia – Biography. 4. Low-carbohydrate diet. I. Saxelby, Catherine. II. Australian Women's Weekly.
III. Title.

641.092
© ACP Publishing Pty Limited 2005

CONTENTS

INTRODUCTION

WHO DOESN'T WANT TO LOOK GOOD, have more energy, and feel healthy?
I certainly do. That's why, when I heard about this great new way of eating
and losing weight, I was eager to give it a try. I couldn't believe how easy
and delicious it is – and it really works.

This is *The Easy Australian Diet*. After years of overseeing all the
fabulous food that goes into our magazines and cookbooks, Pamela decided
to lose weight. Drawing on her vast knowledge, she devised a clever
low-carbohydrate, low-fat eating plan and, over the a six month period,
despite constant tastings, she managed to lose an amazing 20 kilos (3 stone).

Due to popular demand, we published our secret. To make sure that
it's nutritionally sound, we commissioned respected nutritionist Catherine
Saxelby to review the diet so that you are guaranteed an eating plan that's a
surefire winner. You will see her comments throughout the book.

The Easy Australian Diet is a way of eating that is deliciously tasty,
astonishingly simple, and easily adapted to suit family needs (just add extra
carbohydrates such as pasta and rice for children and those not looking to
lose weight).

Pamela's story of how she came to develop *The Easy Australian Diet*
is as interesting as the diet itself. Read that before you turn to the menu
planners on pages 41–45. As well as more than 50 great recipes, there are
quick and easy meal ideas, a pantry list, and a carb, fat and kilojoule/calorie
counter.

Good luck. Here's to a healthier (and slimmer) new you!

Deborah Thomas
Editor-in-Chief, The Australian Women's Weekly

PAMELA'S STORY

it works for me – it can work for you too!

I've lost a total of 20 kilos in 31 weeks, have gone from a size 18 to a size 12 and I feel absolutely fantastic. I've got more energy, I'm sleeping better than ever, and I am healthier and happier all round. Like a lot of you, I've tried to lose weight so often that I've made yo-yo dieting an art form, but this is without doubt the easiest diet I've ever followed. Even better, I've never been bored, felt deprived or lost heart while I've been on it.

What's the secret? It's unbelievably simple. All I've done is cut out refined carbohydrates such as bread, rice, pasta and noodles from my diet – basically anything that contains processed grains.

I have to stress that this is not one of those fad no-carb diets you've probably heard about; I've only restricted certain 'bad' carbohydrates. I'm getting my 'good' carbs from the mountains of fresh fruit and vegies I eat every day. My diet is also low in fat so that helps too. It follows that if you're not eating bread, then you're not eating a spread. If you drop pasta, rice and noodles, you're not eating rich creamy sauces. And, although I love starchy vegies such as potatoes or sweet potato mashed with oodles of milk, cream and butter, I've steered clear of that combination too for now!

I've been a food editor most of my career, and I love food – it's my work and my life; everything revolves around it. In my job, I'm constantly being tempted by yummy things!

The downside is that I have a constant battle with my weight.

A lot of people in the food business choose to exercise vigorously to make up for the amount of food they eat; but that's just not me. Repetitive exercise bores me silly. I'd rather take long walks with my dog and get my exercise that way. I believe this is one of the main reasons this diet works so well: it suits my lifestyle, my career, and my personal likes and dislikes perfectly! After all, if you're trying to follow a diet or exercise regime that doesn't suit you, it's doomed to fail before you begin. And haven't we all been there?

don't wait till tomorrow

If losing weight is truly what you want, you simply have to stop procrastinating, stop making excuses, stop waiting for the mythical 'right' time to come. The right time is now. I promise you, if I can do it, given my line of work and history of failed diets, then you can too. I also promise that you'll not only look better and be healthier, but your self-esteem and confidence will skyrocket. Mine has.

to use this book

I have suggested some recipes to interest your appetite, along with all of the relevant nutritional information. There is also a glossary at the back to explain some of the ingredients. Happy cooking!

CHAPTER ONE:
MY DIETING HISTORY

Apart from following most of the diets ever published, I've done juice and water fasts too, but always under controlled conditions. I've toyed with vegetarianism; if it's done correctly, it's a great way to eat, but it's an impossible regime for me to follow, given my career choice.

Every single diet or eating regime I have ever followed has failed for me when I have gone off the diet. I always, always, always put the weight back on – usually with a few more kilos as a bonus.

I've read everything I could lay my hands on about diets, always looking for the easy way out, just like I was always on the lookout for an outfit that was going to make me look younger, thinner and taller. The fact is, I ate too much and exercised too little. And because I chose to go into an industry where I was surrounded by food every day, temptation was, and still is, never far away. The odds of me ever being slim were seriously stacked against me.

These days, I know that I should be aspiring not to a skinny body, but to a healthy, albeit short and stocky, body.

the reasons for my diet

There were three reasons why I decided it was time for me to lose some weight.

Firstly, I couldn't bear the indigestion I was starting to experience. I have a low tolerance for discomfort and pain. Secondly, I was staying with friends in the country last year, and one of them said he wanted to lose six kilos before

Catherine says:

dieting – the long road ahead

Like most overweight people, Pamela has tried many diets in the past. She has realised that there is no short cut or 'magic bullet' to miraculously melt fat away. She calls it the "easy way out" and it doesn't exist. She has now discovered a healthy way of eating that she can stick to for more than a few days and that suits her rather unusual eating lifestyle.

She admits, though, that temptation is still a problem. It's hard to reverse the habits of a lifetime and she's facing it every day. Psychologists say that it takes three weeks to break a habit and it usually takes much longer to achieve permanent weight loss.

Christmas, and that made me want to lose weight too. But lastly, an important birthday was coming up and a big celebration was being organised. What on earth was I going to wear? More to the point, what did I have that would still fit?

The answer to the last question was that nothing much in the wardrobe fitted me any more, and I really didn't have the time or the inclination to buy anything new. I had three weeks in which to do something before the party. I thought that even if I lost only a few kilos, then my gorgeous green lacy top would fit and, teamed with a pair of trusty black trousers, I'd look just fine.

why a low-carb diet?

The main reason I chose low carb is that I've tried so many other diets and failed. Being curious about all food-related issues, I was interested to see how the low-carb approach would work for me.

Some people following the low-carb craze have eliminated all carbs, including fruit and vegies. I have a real problem with the notion of eating a high-fat, high-protein diet without fruit and vegetables. It is contrary to everything I know about how food makes you feel. So, I decided I'd simply drop the grain-based food that I ate every day, and not worry about the rest of the food I ate. I lost over four kilos without any effort in those first three weeks, so, I thought, why not continue? And what a breeze it's been. The funny thing about this diet is that I don't have cravings for sweet or fatty foods at all. It's a wonderful bonus I didn't expect.

Normally, when I've done something like this before, I return to my errant ways with food. The dangerous thing for me is to have no goal, so I decided that I would continue to eat this way until Christmas, the target being to lose the six kilos my friend was also going to lose. I'd then release myself from the diet over the Christmas period, and think about things in the new year.

However, by Christmas Day I'd been on my diet for 14 weeks and had lost 11 kilos. I was fairly pleased with myself and the way I felt, so I thought, "I can do Christmas dinner without grains", and I did, no hardship at all.

When I returned to the office after the Christmas break, people really began to notice and comment on my weight loss. I found myself committed to the diet because of this book, but that was okay, I was still well and happy with the way things were.

By the end of February, the weight loss had slowed down, though certainly not stopped. The good news was that I had already dropped two sizes in clothes. I was sick and tired of my wardrobe anyway; I'd been hanging on to things for years in the hope that one day I would fit into them again. I decided to set my sights to lose 20 kilos in total over 31 weeks.

In 14 weeks I had lost 11 kilos

Catherine says:

how much should you aim to lose?

Fad diets promise rapid weight loss: "Drop a dress size over the weekend" or "One week to a new you". Usually your weight comes off quickly (while you're motivated and on track), but you can't sustain it. Once you finish the diet, the kilos come straight back on. Mostly what you've lost is fluid (plus a little fat), especially on the high-protein no-carb diets.

This is what happens. You start on a really strict diet or a juice-only fast, only to find that you feel tired and have no energy. Surprisingly, you don't shed that much weight, even though you're not eating much at all. This is because your body thinks it has hit a famine and goes into crisis mode. It shuts down all unnecessary energy expenditure to try to conserve kilojoules for the 'famine' (diet), which is what our bodies have done for thousands of years during the evolution of the human race. Our ancestors were hunter-gatherers and there were many times when food was scarce. Those people who could conserve their fat stores during lean times were best able to survive. Your body is hanging on to every spare gram of fat to enable you to survive.

If your weight loss is more gradual, it won't trigger your body's famine-starvation mode. Nutritionists recommend that you aim to lose half to one kilo a week. This is what Pamela achieved. Over the first 14 weeks, she lost 11 kilos, and the weight has stayed off.

The obesity epidemic

Pamela is not alone in her weight problem, although her circumstances are certainly different from those of most of us.
Britain is in the grip of an epidemic of obesity. Remember smallpox and bubonic plague? They spread throughout the world and killed hundreds of thousands of people before they disappeared. Researchers have called our expanding girth an epidemic because it too has appeared – as if from nowhere – and now plagues almost every Westernised country.

We like to think of themselves as a nation of fit and active people. But while we may watch a lot of sport on television, we certainly don't play enough of it ourselves.

Prevention is the best advice

Public health programs are now trying to prevent weight gain, rather than direct funds to treating obesity. It is easier and less expensive to stop people putting on weight in the first place than to try to get them to lose weight once it is fully established.

It is so difficult to get people to keep off the weight they've lost in the long term (over 12 months). Study after study shows that people initially lose weight driven by the motivation and euphoria of a new diet and exercise regime but, once that wears off, they gradually put it all back on again, and sometimes more.

If people can be helped to lose and then maintain their weight, their chances of getting type 2 diabetes and heart disease in five or 10 years' time can be lessened – and we can save on our already-soaring health-care costs.

Why we're getting fatter

There are many reasons why more and more people are overweight these days:

- Labour-saving gadgets
- Drop in day-to-day exercise
- Driving everywhere in the car
- Less walking and cycling due to increased concerns about safety
- Less manual work, more technology and mechanisation
- Decline in cooking skills
- Lack of time to cook healthy meals
- Wide availability of cheap junk food and soft drinks
- Bigger portion sizes
- Marketing of high-kilojoule nutrient-poor drinks and high-fat takeaways
- Poor quality fresh vegetables in rural areas
- Too much time spent in front of a screen of some sort – watching TV, DVDs or movies, playing computer games or on the internet

Remember, we live in an 'obesogenic world' where everything is contrived to make you put on weight. We have to fight it!

Go your own way

Losing weight successfully, and keeping it off, is a long process that requires patience. As we've seen, no one method suits everyone but there are some things you can do to help make it easier. Try some of the following options:

- Enlist a friend as a 'diet buddy' to stay motivated.
- Join a gym or club that offers activities you love.
- Book a personal trainer to show you the right way to exercise and keep you inspired.

- Try to fit in an hour-long walk every day.
- Make an appointment with an accredited practising dietitian and work out a personalised diet plan.
- Order home-delivered diet meals so you don't have to prepare food and everything is portion controlled.
- Substitute a shake for one meal a day when you're at your busiest. There's a large range of 'meal replacement' shakes and bars at supermarket and health food shops. They're nutritious and convenient if you're on the run.
- Join a diet club where you are weighed each week and have the support of the group – it's a great way to meet new friends, too.

tips for success

The US National Weight Control Registry keeps a record of those dieters aged 18 and over who have successfully lost 14kg or more in weight and kept it off for more than one year. There are more than 3000 'successful losers' registered. Through detailed interviews with them, researchers found five factors that contributed to their success. Successful dieters:

1 exercised regularly and often
2 ate a low-fat diet
3 monitored themselves
4 found ways to cope with stress
5 ate breakfast

CHAPTER TWO:
MY FAMILY LIFE AND CAREER

I was born heavy, over 4kg, and I haven't looked back since. Both my sisters were big babies and they too have battled weight, but not as much as me (mind you, they've never worked in a test kitchen).

I spent most of my pre-school years in Vanuatu where my father worked. My mother used to chat on the two-way radio with other ex-pat mothers about their kids' health. Apparently, most of the other kids didn't respond well to the tropics or the food; they were thin and sickly. Guess who thrived?

In those days, the only contact we had with the outside world was the Burns Philp ship which called in every six weeks, bringing fresh food and other goodies. We had kerosene refrigerators as there was no electricity or gas, so the fresh food didn't last too long.

There was canned food, of course, but a limited range, and my mother held a fairly dim view of canned food anyway, so she fed me whatever was in season on the island. There was a lot of seafood, mostly fish and lobster, and any amount of fresh fruit: papayas, mangoes, mandarins, the sweetest pineapples on earth, bananas, plus coconuts and sugarcane.

The local vegies were some unidentifiable green leafy things, plus taro, manioc, sweet potatoes, yams and anything else the non-locals grew in their vegetable gardens. The seeds we planted came from Australia, which meant they probably originated in Europe, hardly suitable for the tropics. I remember huge watery vegies with hardly any taste. Anyway, despite my diet and the hot humid weather, I thrived and put on weight easily.

With only a few exceptions, both sides of my family are short and stocky; we all like our food. I remember my mother saying she used to wake up in the morning plotting and

Catherine says:
it's in the genes

It sounds as if Pamela inherited her tendency to gain weight easily. In hunter-gatherer days, this would have conferred an evolutionary advantage (as her family would have been able to survive for longer on a meagre supply of food). But today, in a world where food is relatively inexpensive and plentiful, there is no need to carry our 'provisions' around on our hips and thighs.

Researchers estimate that between 40 and 60 per cent of our body shape is determined by our genes. With that percentage in mind, there's only so much diet and exercise we can do to change our body shape. Pamela accepts that, no matter how hard she diets and exercises, she will never be tall and thin. Her body shape will always be more solid, but she can aim to be the best weight for her height and build, and reach a weight at which she feels good about herself and one that's healthy for her.

planning what she'd cook us for breakfast. We weren't allowed out of the door until we'd been properly fed and watered.

Many of you will sympathise with me when I tell you about the eating habits established in my childhood. You could say our lives revolved around the next meal. My mother was a wonderful cook, and she didn't go to work, so we had large home-cooked meals every night, not forgetting breakfast, packed lunches and weekend picnics, and barbecues.

As a family, we ate large meals, there is no doubt about that. We always ate the evening meal together; mostly it consisted of the traditional meat and three veg. We always had dessert of some kind, and Mum's apple pies were legendary.

I well remember when Mum first made coleslaw using new ingredients like peppers and garlic. She made a curry every couple of weeks and we ate fish once a week on Friday. It was usually salmon (canned, of course) mornay, salmon patties, smoked fish, or fresh fish, battered or crumbed and fried; we loved it with Mum's homemade chips and coleslaw. Chicken and pork were reserved for special occasions, and a roast dinner, usually a leg of lamb, on Sunday was the norm.

Just in case we were not filled to capacity, there was always bread at every meal.

As a result of my rather firm but deliciously satisfying upbringing, I never made my son eat anything he didn't want to eat. I couldn't stand the drama of force-feeding him, so I just

Catherine says:
dripping, scones and pud

Pamela's early years reflect the attitudes prevalent at the time. Good family meals, sunshine and outdoor play were the cornerstones of bringing up healthy kids. She recalls the meat and vegie dinners always followed by pudding – big meals which meant her stomach was programmed for big volumes of food.

But there were few between-meal snacks (unlike today) and kids were much more active. There were no muesli bars, premium ice-creams, thickshakes or happy meals. Soft drink was reserved for special occasions.

The food back then was not the most nutritious. Often the meat was fatty, roasts were cooked in dripping, bread was mainly white, and there wasn't the variety of fresh fruit and vegetables that we are accustomed to today. And scones, cakes and puddings were baked regularly. Despite this, we were bronzed, fit Aussies who were active and lean.

let him have his way. He didn't starve; I just offered him something else when he turned his nose up at certain things. Having said that, he was an easy child to feed, placid by nature, and quite willing to try most things from an early age. I do sympathise with mothers who worry about their children's diet; I think it has a lot to do with luck and not much else. My son today is of normal build, not what I'd call overweight. (By the way, he loves to cook.)

this is not a new diet

My nanna (my maternal grandmother) had a lifelong battle with weight. She was a keen cook and influenced me in my career choice; we were great fans of each other. I remember her saying quite often that she had to stop eating bread and potatoes because she had put on weight; she also stopped eating cakes, biscuits and pastry. This is not very different from what I'm doing now. In those days, pasta was a new food, except for canned spaghetti; rice was eaten mainly as a dessert, hardly ever as a savoury accompaniment; and noodles were virtually unknown. So, really, Nanna was on my low-grain/low-carb diet all those years ago without ever knowing it.

school days

In high school my favourite subject soon became Home Science. I really loved it.

I liked to cook, and even did a cake-decorating course in the evenings at the local technical college. My Home Science teacher inspired and encouraged me and, as they say, the rest is history. I knew when I was 11 that I wanted to work somewhere in the food industry. Weight-wise, it was probably the worst career path for me, but I wouldn't have missed any part of it for anything.

first jobs in food

I have been in the food industry since I left school at age 17 in the early 1960s. I had a couple of positions in the home economics field at the AGL (then called the Australian Gas Light Company) and at the St George County Council. During the seven years I was at the Council, we worked at the Sydney Royal Easter Show each year, and I became quite friendly with a girl who ended up working in *The Australian Women's Weekly* Test Kitchen (*AWW* TK). One fateful day she phoned and told me the senior position in the Test Kitchen was up for grabs. Ellen Sinclair was the food editor then, and we liked each other straight away. I started work here in September 1969.

the australian women's test kitchen

Working away in the *AWW* TK, making up and cooking endless recipes every day, did nothing for my figure. It's an eatathon here, but I love it. In those days, the Test Kitchen was called the Leila Howard Test Kitchen. Leila never existed, it was just a name. Later, in the 1970s, Ellen Sinclair's name finally appeared in the pages of the magazine. In 1976, the first in the now-internationally famous series of *AWW* cookbooks hit the market. They were, and still are, a phenomenal success.

The Test Kitchen is a unique place situated in an office building in the heart of Sydney, and creates and tests recipes for The *Australian Women's Weekly, Woman's Day* and *The Australian Women's Weekly* cookbooks. This amounts to testing and tasting literally thousands of recipes every year.

There are 12 work stations or bays in the TK; each bay has a regular domestic stove set in a stainless steel bench, then two team members share a sink and microwave oven. Each person has his or her own knives, boards and various basic kitchen equipment.

The members of the team here have varied backgrounds, the common thread being a passion for food, a creative bent, excellent cooking skills, and the ability to carefully write the recipes they have created so they can be replicated by you at home. The TK is famous for triple-testing recipes; this is why our work is so respected throughout the world – the recipes do work. We don't go in for anything too fancy; we are, after all, making up recipes for normal people and their families, just like you and me.

The team in the Test Kitchen try to organise themselves around presenting food for tastings twice a day at 12 noon and 3pm, but there is always something that messes up the system, and sometimes there are more, or sometimes fewer, tastings. Often six people could have cooked at least three things each for one tasting – that's 18 recipes for all of us to try in one hit. Small wonder I have a weight problem. Tricky things like omelettes and soufflés, things that simply won't tolerate waiting, are served and eaten whenever the cook calls. Picky eaters don't survive here!

Catherine says:

good carbs, bad carbs, right carbs, wrong carbs

Pamela's diet cuts out most refined starchy carbohydrates such as bread, pasta, rice, cereal (apart from muesli) and restricts starchy vegetables like potatoes, pumpkin and peas.

The difference between Pamela's way of eating and that of an average person wanting to lose weight is that her Test Kitchen tastings include a variety of carbs that an average person wouldn't consume in this way. Therefore, rather than cut back on the carbohydrates as drastically as she has done, to keep to a healthy way of eating, you should ensure that you include good carbs in your diet every day.

What is a good carb exactly? While I don't necessarily believe in labelling food good or bad, there's no doubt that certain carbs are better for you than others. It's worth having a look at how different carbohydrates work and what effect they have on our bodies.

Modern carbs

Our modern staples like white bread, white rice and many breakfast cereals:

- are refined – a percentage of their original nutrients have been removed
- are kilojoule-dense – 100 grams of cooked brown rice packs in 600kJ while 100 grams of fish contains 500kJ and one large orange (weighing 300 grams) has only 450kJ
- are easy to overconsume (they don't 'fill you up')

- have a high glycaemic index (GI) – they are digested and absorbed quickly (see page 54)
- are often a 'vehicle' for carrying fat – Pamela has already pointed out how much butter, oil, cheese or cream you can add to potato mash
- may carry a great deal of 'hidden fat' – think of biscuits, croissants, doughnuts and potato chips

Why the wrong carbs make you fatter

Think of a loaf of white bread or a hamburger bun. It's soft, nice to eat and easy to swallow. You can probably wolf down two or three slices with butter or jam in a couple of minutes – no worries. That's the problem.

The modern carbs are too easy to eat. They've had their fibre removed so they require no chewing. Before you know it, you've swallowed 800kJ.

These carbs enter the bloodstream rapidly, causing your blood sugar levels to do a sudden spike, which then triggers a surge of insulin. Insulin is a hormone that turns a key in the cells of your muscles, allowing all that sugar to get into the muscles and power them with fuel. But it also directs any unused sugar into storage – in your fat cells. The end result? You eat more than you realise but you don't feel satisfied, so you're looking for a snack an hour later. Your body has had to call on more insulin than it needed and so a little more fat has been laid down.

What this means is that, if you are on a diet, you would do far better on wholegrain or low-GI carbohydrate foods, such as grainy bread, brown rice or a jacket potato with skin. These good carbohydrates will make you feel fuller before you've overeaten and they will 'stick with you' for longer. Pamela's decided to cut out most starchy foods, but you don't have to completely eliminate them in order to lose weight. Just choose small quantities of those that help your diet efforts.

Ideally, a good carb should be:

- nutrient-dense (meaning it's packed full of essential vitamins, minerals and fibre)
- wholegrain OR slowly absorbed (with a low-GI number of 55 or less) which helps counter obesity

Examples of good carbs are: oats; barley; breads – mixed grain, wholemeal, dark rye, linseed and soy, fruit loaf - the less smooth, the better; cereals – wholegrain, bran, high fibre; legumes – beans, lentils, spilt peas; fruits; starchy vegetables – corn, peas, carrots, sweet potato; pasta, noodles; rice – basmati rice; yogurt; ice-cream – low-GI varieties.

How many good carbs should you eat each day?

Aim to eat three servings of good carbs every day. You can choose from:

- one slice of a dense grainy bread or pumpernickel
- one bowl of muesli (try Pamela's recipe on page 17) or porridge
- 60g legumes (soy beans, lentils, baked beans, broad beans)
- 60g pasta, brown rice, barley or buckwheat
- 60g pumpkin, peas, carrot or potato

If you prefer, you can replace one or two good carb servings with an extra serving of fruit, eg: a medium apple, pear or orange; 120g fruit salad; a small bunch of grapes; 20 cherries.

Ways to change from bad to good

Here are a few easy ways you can decrease your intake of bad carbs and increase the good carbs in your diet.

1 Avoid the 'junk' carbs like soft drinks, sweets, cakes and biscuits.
2 Swap your regular white bread for a nutritious grainy or chewy wholemeal loaf.
3 Swap your breakfast cereal to one made from oats (muesli or porridge), wholewheat (wheatflake biscuits, wheat flakes) or bran (All-Bran, bran flakes). A bowl at breakfast will keep your bowels working well.
4 Check how much potato and rice you serve for dinner. One medium potato or 60g of rice is plenty and won't overload you with carbs. Certain vegetables contain higher carbohydrate values but are still nutritious. Just have a small serving of pumpkin, carrots, corn or peas.
5 Skip juice which has had its fibre removed and is too easy to overconsume. Drink water and eat the whole fruit instead.

CHAPTER THREE: MY DIET IN DETAIL

breakfast

I used to eat breakfast when I woke up, whether I wanted it or not. Since I'm used to eating on command with my job, I did it without thinking. But I decided to try a different approach when I began my diet. Now, I take myself and the dog for a walk first thing. I love plotting and planning the day in peace this way. After I've showered, I treat myself to my one cup of really strong coffee for the day. Then I wait until I hit the office around 8.30am to eat breakfast. Since I've been on the diet, breakfast usually consists of fruit (whatever is in season) and yogurt, or a handful of dried fruit and nuts. On the weekend, I love a good fry-up (see page 52) with eggs. I have to confess though, I'm particularly partial to my own homemade muesli which I eat with skim milk and yogurt. Here's the recipe (see opposite page).

Catherine says:

breakfast

You've heard it before and Pamela has confirmed it. If you're dieting, breakfast is important and not a meal to skip. It stops you picking mid-morning at biscuits or a pastry and it appears to boost your metabolic rate for the day – our body clocks seem to be set to burn more in the morning hours and less in the afternoon and evening. Shift workers and nurses agree: once you swap your working hours for the night shift, you somehow start to gain weight.

I'm not one to force people to eat when they don't feel hungry, but if you can't eat anything first thing, make sure you plan to have something healthy by 10am. The reason? Sales of pastry, doughnuts, pizza and hot chips shoot up at around 10am. All the hungry people who skipped breakfast are by now ready to eat, but there's nothing quick and healthy, so they grab a cappuccino and a danish pastry. Not good for your health or your weight.

Here's my assessment of Pamela's breakfast choices:

Pamela's muesli, skim milk and yogurt
A great way to start the day. High in fibre, natural and low GI, so it sticks with you for the morning. It can take you to lunch. This muesli gets my vote.

Fruit
Healthy; the addition of a small tub of yogurt offers a balance of protein and calcium.

Eggs
High in protein with a range of vitamins and minerals. As long as you don't fry them in oodles of butter, they're one of nature's perfect whole foods. And they're even more delicious teamed with a slice of wholegrain toast.

toasted muesli

PREPARATION TIME: 10 minutes
COOKING TIME: 10 minutes

2 tablespoons golden syrup
2 tablespoons walnut oil
90g rolled oats
160g coarsely chopped blanched almonds
120g coarsely chopped roasted hazelnuts
160g pepitas (pumpkin seed kernels)
220g sunflower seed kernels
70g linseed, sunflower and almond blend (LSA)
55g finely chopped dried seeded dates
75g finely chopped dried apricots

1 Preheat oven to moderate.

2 Combine syrup and oil in small bowl.

3 Combine oats and nuts in shallow baking dish; drizzle with syrup mixture. Toast, uncovered, in moderate oven about 10 minutes or until browned lightly, stirring halfway through cooking time. Cool 10 minutes.

4 Stir pepitas, kernels, LSA blend and dried fruit into muesli mixture; cool.

SERVES 20 (35g PER SERVING)

PER SERVING 11.4g carbohydrate; 21.1g total fat (2.1g saturated fat); 1112kJ (266 cal); 8.6g protein

slow it down

Slowing down your rate of eating and not finishing everything that's on your plate are two excellent techniques for weight control. They both have the same result – they make you listen to your body's own sense of hunger so you stop eating when you're satisfied, but not too full.

If you overeat just 200 kilojoules a day (the amount in just one choc-chip cookie), you'll end up 2kg heavier by the end of a year. Not a lot, but this is precisely how our excess weight creeps on over time, in amounts so small and so gradual that you hardly notice. A study tracking a group of Australian men and women over 25 years found that, since 1976, the men had gained on average 8kg, while the women had put on 12kg. That translates to a mere 320g a year for the men and 480g a year for the women. That's the obesity epidemic.

lunch

I usually take a salad to the office with me each day (see box on following page). I could easily make something to eat in the Test Kitchen, but, I know me, I'd be in that coolroom trimming the edges off everything in sight, and finishing off bits and pieces. Scraps are wonderful and I can easily convince myself that eating them quickly doesn't count! I do try to eat more slowly these days, but old habits die hard. I love the texture of food, and there are not too many flavours that I really dislike. If you can teach yourself to eat and chew your food more slowly and thoroughly, your digestive system will thank you for it.

I change the combination of my lunch ingredients quite a bit. For a dressing, I always squeeze half a juicy lemon or lime over everything, then I top it all with a mix of fresh herbs, and sometimes a dollop of yogurt. I have to confess to preferring the high-fat variety of yogurt. I'm not into deprivation. About every third day, I make a mix of fresh herbs (see page 39). My current favourite herb combo consists of flat-leaf parsley, basil and coriander or tarragon (home-grown French tarragon). Sometimes I throw in some mint. I love mint if I'm eating lamb and yogurt.

After washing and drying the herbs in a lettuce spinner, I toss them into the food processor with, say, about six trimmed green onions. Sometimes I throw in a small clove of garlic too, or garlic chives, or, better still, a shallot; I'm mad about those. I process them until they're coarsely chopped, then put them into a plastic container, ready for the early morning rush hour, which includes making my lunch. The last thing I do is toss about 60g of the herb mixture onto the salad, and off I go.

If I feel hungry after my salad, I eat some fruit, fresh or dried, and I eat a handful of nuts every day. I've taken a great liking to raw cashews. They are a low-GI food and, although high in oil, and therefore high in kilojoules, they make your digestive system work hard. And the oil is one of the good mono-unsaturated oils that actually help to lower cholesterol in the body. Pecans are another favourite nut of mine, followed closely by walnuts and almonds. Stay away from salted nuts; you really don't need all that salt. Dry roasted nuts are good but you can't always be sure what kind of oil has been added for regular roasting; it could be palm oil which is high in 'bad' saturated fat (see pages 22-23). If you crave something sweet as a dessert replacement, eat some muscatels, dates or dried pears.

the main meal of the day

From Monday to Friday I eat a simple meal in the evening, something quick and easy to prepare, because I really only want to relax in front of the TV or read a book, just quietly closing down for the night. I always have some form of protein with vegetables or salad. I eat fish at least twice a week. I usually grill or barbecue the fish and eat it with a good squeeze of lemon or lime juice. Grilled or barbecued chicken thigh fillets or cutlets are another favourite stand-by.

Once a week, I'll have a steak, a decent-sized piece, and I trim the excess fat before I cook it. Mostly I barbecue it, or cook it in a griddle pan, over a really high heat, until it's barely done. Then I wrap it in foil to rest before I eat it.

During the weekend, I'm likely to cook something more fancy for friends or family. For inspiration, just feast your eyes on the wonderful recipes in this book.

If you're the only member of the family on a diet, you'll know there's no fun in having to prepare different meals for other family members. All the main courses in this book can be eaten by the non-dieters and I've suggested what carbs you could add to the meal.

Catherine says:

lunch

A large salad is an excellent lunch for anyone, but particularly for a dieter. Salads have a great many benefits, as Pamela has discovered. They:

- have virtually no fat
- are very low in kilojoules
- give you lots of fibre which fills you up and stops you snacking in the afternoon
- are packed full of vitamins, antioxidants and minerals
- have endless variations, as Pamela has shown
- can use a dressing to add not only heart-friendly oils but also acidity in the form of lemon juice or vinegar which slows down digestion.

dinner

Eat breakfast like a king, lunch like a prince and dinner like a pauper – there is a lot of nutritional wisdom in this old saying which rearranges the size of our meals in reverse order to the way we currently eat them. Eating our biggest meal at the end of the day when we are least active is a formula for putting on weight. We're taking in most of our kilojoules when our bodies have no way of burning them off.

Some research shows that switching lunch and dinner around helps many people shed weight. This is the meal pattern of days gone by – the main meal in the middle of the day to give you fuel for more physical work in the afternoon.

alcohol

I'm not much of a drinker but I sometimes have a glass of wine with my main meal. If you choose to have a drink, remember that many, such as beer and mixer drinks, are loaded with sugar (ie, empty carbs) and can undo your efforts.

tea and coffee

I have one really strong cup of coffee in the morning and that's enough for me. I tend to drink tea during the day, two or three cups with a splash of skim milk. I also like most herbal teas, particularly the lemon and mint varieties. Iced tea with mint on a hot summer's day is wonderful, too.

Catherine says:

alcohol – a problem for many

Too much alcohol is often a hidden reason behind weight problems. It's easy to sip, it helps you relax and socialise, but it can pile on the weight. Alcohol also weakens your resolve, so you munch on junk food you would normally resist. Being a light drinker has helped Pamela's dieting efforts. If you're trying to lose weight, having alcohol-free days saves kilojoules, gives the liver a chance to recover, and lessens the risk of breast cancer for women.

caffeine pros and cons

One strong cup of coffee a day is fine and obviously gives Pamela the hit she likes. You'll know if you've had too much – you get the shakiness, anxiousness and irritability of caffeine overload, accompanied by heart palpitations and sleeplessness if you really overdo it.

Tea also contains caffeine but at concentrations that are only half or one-third of those in coffee. In terms of weight loss, caffeine can mobilise fatty acids out of storage and into the bloodstream, giving you a short-term supply of fuel when you're eating little, something models and gymnasts figured out long ago!

water and salt

Thirst is not so very different from hunger, just listen to your body and it will tell you when to eat and drink. I'm not one for downing litres of water every day just for the sake of it, but it is without doubt the best thirst-quencher there is.

If you are used to eating a lot of highly salted food, try to break the habit, or at least reduce the amount of salt you eat. Sometimes you need salt at the beginning of the cooking process, but it's best to season your food at the table. Instead of salt, try fresh herbs, spices and fresh lime or lemon juice.

fats

It's hard to stick to a strict low-fat diet in my job. There's a plethora of low-fat/lite/light products in the marketplace, many of which I dislike, and if I can't have the product with the full flavour, I'd rather go without. Amazingly though, despite the number of low-fat products available, as a nation we've never been heavier, so what's gone wrong? But just as some carbs are better than others, so are some fats better than others. We need to know how to separate the good guys from the bad guys.

fluid needs

We tend to underestimate how important water is for us to function. We need water to:

- transport nutrients around the body
- remove wastes
- serve as a medium for the countless biochemical reactions that take place in the body
- moisten our food to facilitate chewing
- maintain body temperature – when we sweat, heat is released as the sweat evaporates and this cools us down

Research has also linked lack of fluid over a lifetime with an increased risk of kidney stones and bladder cancer in later years.

Thirst is not a reliable guide to our fluid needs as we are usually dehydrated by the time we experience it. To ensure we are well hydrated, guidelines suggest we have at least eight glasses or two litres of fluid each day, and more in hot, humid weather.

Not all fluids are equal in the hydration stakes. Aim to drink water, the ideal fluid. Then you can count tea, clear soup, milk and juice towards your day's total.

Catherine says:

the facts on fat

Pamela is right: we need to become more fat smart, not fat obsessed. It is an essential nutrient in our diet, but it pays to know what's what. Just because something is labelled 'low fat' for example, doesn't mean you can eat it with abandon. Most foods labelled 'low fat' or '97% fat free' have similar kilojoule counts to their full-fat cousins because they contain higher amounts of sugar or starch to make up for the missing fat.

Low-fat and light products generally contain 25 or 30 per cent less fat than the regular product. For dieters, some of these – such as yogurts, dairy desserts, milks and margarine spreads – offer genuine reductions in fat and kilojoules without compromising taste, and are valuable diet foods. But with other products, there is little or no saving in kilojoules – think of light olive oil (light in flavour but not fat) or light crisps (lightly salted). To avoid the pitfalls, you need to become an avid reader of labels on products like muesli bars, breakfast bars, biscuits and muffins.

Fat is very easy to overconsume and packs in a hefty number of kilojoules per gram. Fat balance in the body is poorly regulated too, so, if you overeat, it'll show up before very long in an increase in body fat!

types of fat

Mono-unsaturated

Mono-unsaturated fats are 'good' fats and lower cholesterol when they displace saturated fats in the diet, although not as effectively as polyunsaturates. They are found in all fats but are high in olive, canola, macadamia and peanut oils, avocados and most nuts.

Polyunsaturated

Polyunsaturated fats reduce the risk of heart disease. They are found in all fats and exist as two distinct types:

- Omega-3 fats such as alpha-linolenic acid and its derivatives eicosapentaenoic acid (EPA) and docosahexaenoic acid (DHA) are primarily found in the fats of fish, particularly deep-sea oily fish. These are important for your heart.
- Omega-6 fats like linoleic acid are the main polyunsaturated fatty acids of common vegetable oils (sunflower, safflower, maize, cottonseed and grapeseed), polyunsaturated margarines and some nuts. Eat them in moderation.

Saturated

These are the 'bad' fats that tend to raise cholesterol and be deposited as body fat. They are found in animal fats such as butter, cream, cheese, fat on meat, deli meats (salami, bacon, sausages) and in cakes, biscuits, pastries, confectionery and fried take-aways. Coconut and palm oils are also high in saturated fat.

dairy foods

I'm partial to dairy foods of all kinds. When I devised this diet, I deliberately chose to include them. In most cases, I prefer the full-fat dairy foods, but I only have tiny quantities. If you like the reduced/low/no-fat and skim products, you should use them as you will be reducing your fat intake even more.

milk

I prefer full-fat milk in coffee, but I only have one cup of coffee each day, so there's no big deal about the quantity of full-fat milk I drink. I prefer to drink skim milk on its own and I have a little on muesli and in tea.

cheese

I enjoy eating a little cheese, probably about three or four times a week. I love parmesan, freshly grated over all sorts of things. I often mix it with fresh coarsely chopped herbs, combined with finely chopped green onions.

yogurt

This is a wonderful nutrient-packed food; I think it should be eaten at least once a day. I buy the plain variety, so I can use it with either savoury or sweet foods. My favourite indulgence is a teaspoon of my homemade Seville orange marmalade stirred through yogurt; the combination of bitter and sweet teamed with velvety creaminess is amazing.

buttermilk

If I'm making something like a curry, I like to use buttermilk instead of yogurt. Some people like to drink buttermilk; I'm not one of them, but it's a great source of calcium, and is quite low in fat and kilojoules.

cream

I'm avoiding cream in all its forms while I'm on this diet. While I like it – a lot – I made the decision not to eat it from day one. I make an exception when I have to taste something made in the Test Kitchen which has cream as an ingredient.

quality and cost of food

Eat the freshest, best quality, cleanest food you can afford. This applies to meat and seafood as well as fruit and vegies. If you have the luxury of having a space to grow at least some of your own fruit, herbs and vegies, then you're way ahead.

People are strange, they baulk at paying a dollar for a beautiful apple or peach, but think nothing of paying a similar amount for a candy bar or a packet of crisps.

Nuts are a fantastic snack food; they may be high in kilojoules but they contain mono-unsaturated fats which are wonderfully good for you. I eat a big handful every day.

Avocado is another vitamin-packed, filling food. I eat half an avocado a day, with a squeeze of lemon or lime juice. I can easily polish off a whole avocado in one sitting, as I just love their flavour and texture, but I'm trying to exercise restraint.

counting kilojoules

I haven't concerned myself with this exercise; how could I, as my job involves tasting the weirdest combinations of things at one sitting. I would drive myself crazy if I tried to work out how many kilojoules I got through in a day. It would be a terrifying total, which makes me wonder about kilojoules. It must be that the different types of food and their kilojoules affect my body in different ways. I do know there is some discussion about this subject in scientific circles. Obviously, we still have a lot to learn about food and the way it impacts on our health, weight and wellbeing. Having said all that, if we eat a wide variety of food, surely we'll have all bases covered.

There is a lot of information to be absorbed out there: theories that come and go; myths are often exploded; then someone dredges up a forbidden fruit from the past, only to say how wonderful it is now. It's this minefield of data that sets the mind spinning; it is no wonder that people have become confused and need advice about the way to live. I believe you have to work through the details and make up your own mind about which paths to follow. We should all take responsibility for what we eat and drink, and feed to our families.

weight maintenance

This is the hard bit but, now that I know this way of eating works for me, I've slowly begun reintroducing small helpings of low-GI grain-based foods. They fill me up and keep me from feeling hungry and therefore snacking indiscriminately. It's so easy I wish I'd discovered it years ago! The low-GI foods I'm talking about are rice, in particular basmati, (a variety with the lowest GI), slightly undercooked (al dente) pasta and some good wholegrain bread. In winter, I include more pulses and starchy root vegetables. Other than these small additions, I intend sticking to this way of eating for good. (For more detailed information on GI foods, see page 34.)

a note on adapting my diet for non-dieters

The recipes in this book are really delicious, the flavours are fresh, and the combination of ingredients nutritionally sound. All that is missing is the carbohydrate element. If you're going to add carbs to the recipes for some or all members of the family, think about the type you're adding, and why.

Consider if the people who are going to eat the meals lead sedentary or active lives; don't overload them with energy foods their bodies can't use. I don't want you to think I am never going to eat carbs again. I am. I really like the starchy texture of grains. But because I don't expect my job or life to change very much over the next few years, I know I only need small amounts of carbs. Unless you're cooking for a marathon runner or someone who burns up excessive amounts of energy on a daily basis, almost everyone can do well following an eating plan based on and around this one.

using recipes in this book

If you look through the recipes in this book and *The Australian Women's Weekly* cookbooks, *Low-Carb Low-Fat* and *501 Low-Carb Recipes*, you will notice we have supplied you with carb, fat, protein, kilojoule and calorie counts at the end of each recipe. You will also notice the big range of nutritional counts from lowest to highest. This is quite deliberate – I really want you to mix up the food you eat. In order to do this, you'll need to work out a weekly or monthly menu for yourself (and your family if you like). I've worked one out to get you kick-started (see page 41), but you will have to try the recipes to determine your favourites. Once you've mastered all the recipes in this book, you'll be easily able to make up your own for this way of eating. Balance is everything: if you choose to eat a really low-fat soup for one meal, you can choose something higher in fat for the next meal.

getting stocked and started

With any diet, it's easier if you get organised. That's also true if you're adding carbs for the non-dieters in the family. To help you along, I've suggested carb additions for every recipe.

If you're an active person and you think you need the power boost of muesli in the morning, make a batch for yourself. Try it on the family too, it's not cheap to make, but you don't need heaps of it. Most people who've tried it simply love it. Keep it in an airtight container in the fridge and it will stay fresh for up to three months.

Your pantry needs to contain stand-bys for when your mind goes blank about what to eat. I haven't specified particular types of any food. I've left that up to you. For example, if you don't like tuna canned in water, buy the variety canned in oil – but drain it *really* well before using it.

I shop once a week and I'm fussy about how I store food, as it's too expensive to waste (see my pantry list, page 106).

unrestricted vegetables (lower in carbs)

Eat as much as you like, any time you like. Eat as many raw as you can; steam, boil, stir-fry or microwave the ones that need cooking. Don't use oil, butter or margarine for cooking; a light coating of spray oil is fine for stir-frying.

Asparagus, all varieties and colours, lightly cooked

Broccoli and **broccolini**, lightly cooked

Cabbage, all varieties and colours, lightly cooked and raw

Cauliflower, raw or cooked

Celery, raw or cooked

Chillies, lemon grass, ginger, lime leaves, curry, garlic, use for flavouring

Courgette (Zucchini), squash, all varieties and colours, lightly cooked with skin on

Cucumbers, all varieties, raw

Greens, leafy greens, all lettuce, Asian greens, rocket, spinach, Swiss chard, watercress, eat raw and cooked

Herbs, all types, raw, use for flavouring, add at end of cooking

Mushrooms, all types, raw or cooked

Onions, all colours, **leeks**, **spring onions**, **chives**, use for flavouring, cooked or raw

Peppers, all colours (red has the most vitamin C), eat raw most of the time, cooked occasionally

Radishes, all varieties, including daikon, raw

Sprouts and **shoots**, all types, raw or added after cooking

Tomatoes, eat raw most of the time, cooked occasionally (twice a week, no more)

restricted vegetables (higher in carbs)

Choose two servings **per week** from the list below. Boil, steam or microwave these vegetables. Eat 250g per serving (see carb, fat and kilojoule counter, page 107).

Beans, all types and colours, lightly cooked

Beetroot, all colours, raw or cooked

Carrots, eat raw most of the time, cooked occasionally

Celeriac, raw or cooked

Corn, all types, lightly cooked

Peas, all types including snow and sugar snap, raw or cooked

Potatoes, all types, cooked

Pulses, all types and colours, dried and cooked or canned, including **lentils**, **chickpeas** and **beans**

Pumpkin, all types, cooked

Swedes, **parsnips** and **turnips** cooked

Sweet potato, all types, cooked

fruit

Eat a maximum of five servings of fresh fruit each day.

With cherries, grapes, berries, pineapple, etc, consider 250g equivalent to one serving. Eat as much melon you like. Eat half an avocado a day and about 55g dried fruit a day.

protein

Eat eggs, all lean meat including chicken, and seafood of all types (for quantities, see meal ideas on pages 41 to 45).

dairy foods

Eat three servings per day (25g cheese, 250ml milk or 95g yogurt per serving).

nuts

Eat about 55g per day (almonds, macadamia, pecans, raw cashews, walnuts).

exercise

I'm sure we're all very different in terms of what we need to eat and drink to be healthy; I think the same goes for exercise. I feel so much better, both physically and mentally, if I exercise in a moderate way. I love to walk and swim, but hate someone telling me what I should do in group exercises; as for gyms, I really can't think of anything worse. Walking and swimming allow me time to think of other things; I let my mind wander and quietly enjoy myself.

Being on this diet has definitely made me more energetic. I wake up earlier with more get-up-and-go. These days I hit the floor at 5.30am and take my dog for a walk around the neighbourhood for 30 minutes to an hour. If it's raining, I simply don't go. I refuse to become fanatical or feel guilty about anything to do with diet or exercise.

An inexpensive pedometer, available from your local chemist or sports store, is a handy gadget to have as it counts the steps you take. Some even count the kilojoules you burn, too. Experts recommend we take about 10,000 steps each day, which equates to about eight kilometres. I know that sounds impossible but it's amazing how quickly the steps add up!

I really enjoy swimming. It's great because no one can see your unfortunate bits under the water, it makes you feel good, you can't hurt yourself as the water cushions you against any impact, you can do it at your own pace, and it's such a fantastic all-over workout, not to mention the breathing exercise it gives you.

Catherine says:

the benefits of exercise

Pamela has shown what we all know – exercise is important for permanent weight loss. There are two ways to exercise more. Firstly, you can schedule a time to exercise by walking or going to the gym. Or you can get more 'incidental' exercise. That simply means moving more in your daily life: get up to turn off the TV rather than use the remote; walk to the shops rather than take the car; walk to a colleague's office rather than send an email.

Just how important this 'moving' is for weight control was demonstrated by researchers from the University of Alabama in the US. They tracked a group of 61 healthy-weight premenopausal women at the beginning and end of a one-year period and discovered two distinct groups: gainers – those who

If you're at all aquatic, but think you're lacking in swimming skills, find a teacher and you'll quickly become proficient in the water. Aqua aerobics is another great way to exercise, in a class or even by yourself. Learn how to do it in deep water, as this is the most demanding on your body.

There will be days when you won't feel like exercising, but, believe me, expending energy by exercising is the only way you're going to get more energy. Remember, the less you do, the less you want to do, so you must break that pattern – get out there and get motivated!

put on more than six kilograms – and maintainers – those who put on less than two kilograms.

The researchers found the most important difference between these two groups was how much physical activity they did and the amount of muscle mass they had. All the women studied were sedentary, so these differences in activity really came down to who climbed the stairs and who didn't.

Exercise also makes the greatest impact on your metabolism, turning your body from a 'slow simmer' to a 'rapid boil'. You can notice this yourself – when you finish an exercise session, your body feels warm for some hours afterwards. The engine's fired up and glowing with heat (a form of energy). Becoming more active is the best way to boost your metabolism. Don't forget that crash diets slow your metabolic rate and cause you to lose lean muscle.

nutritional assessment of pamela's diet

On the whole, Pamela's diet meets almost all her nutritional needs for her age and activity level. With its high levels of vegetables, fruits, lean meat, fish and nuts, it is a healthy option and rates much better than the 'average' diet.

Her eating plan has five features in common with other sensible weight-loss plans. It:

- cuts back on the bad saturated fats
- concentrates on healthy unsaturated fats from nuts, avocado and a little oil

- is high in protein, which is filling and satisfying, so she doesn't feel hungry between meals
- can be followed for weeks without resulting in Pamela being tired, constipated, lacking in nutrients or constantly thinking about food (a common complaint on most fad diets)
- covers her body's needs for essential vitamins and minerals

ten things Pamela did which helped her win the weight-loss war

1. She exercised – not a lot, but enough to make a difference to her efforts.
2. She didn't try for the quick fix or short cut. She went in thinking weeks and months, not days.
3. She ate large helpings of salad and vegetables.
4. She snacked on fruit and nuts, not junk.
5. She allowed herself small indulgences so she didn't break out and have a big binge from deprivation.
6. She weighed herself only once a week.
7. She tailored her diet to her own food preferences and her somewhat unusual occupational hazard.
8. She always planned her meals ahead of time.
9. She kept alcohol to a minimum.
10. She still ate out at restaurants and chose things from the menu to suit her diet.

CHAPTER FOUR: AVOIDING THE PITFALLS

emotion-driven eating

I have to confess to overeating when I'm stressed or unhappy; I can't imagine where that 'fat and happy' saying came from, as from my experience the reverse is true. Eating food for comfort is very common, so if this sounds like you too, don't feel that you're unique. Isn't it odd though that we don't overindulge in healthy food? It's always the fattening stuff we crave, never a worthy salad! Of course, after you've wolfed down a whole packet of biscuits, or a big bag of crisps, you feel worse, physically and psychologically.

Most people who comfort eat tend to eat alone, since they're too ashamed to eat in front of friends or family. I don't pretend to know the answers. All I can say is that my new eating regime makes me feel good, I feel in control and it's easy for me to do. If I had to eat certain prescribed foods and specific amounts, it would send me into a tailspin.

I can also tell you that I have never once felt hungry on this diet. If you do feel hungry at any time while you're following it, grab some protein – cold meat, a couple of hard-boiled eggs, or a big bowl of soup.

As for cravings, mine have pretty much subsided. I once told Rosemary Stanton, a long-time friend and colleague, that I had a sweet tooth. She told me I was wrong, that I had a 'fat' tooth, and it was coincidence the things I craved, such as chocolate and ice-cream, were sweet. They are, of course, also high in fat. Pre-diet, I used to crave salty things like chips, peanuts and potato crisps. They're high in fat too, so maybe Rosemary is right. Now, whenever I fancy something sweet, as I've already suggested you do, I eat some dried fruit. My favourites are dates, prunes, muscatels, apricots, figs and pears. I eat a handful each day, often teamed with the handful of nuts I love.

eating out

I have to eat out quite often at work-related functions, lunches, dinners, product launches, all sorts of things. So far I have had no difficulty avoiding grain-based, high-carb foods. Most restaurants are diet-sympathetic these days so, if there is nothing that suits you on the menu, either forget the diet, or ask the waiter if the chef could re-jig something on the menu just for you. If you know when and where you're going to eat, phone ahead, explain your diet, and I'm sure that they'll be happy to help.

Take-away food is quite another matter. You should definitely avoid pizzas, fried fish and chips, burgers, and all high-fat junk foods. However, there's usually something that you can eat on the menu of the average take-away shop, or that you can deconstruct to suit your needs. Bunless hamburgers are growing in popularity and most fish and chip shops will grill fish for you, so have two pieces of fish with lemon, and avoid the fried chips. If they do non-creamy salads, have one of those. It's really not hard, just make sensible choices.

Catherine says:

comfort eating and cravings

Eating when under stress is one of the main reasons many women stay overweight. But using food to cope with emotional problems is not the best way in the long run. You need to find other non-food ways to comfort and calm yourself when you're upset.

Pamela's idea of increasing the amount of protein in your diet is a good one, as it will help you feel fuller for longer, and also help keep cravings at bay.

There are many theories about why we crave certain foods, some based on what our bodies might be lacking, others purely psychological. Any diet that reduces cravings will be a winner as comfort eating and cravings can undo all your good diet and exercise intentions. Think of it like this: just one 50g bar of plain milk chocolate will set your diet efforts back by 1080 kilojoules, 13g fat and 31g carbohydrate.

dining out

A good meal out is one of life's treats and a way to relax and enjoy yourself, but it's worth keeping these tips in mind:

- Order carefully – choose something light and fresh.
- Think small – forgo an entrée or share one.
- Order vegetables or salad with your main course.
- Just eat enough to feel satisfied – you don't have to finish everything on your plate.
- Eat slowly and pace yourself – be the last to finish.
- Keep your alcohol to a minimum – order one glass of wine and drink lots of water.

Best cuisines: modern British, seafood, Japanese, Vietnamese (but watch out for fried entrées).

eating a variety of food

It's important to eat as wide a variety of food as possible. Try fruits and vegetables you've never tried before, experiment with fresh herbs, different varieties of chillies, and, of course, spices. If you have Asian food stores near you, it's worthwhile trying their vegies, as they're always fresh, of good quality and often inexpensive. If you can buy from growers' markets or roadside stalls where produce is homegrown, then do so; fresh is best, there is no doubt about that.

If you eat a lot of different foods, and presuming you're healthy, you probably won't need any vitamin and mineral supplements while you're on this diet. I know this is a controversial issue, but many nutritionists will tell you that you can get everything your body needs from a wide and varied diet of the good food that abounds in this country.

One day, write down everything you eat. If you're not eating between 25 and 30 different foods a day, you need to increase the variety in your diet.

my three-day theory

From my vast experience with dieting I have developed a three-day theory. I think if you can cope with the first three days of any radical change you make to your body, you're well on the way to success. I used to be a heavy smoker, never one to do anything by halves. I haven't smoked since July 1978.

One day, I thought to myself, what's so scary about giving up smoking forever? Of course I was afraid of the withdrawal symptoms, but it's not as if they are life-threatening, so I gave it up. The first three days were frightful. I was addicted not only to the nicotine, but to the habit of reaching for a cigarette whenever I had a coffee, or a meal. The point I'm making is that those first three days were the worst; after that, it became easier and easier every day, and it will for you, too.

the dreaded 'o' word

Obesity is a dreadful word. I hate it with a passion. All my life I battled with my weight but I never considered myself actually 'obese'. Imagine my horror and shame at being told I was indeed obese when I went to visit a doctor about six years ago. I share this story with you to show you that even though there are times when your self-esteem takes a real battering, you can always rise above it. Sometimes, we have to listen to things we don't want to hear, but it's often a great way to learn and grow.

My confession is this: I had been well-endowed in the breast department, and always hated them. I developed before anyone else at school and was wearing a 34B bra at age 11.

I soldiered on through life, trying to find clothes that would fit; garments that buttoned down the front were out of the question, and buying a swimming costume was a nightmare. One day I was in a store looking at the bras, when a resident expert appeared. She asked my size, I told her (36DD), so in we went to the fitting room armed with six different styles of bra. After we'd rejected about four bras, she announced I was an E cup. I was devastated. That's when I made another decision that transformed my life. The boobs had to go.

I had always rejected the idea of breast reduction surgery, thinking it was something only vain people did. But then I started thinking about the furrows in my shoulders from bra straps and the almost-constant niggling neck, back and shoulder pain I suffered. I made an appointment with my GP who sent me for a consultation with a surgeon.

That's when I was told I was obese. They would only do the surgery if I lost 20 kilos. I was so offended. I left the surgery swearing I'd never go back. But I swallowed my pride and went back. I'd only lost a couple of kilos by that time but, after I explained the constraints of my job, the doctor agreed to perform the surgery. It was a great success. She removed three kilos of breast tissue and I have minimal scarring. That might not sound a lot, but it's made a world of difference to my self-esteem and my life in general. I have no more back or neck pain. I now wish I'd done it years ago. It's a radical way to lose three kilos, but it was also a real wake-up call about my weight and my health.

cholesterol and blood pressure

Fortunately, my blood pressure has always been on the average to low side, while my cholesterol levels are a bit high, and were particularly at the beginning of this diet, when I was at my all-time heaviest and unfittest. It's really important to know and understand your blood pressure and cholesterol. Ask your doctor to explain in detail what it all means.

Catherine says:

the glycaemic index and your weight

What is the Glycaemic Index?

The Glycaemic Index (or GI) is a ranking of foods from 0 to 100 that tells us whether a carbohydrate food will raise blood sugar (glucose) levels dramatically, moderately or just a little. It is a measure of how a carbohydrate will affect blood sugar levels.

Carbohydrates that are digested and absorbed slowly (such as lentils or pasta) release glucose into the bloodstream gradually – these are low-GI carbohydrate foods. They have a GI value of 55 or less.

Carbohydrates that are digested and absorbed quickly (like white bread and potato) cause a fast release of glucose – these carbohydrate foods are high GI. Their GI figures are over 70.

Carbohydrates that fall in between these two extremes, with values ranging from 56 to 69, are classified as moderate GI. Examples are long-grain rice, sugar and raisins.

Go slow, go low GI

Too much processed food – particularly carbohydrates – is now believed to be a key factor in the rising numbers of overweight and obese Australian adults and children.

Highly processed carbohydrates are usually high GI, but not always. They enter the bloodstream quickly, raising blood sugar levels and triggering a surge of insulin. They flow through our bodies quickly but leave us feeling hungry soon after.

If you eat a lot of these, it will be hard for you to lose weight as you'll probably be feeling hungry much of the time. The solution? Swap your carbohydrates from high-GI to low-GI

types. It will make your diet more satisfying and filling without adding extra kilojoules (see table for easy swaps). For example, a potato has around the same amount of carbohydrate and kilojoules as pasta but the pasta takes longer to be digested so delays the return of hunger before the next meal.

What to aim for
Low GI choices

High GI (quickly digested)	Lower GI alternative (slowly digested)
Refined breakfast cereals (ie, puffed rice, corn flakes or wheat flakes)	Rolled oats (not instant) OR oat-based cereal like muesli Bran-based cereal OR sprinkle rice bran or oat bran over your usual cereal
Bread (white or fine wholemeal)	Bread with whole grains, like oat bran with barley, heavy rye (black bread) and pumpernickel Pitta bread Sourdough or stoneground flour breads
Puffed crispbreads and water crackers	Wholegrain crispbreads
Rice (calrose and jasmine)	rice or basmati rice Pearl barley, cracked wheat, buckwheat
Potato *	Pasta**, noodles, sweet potato, legumes

* baby new potatoes cooked until just tender are low GI

** cooked al dente

Not every carbohydrate you eat needs to be a 'slow carb'. Just aim for one low-GI food at each meal and you will significantly lower the GI of your total diet and improve heart health. For example, at dinner add some soy beans to your lamb curry or cook pasta in place of potato.

A new food-labelling program has recently been launched to help consumers identify the GI values of foods in the supermarket. Known as The Glycemic Index Symbol Program, it aims to help people make informed food choices via the use of an easily recognisable GI symbol on foods. To find out more, visit the website at www.gisymbol.com

---

How to work out the GI

There is no way of estimating what GI figure a food will have, as many factors influence the GI, including:

- the type of starch in the carbohydrate (amylose is more slowly digested than amylopectin)
- the type of sugar (glucose is rapidly absorbed, whereas sucrose raises blood sugar levels moderately)
- whether the food is processed and by what method it is cooked
- whether there is any fat accompanying the carbohydrate, as fat slows the rate of stomach emptying and so slows digestion
- the presence of any viscous fibre accompanying the carbohydrate. This increases the viscosity of the contents of the intestines, slowing down the interaction between digestive enzymes and starch and so slowing digestion
- the acidity of the food. Acid foods such as vinegar, lemon juice, vinaigrette dressing and acidic fruits slow down the process of emptying the stomach.

CHAPTER FIVE: THE LAST WORD

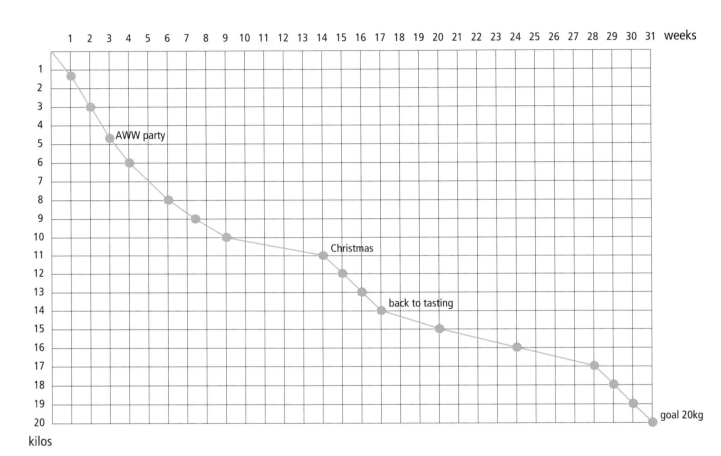

Above is a chart showing (in blue) Pamela's progress from the day she started her diet, until the day day she completed the book. The chart depicts a steady and gradual loss of weight, which is the healthiest way to achieve a long-term weight loss.

Having lost the 20 kilos I set out to lose when I started this diet (it took Pamela 31 weeks to lose this amount of weight), I'm feeling pretty fine. If you look at the graph above, you can see the progress I made. The loss averages 0.645 of a kilo per week, which is only a little bit more than the old-fashioned idea of losing a pound a week (ie, one pound equals 0.45kg).

I have always studiously avoided looking in mirrors, particularly those column-length ones in large stores. At home I'm used to the way I look in my mirrors, but the ones in changing rooms are seriously frightful. Now, I just get a shock if I accidentally see the new thinner me. Another great, if trivial, thing I've noticed about being thinner is that I can cross my legs now. I've always been amazed how women with long slim legs can wind them about each other, not once but twice. I may never get there, but that's okay!

Since beginning this book, I've been even more alert to stories in the press about obesity. No miracle drug has been found recently to help us beat the problem for good. There are stop-gap measures, pills and potions, but

I do know there are no magic formulas or amazingly different or weird combinations of food that are going to make us slimmer, and therefore healthier, in the long term. It's all about eating and exercising in a way that works for you.

I really do know how it feels to be overweight. I'm on your side and, from sharing just about everything I know about fat and dieting, I hope my story can help you achieve a slimmer, healthier, more positive you.

I haven't found this book easy to write; however, it has been an amazingly cleansing and comforting experience for me. By giving voice to some of my little faults and foibles, they're no longer such huge issues for me to deal with. A long time ago I read about the therapy people found when they wrote troublesome things down on paper. At the time, I thought it was probably what I call psycho-babble but, if you're anything like me, perhaps you should give the idea of writing things down a go. That's if you've got time, what with the exercising, the cooking, the eating, and all the shopping for your wardrobe of new clothes!

MY QUICK AND EASY MEAL IDEAS

Here are some really simple weeknight meals that I cook for myself – not proper recipes, just quick and easy ideas. Any of these ideas can be substituted for the main-course recipes I've suggested in the Meal Planner on pages 41-45. The meals below will serve one person.

beef

200g of your favourite lean steak (fillet, rump, rib-eye, any grilling or barbecuing quality cut). Grill, barbecue or pan-fry (grease the pan with a little spray oil) until cooked as desired. Wrap beef in foil, stand 5 minutes before serving. Lean mince is fine too, made into burgers, patties, rissoles or sauces such as bolognese.

chicken

200g of your favourite lean skinless cuts (thigh cutlets or fillets, breast fillets or breast on the bone, schnitzels, drumsticks, drumettes). Grill, barbecue, pan-fry or stir-fry (grease the pan or wok with a little spray oil), microwave, poach, steam (foil-wrapped in the oven is fine) or bake until cooked through.

eggs

Eggs are a wonderful source of protein. I've been eating, on average, eight eggs per week either boiled for lunch, or in the form of an omelette or frittata.

fish

200g of your favourite fish (cutlets, steaks or fillets). Grill, barbecue, pan-fry (grease the pan with a little spray oil) microwave, poach or steam (foil-wrapped in the oven is fine) until just barely cooked. Wrap the fish in foil, stand 5 minutes before serving. Serve fish topped with chopped herbs (see opposite) plus a good squeeze of lemon or lime juice.

lamb

200g of your favourite lean cut (chops of any kind, cutlets, backstrap, fillets or steaks). Grill, barbecue or pan-fry (grease the pan with a little spray oil) until cooked as desired. Wrap lamb in foil, stand 5 minutes before serving.

pork

200g of your favourite lean cut (chops of any kind, fillet, schnitzels, steaks). Grill, barbecue or pan-fry (grease the pan with a little spray oil) until just barely cooked. Wrap pork in foil, stand 5 minutes before serving.

veal

200g of your favourite lean cut (chops, cutlets, fillet, schnitzels, steaks). Grill, barbecue or pan-fry (grease the pan with a little spray oil) until just barely cooked. Wrap veal in foil, stand 5 minutes before serving.

accompaniments from the unrestricted list

If you're not using any of the recipes in this book for your main course, and you decide to cook something from the suggestions I've just made, choose two of these accompaniments. Don't forget to add a fresh herb mix, too (see column, right).

Asian greens: Chinese broccoli, choy sum, bok choy and tat soi are all delicious; eat all of the vegetables – stems, leaves, the lot. Stir-fry, microwave or steam for the best results.

Asparagus: Snap the tough ends off, then wash and microwave. They'll take 1 minute to cook on HIGH (100%).

Broccoli, cauliflower and broccolini: Eat as much of these as you like. Steam or microwave them until they're barely cooked, around 2 minutes on HIGH (100%).

Cabbage: Cook a rasher of chopped lean bacon in a saucepan until it's crisp, add a clove of crushed garlic and two finely chopped green onions. Add about 240g finely shredded cabbage, cover the pan with a tight-fitting lid and cook over a high heat, shaking the pan occasionally, for about 2 minutes, or until the cabbage is barely wilted.

Coleslaw: You need about 240g finely shredded cabbage of any kind, add one small grated carrot, half a small chopped red pepper, two finely chopped green onions, 35g finely chopped parsley (and/or mint and coriander). Mix in the juice of half a lemon combined with 2 teaspoons olive oil.

Courgette: Coarsely grate two medium (any colour) courgettes; finely grate about 1 teaspoon lemon rind; crush a clove of garlic. Heat a large frying pan, coat it with a little spray oil, then spread the courgettes, rind and garlic over the base of the hot pan. Cook over a high heat for 2 minutes, moving about with a fork all the time, until just wilted. Serve immediately.

Fresh herb mix: I've talked about this often enough, so I'd better tell you precisely what I do. This is a typical mix for me. I wash and dry a large bunch of flat-leaf parsley, chop off all the leafy top part of the bunch, along with some stalks, toss them into a food processor with six trimmed green onions, process them until they're coarsely chopped, then put them into a small plastic airtight container and keep them in the fridge; they will last three to four days. I add other freshly chopped herbs to this mix depending on what I'm eating. If it's lamb, I add rosemary, mint and/or basil; if it's chicken I add tarragon, basil or coriander; if it's fish, I add coriander, dill or tarragon; if it's beef, I add basil or coriander; if it's veal and pork, I add coriander and/or basil. So much depends on which cuisines I'm visiting at the time. I think herbs are a wonderful addition to any meal; they just tie the flavours together and give plain food such a boost. Sometimes I add finely chopped celery, garlic, garlic chives, chilli or some finely shredded lime leaves; it just depends on what I feel like. These herbs are my favourites, as I like their fresh flavours, but you can use whatever you prefer. You should always try to think of herbs as an additional vegetable for the meal, not just a garnish.

Mushrooms: You need about 100g mushrooms, whatever type and size you like; I leave the baby ones whole and coarsely chop the larger ones. Chop a small brown onion, crush a clove of garlic, and cook in a saucepan with 1 teaspoon olive oil or butter. When the onion is soft, add the mushrooms, cover the pan with a tight-fitting lid, and cook over a low heat for about 10 minutes, or until the mushrooms are as soft as you like them. Remove the lid and continue to cook until any liquid evaporates; toss in a handful of chopped parsley.

Quick ratatouille: I used to be dedicated to making 'rat' the proper slow way, but these days I throw all the components into a saucepan, or a casserole dish, and just let them stew away for at least 30 minutes; longer, up to an hour, if I have the time. All the ingredients are coarsely chopped: they are two medium brown onions, three peppers (any colours), one large peeled aubergine, 1kg fresh tomatoes, a 440g can crushed tomatoes, three medium courgettes (I half peel these, in stripes). If I decide to cook the 'rat' in the oven, I cook it in a moderately slow oven in a covered casserole dish for about 1½ hours. Once it's cooked, I add two cloves crushed garlic and season it. Keep the ratatouille in an airtight container in the refrigerator for up to a week.

Salads: Make as large a salad as you like from the Unrestricted list of goodies. If you like a dressing on your salad, an easy, low-fat one can be whipped up quickly. Combine 80ml lemon or lime juice in a jar with a crushed clove of garlic, 1 teaspoon dijon mustard, 1 teaspoon olive oil, a tiny pinch of sugar and a little salt and pepper. Give the jar a good shake, then toss the dressing through the salad just before you eat.

Stir-fry: I often stir-fry vegies and add some Asian flavourings; you can eat quite a wide variety of vegies at one meal this way. Choose anything you like from the Unrestricted list, but here's a combination I like. Make sure you have everything ready – all the vegies prepared before you start to cook – as the actual cooking time will only be about 5 minutes. Coat a wok with cooking oil spray, heat 1 teaspoon sesame oil in the wok, add a clove of crushed garlic, 1 teaspoon grated fresh ginger, two finely chopped spring onions, a tiny pinch of sugar, salt, pepper and a small brown onion; stir-fry until the onion is barely soft. Add half a small red pepper, half a small green pepper, one stick of celery, quarter of a bunch of broccolini (or cauliflower or broccoli florets) and a handful of baby mushrooms; stir-fry until the broccolini is barely tender. Finally, add about 60g bean sprouts (or finely shredded Chinese cabbage). Add a dash of soy sauce if you like.

Tomato and onion sauce: If I feel like something saucy over steak, chops or chicken, I slice a medium brown onion, cook it in 1 teaspoon olive oil, in a saucepan with the lid on, until it's really soft; this takes at least 10 minutes. Then I toss in three medium chopped flavoursome tomatoes; sometimes I take the skins off, other times I don't bother. Cook these with the lid on until the mixture is really soft and pulpy, a good 30 minutes, or longer if you have the time. Then add a clove of crushed garlic, salt and pepper, and 2 teaspoons tomato sauce. The sugar in the tomato sauce rounds out any sharpness or acidity in the sauce. Finally, add some finely shredded basil, about 2 tablespoons. Even though tomatoes are at their best, nutritionally speaking, eaten raw, they're just lovely this way.

MENU PLANNERS

Week 1

	MONDAY	TUESDAY	WEDNESDAY	THURSDAY	FRIDAY	SATURDAY	SUNDAY
breakfast	55g low-carb muesli, topped with a heaped teaspoon yogurt, add enough skim milk to moisten muesli, top with a little dried, fresh or stewed fruit taken out of your daily ration of the equivalent of five pieces of fresh fruit per day and 55g dried fruit of your choice. Tea or coffee					Tropical fruit salad, p53	Breakfast fry-up, p52
snack	Two pieces of fresh fruit from your daily ration of the equivalent of five pieces of fresh fruit per day. OR dried fruit of your choice, from your ration of 55g per day and/or 55g nuts of your choice (see page 27 for more information on nuts).						
lunch	Lunchbox salad (see page 27 for ideas and variations).					Sweet chilli and lime mixed vegetable salad, p63	Thai char-grilled beef salad, p60
snack	Same as morning snack, eat fruit and/or nuts from your daily rations.						
dinner	Lamb (see meal ideas on p38) OR Teriyaki lamb stir-fry, p86	Fish (see meal ideas on p38) OR Fish Provençale with herbed fresh tomato, p71	Chicken (see meal ideas on p38) OR Tarragon chicken with carrot mash and leek, p78	Pork or beef (see meal ideas on p38) OR Roasted pork fillets with orange salad, p84	Fish (see meal ideas on p38) OR Salmon steaks with fennel salad, p75	Vietnamese beef, chicken and tofu soup, p98	Vegetable curry with yogurt, p105
snack	Eat whatever is left from the day's rations of fresh fruit, dried fruit and nuts.						

Week 2

	MONDAY	TUESDAY	WEDNESDAY	THURSDAY	FRIDAY	SATURDAY	SUNDAY
breakfast	As for week 1					Spiced plums with yogurt, p54	Bacon and asparagus frittata, p47
snack	As for week 1						
lunch	As for week 1					Chicken and vegetable soup, p56	Salade niçoise, p58
snack	As for week 1						
dinner	Veal or beef OR Veal and mushroom casserole, p95	Fish OR Prawn, scallop and asparagus salad with ginger dressing, p67	Beef OR Beef steaks with green pepper salsa, p101	Pork or lamb OR Pork and broccolini stir-fry, p82	Fish OR Fish and spinach with olive and basil sauce, p69	Lamb shanks in five-spice, tamarind and ginger, p90	Portuguese-style chicken thighs, p79
snack	As for week 1						

Week 3

	MONDAY	TUESDAY	WEDNESDAY	THURSDAY	FRIDAY	SATURDAY	SUNDAY
breakfast	As for week 1					Scrambled eggs with dill and smoked salmon, p50	Baked ricotta with roasted tomato, page 51
snack	As for week 1						
lunch	As for week 1					Mussels with basil and lemon grass, p59	Sang choy bow, p61
snack	As for week 1						
dinner	Fish OR Swordfish with Thai dressing, p72	Beef OR Ginger beef stir-fry, p103	Fish or lamb OR Fish fillets with pancetta and caper herb butter, p70	Pork or chicken OR Chilli pork with oyster sauce, p81	Veal OR Veal steaks with lemon thyme sauce, p93	Lamb steaks with walnut gremolata tomatoes, p87	Lemon pepper chicken with courgette salad, p80
snack	As for week 1						

Week 4

	MONDAY	TUESDAY	WEDNESDAY	THURSDAY	FRIDAY	SATURDAY	SUNDAY
breakfast	As for week 1					Egg-white omelette, p48	Poached eggs with bacon, spinach and pecorino, p49
snack	As for week 1						
lunch	As for week 1					Stir-fried aubergine and tofu, p62	Smoked salmon and roasted vegetables, p57
snack	As for week 1						
dinner	Pork OR Pork, lime and peanut salad, p83	Fish OR Mixed vegetable and herb frittata, p104	Lamb OR Grilled lamb steak with ratatouille, p92	Fish OR Tuna with peas and spring onion, p73	Chicken OR Chicken and Thai basil stir-fry, p77	Beef and vegetable teppanyaki, p96	Barbecued balsamic and garlic octopus, p65
snack	As for week 1						

BREAKFAST RECIPES

bacon and asparagus frittata

PREPARATION TIME: 15 minutes
COOKING TIME: 45 minutes

4 bacon rashers (280g), rind removed, sliced thickly
1 large red onion (300g), sliced thinly
170g asparagus, trimmed, halved lengthways
4 eggs
4 egg whites
250ml buttermilk

1   Preheat oven to moderate. Oil deep 19cm-square cake pan; line base and sides with baking paper.

2   Cook bacon, stirring, in small heated frying pan until crisp; drain on absorbent paper. Add onion to same pan; cook, stirring, until soft. Layer bacon, onion and asparagus in prepared pan.

3   Whisk eggs, egg whites and buttermilk in medium jug; pour into pan. Cook, uncovered, in moderate oven about 35 minutes or until frittata is set. Stand 10 minutes before serving.

SERVES 4

PER SERVING   8.5g carbohydrate; 11.6g total fat (4.3g sat. fat); 1349kJ (322 cal); 45.6g protein

CARB TIP   Serve with toasted sourdough.

egg-white omelette

PREPARATION TIME: 25 minutes
COOKING TIME: 20 minutes

12 egg whites
4 spring onions, chopped finely
2 tablespoons finely chopped fresh chives
2 tablespoons finely chopped fresh chervil
2 tablespoons finely chopped fresh flat-leaf parsley
60g coarsely grated cheddar cheese
60g coarsely grated mozzarella cheese

1 Beat a quarter of the egg whites in small bowl with electric mixer until soft peaks form; fold in a quarter of the combined onion and herbs.

2 Pour mixture into 20cm heated oiled frying pan; cook, uncovered, over medium heat until omelette is just browned lightly on the bottom.

3 Sprinkle a quarter of the combined cheeses on half of the omelette. Place pan under preheated grill until cheese begins to melt and omelette sets; fold omelette over to completely cover cheese. Carefully slide omelette onto serving plate; cover to keep warm.

4 Repeat process three times with remaining egg white, onion and herb mixture, and cheese.

SERVES 4

PER SERVING 1.1g carbohydrate; 7.9g total fat (5g sat. fat);
620kJ (148 cal); 18.2g protein

CARB TIP Serve with roasted tomatoes and toast.

poached eggs with
bacon, spinach & pecorino

PREPARATION TIME: 5 minutes
COOKING TIME: 10 minutes

600g spinach, trimmed, chopped coarsely
4 bacon rashers (280g), rind removed
4 eggs
40g shaved pecorino cheese

1 Boil, steam or microwave spinach until just wilted; drain. Cover to keep warm.

2 Meanwhile, cook bacon in heated large frying pan until crisp; drain on absorbent paper. Cover to keep warm.

3 Half-fill the same pan with water; bring to a boil. Break eggs into cup, one at a time, then slide into pan. When all eggs are in pan, allow water to return to a boil. Cover pan, turn off heat; stand about 4 minutes or until a light film of egg white sets over yolks. Remove eggs, one at a time, using slotted spoon; place spoon on absorbent-paper-lined saucer to blot up poaching liquid.

4 Divide spinach among serving plates; top spinach with bacon, egg then cheese.

SERVES 4

PER SERVING   0.8g carbohydrate; 13.1g total fat (5.2g sat. fat); 813kJ (194 cal); 18.5g protein

CARB TIP   Serve on toasted Turkish bread.

scrambled eggs
with dill and smoked salmon

PREPARATION TIME: 5 minutes
COOKING TIME: 5 minutes

8 eggs
125ml milk
1 tablespoon finely chopped fresh dill
10g butter
300g sliced smoked salmon

1 Whisk eggs in medium bowl; add milk and dill, whisk until combined.

2 Melt butter in medium frying pan; cook egg mixture over low heat, stirring gently, until mixture is just set.

3 Serve scrambled eggs with salmon.

SERVES 4

PER SERVING 1.8g carbohydrate; 17.2g total fat (6.1g sat. fat); 1179kJ (282 cal); 31.1g protein

CARB TIP Serve with small buckwheat pancakes, sour cream and finely chopped red onion.

baked ricotta with roasted tomatoes

PREPARATION TIME: 10 minutes
COOKING TIME: 15 minutes

2 teaspoons olive oil
1 tablespoon pine nuts
2 cloves garlic, crushed
100g baby spinach leaves
250g low-fat ricotta cheese
1 egg, beaten lightly
2 tablespoons coarsely chopped fresh chives
500g cherry tomatoes
1 tablespoon balsamic vinegar

1 Preheat oven to hot. Oil four holes of a six-hole $1/3$-cup (80ml) muffin pan.

2 Heat half of the oil in medium frying pan; cook nuts and half of the garlic, stirring over low heat, until fragrant. Add spinach; stir until spinach wilts. Cool 10 minutes.

3 Combine spinach mixture in medium bowl with cheese, egg and chives; divide among prepared holes. Bake, uncovered, in hot oven about 15 minutes or until cheese browns lightly.

4 Meanwhile, combine tomatoes and vinegar with remaining oil and remaining garlic in small shallow baking dish. Roast, uncovered, in hot oven 10 minutes. Serve baked ricotta with roasted tomatoes.

SERVES 4

PER SERVING   4g carbohydrate; 11.8g total fat (4.4g sat. fat);
686kJ (164 cal); 10.5g protein

CARB TIP   Serve with toasted ciabatta.

breakfast fry-up

PREPARATION TIME: 10 minutes
COOKING TIME: 20 minutes

4 medium plum tomatoes (300g), quartered
2 tablespoons balsamic vinegar
cooking-oil spray
300g mushrooms, sliced thickly
2 tablespoons loosely packed fresh basil leaves, torn
2 tablespoons loosely packed fresh coriander leaves
2 tablespoons loosely packed fresh flat-leaf parsley leaves
200g shaved ham

1   Preheat oven to moderately hot.

2   Combine tomato and half of the vinegar in medium shallow oiled
    baking dish; spray with oil. Roast, uncovered, in moderately hot oven
    20 minutes.

3   Meanwhile, combine mushrooms with remaining vinegar in medium bowl.
    Cook mushroom mixture, stirring, in oiled medium frying pan until tender;
    stir in herbs. Transfer to serving dishes; cover to keep warm.

4   Place ham in same pan; heat, stirring gently. Serve ham and tomato with
    mushroom mixture.

SERVES 4

PER SERVING   2.6g carbohydrate; 2.9g total fat (0.7g sat. fat);
                  380kJ (91 cal); 13g protein

CARB TIP   Serve with thick slices of toast.

tropical fruit salad

PREPARATION TIME: 10 minutes
COOKING TIME: 20 minutes (plus refrigeration time)

500ml water
3 cardamom pods, bruised
4cm piece fresh ginger (20g), quartered
1 teaspoon finely grated lemon rind
1 tablespoon lemon juice
1 tablespoon lime juice
1 vanilla bean, split lengthways
½ medium canteloupe (rockmelon) (850g), chopped coarsely
1 small papaya (600g), chopped coarsely
3 medium kiwi fruit (255g), sliced thickly
1 medium mango (430g), chopped coarsely
80ml passionfruit pulp

1   Place the water, cardamom, ginger, rind and juices into medium frying pan. Scrape vanilla seeds into pan then add pod; bring to a boil. Reduce heat; simmer, uncovered, without stirring, 20 minutes. Strain syrup into medium jug; discard spices and pod. Cool 10 minutes. Refrigerate, covered, until syrup is cold.

2   Just before serving, place syrup and remaining ingredients in large bowl; toss gently to combine.

SERVES 4

PER SERVING   30.6g carbohydrate; 0.6g total fat (0g sat. fat); 607kJ (145 cal); 3.4g protein
CARB TIP   Serve with thick Greek-style yogurt.

spiced plums with yogurt

PREPARATION TIME: 10 minutes
COOKING TIME: 10 minutes *(plus cooling time)*

1 litre water
125ml orange juice
75g caster sugar
5cm strip orange rind
2 star anise
4 cloves
1 teaspoon mixed spice
1 cinnamon stick
1 vanilla bean, split lengthways
8 blood (purple) plums (900g), unpeeled
375g yogurt

1   Place the water, juice, sugar, rind and spices in medium frying pan. Scrape vanilla seeds into pan then add pod; cook mixture, stirring, without boiling, until sugar dissolves.

2   Add plums to pan; poach, uncovered, over low heat about 10 minutes or until just tender. Using slotted spoon, place two plums in each of four serving dishes (reserve 2 tablespoons of the poaching liquid). Cool plums 20 minutes.

3   Combine yogurt and reserved poaching liquid in small bowl; serve mixture with plums.

SERVES 4

PER SERVING   39.1g carbohydrate; 3.4g total fat (2.1g sat. fat); 906kJ (217 cal); 57g protein

CARB TIP   Serve with raisin toast.

LUNCH & LIGHT MEAL RECIPES

chicken and vegetable soup

PREPARATION TIME: 25 minutes
COOKING TIME: 20 minutes

500ml water
1.5 litres chicken stock
1 medium carrot (120g), diced into 1cm pieces
2 trimmed celery stalks (200g), sliced thinly
½ small cauliflower (500g), cut into florets
350g chicken breast fillets, sliced thinly
2 large courgettes (300g), cut into 1-cm pieces
150g sugar snaps, trimmed, sliced thinly
3 spring onions, sliced thinly

1   Combine the water and stock in large saucepan; bring to a boil. Add carrot, celery and cauliflower; return to a boil. Reduce heat; simmer, covered, about 10 minutes or until vegetables are just tender.

2   Add chicken and courgettes; cook, covered, about 5 minutes or until chicken is cooked through.

3   Stir in peas and onion.

SERVES 4

PER SERVING   10.2g carbohydrate; 4g total fat (1.3g sat. fat); 794kJ (190 cal); 28.2g protein

CARB TIP   Add macaroni to soup with chicken and courgettes.

smoked salmon and roasted vegetables

PREPARATION TIME: 10 minutes
COOKING TIME: 15 minutes

2 large red peppers (700g)
6 baby aubergines (360g)
4 medium courgettes (480g)
250g rocket leaves
200g sliced smoked salmon
1 teaspoon finely grated lemon rind
2 teaspoons lemon juice

1   Quarter peppers; discard seeds and membranes. Roast under grill or in very hot oven, skin-side up, until skin blisters and blackens. Cover with plastic or paper for 5 minutes; peel away skin. Slice pepper thinly.

2   Meanwhile, slice aubergines and courgettes lengthways. Place aubergines and courgettes, in single layer, on oiled oven trays. Place under hot grill or in very hot oven until browned lightly both sides.

3   Divide roasted vegetables, rocket and salmon among serving plates; sprinkle with rind; drizzle with juice.

SERVES 4

PER SERVING   11g carbohydrate; 3.6g total fat (0.5g sat. fat);
614kJ (147 cal); 17.6g protein

CARB TIP   Serve with lavash.

salade niçoise

PREPARATION TIME: 20 minutes
COOKING TIME: 10 minutes

200g green beans, trimmed, sliced thickly
250g cherry tomatoes, halved
80g seeded black olives
2 cucumbers (260g), sliced thinly
1 medium red onion (170g), sliced thinly
150g mesclun
6 hard-boiled eggs, quartered
425g can tuna in springwater

light vinaigrette
1 teaspoon olive oil
60ml lemon juice
1 clove garlic, crushed
2 teaspoons dijon mustard

1 Boil, steam or microwave beans until just tender; drain. Rinse under cold water; drain.

2 Meanwhile, make light vinaigrette. Place ingredients in screw-top jar; shake well.

3 Place tomato, olives, cucumber, onion, mesclun and eggs in large bowl with vinaigrette; toss gently to combine. Divide salad among serving plates.

4 Carefully turn tuna out of can into colander; cut into wedge-shaped quarters. Place one wedge of tuna on each salad.

SERVES 4

PER SERVING 10.9g carbohydrate; 13.8g total fat (3.2g sat. fat); 1496kJ (358 cal); 46.8g protein

CARB TIP Add a 400g can of rinsed, drained cannellini beans.

mussels with basil and lemon grass

PREPARATION TIME: 20 minutes
COOKING TIME: 10 minutes

1kg large black mussels (approximately 30)

2 teaspoons peanut oil

1 medium brown onion (150g), chopped finely

2 cloves garlic, crushed

10cm stick (20g) thinly sliced fresh lemon grass

1 fresh small red Thai chilli, chopped finely

250ml dry white wine

2 tablespoons lime juice

2 tablespoons fish sauce

60g loosely packed fresh Thai basil leaves

125ml coconut milk

1 fresh small red Thai chilli, sliced thinly

2 spring onions, sliced thinly

1   Scrub mussels under cold water; remove beards.

2   Heat oil in wok; stir-fry brown onion, garlic, lemon grass and chopped chilli until onion softens and mixture is fragrant.

3   Add wine, juice and sauce; bring to a boil. Add mussels, reduce heat; simmer, covered, about 5 minutes or until mussels open (discard any that do not).

4   Meanwhile, shred half of the basil finely. Add shredded basil and coconut milk to wok; stir-fry until heated through. Place mussel mixture in large serving bowl; sprinkle with sliced chilli, green onion and remaining basil.

SERVES 4

PER SERVING   6.7g carbohydrate; 9.8g total fat (6.4g sat. fat); 781kJ (187 cal); 8.2g protein

CARB TIP   Serve with a loaf of ciabatta.

Thai char-grilled beef salad

PREPARATION TIME: 20 minutes *(plus refrigeration and standing time)*
COOKING TIME: 5 minutes

600g piece beef rump steak
2 teaspoons sesame oil
80ml kecap manis (sweet soy sauce)
120g loosely packed fresh mint leaves
120g loosely packed fresh coriander leaves
60g loosely packed fresh Thai basil leaves
6 spring onions, sliced thinly
5 shallots (125g), sliced thinly
250g cherry tomatoes, halved
1 cucumber (400g), seeded, sliced thinly
10 fresh kaffir lime leaves, shredded finely
100g mesclun

sweet and sour dressing
125ml lime juice
60ml fish sauce
1 teaspoon sugar
2 fresh small red Thai
chillies, sliced thinly

1   Place beef in medium shallow dish; brush all over with combined oil and kecap manis. Cover; refrigerate 30 minutes.

2   Meanwhile, place herbs, onion, shallot, tomato and cucumber in large bowl; toss gently to combine.

3   Make sweet and sour dressing. Place ingredients in screw-top jar; shake well.

4   Cook beef on heated oiled grill plate (or grill or barbecue) until cooked as desired. Cover beef; stand 10 minutes. Slice thinly.

5   Place beef, lime leaves and mesclun in bowl with herb mixture and dressing; toss gently to combine.

SERVES 4

PER SERVING   11.3g carbohydrate; 13.1g total fat (4.9g sat. fat); 1354kJ (324 cal); 39g protein

CARB TIP   Serve with bean thread noodles.

sang choy bow

PREPARATION TIME: 15 minutes
COOKING TIME: 10 minutes

1 tablespoon sesame oil

1 medium brown onion (150g), chopped finely

2 cloves garlic, crushed

300g pork mince

300g veal mince

60ml soy sauce

60ml oyster sauce

1 medium red pepper (150g), chopped finely

240g bean sprouts

3 spring onions, chopped coarsely

1 tablespoon toasted sesame seeds

8 large iceberg lettuce leaves

1   Heat oil in wok; cook brown onion and garlic, stirring, until onion softens. Add pork and veal mince; cook, stirring, until mince is just browned.

2   Add sauces and red pepper, reduce heat; simmer, uncovered, stirring occasionally, 3 minutes.

3   Just before serving, stir in sprouts, spring onion and seeds. Divide mince mixture among lettuce leaves. Serve immediately.

SERVES 4

PER SERVING   10.1g carbohydrate; 17.2g total fat (4.9g sat. fat); 1463kJ (350 cal); 37.9g protein

CARB TIP   Serve with fried chow mein noodles.

stir-fried aubergine and tofu

PREPARATION TIME: 15 minutes *(plus standing time)*
COOKING TIME: 15 minutes

1 large aubergine (400g)
1 tablespoon cooking salt
300g fresh firm silken tofu
2 teaspoons peanut oil
1 medium brown onion (150g), cut into thin wedges
1 clove garlic, crushed
2 fresh small red Thai chillies, sliced thinly
1 tablespoon grated palm sugar
850g gai larn (Chinese broccoli), chopped coarsely
2 tablespoons lime juice
80ml soy sauce
35g coarsely chopped fresh Thai basil

1   Cut unpeeled aubergine in half lengthways; cut each half into thin slices. Place aubergine in colander, sprinkle with salt; stand 30 minutes.

2   Meanwhile, pat tofu all over with absorbent paper; cut into 2cm squares. Spread tofu, in single layer, on absorbent-paper-lined tray; cover tofu with more absorbent paper, stand at least 10 minutes.

3   Rinse aubergine under cold water; pat dry with absorbent paper.

4   Heat oil in wok; stir-fry onion, garlic and chilli until onion softens. Add sugar; stir-fry until dissolved. Add aubergine; stir-fry, 1 minute. Add gai larn; stir-fry until just wilted. Add tofu, juice and soy; stir-fry gently, until heated through. Remove from heat; toss basil through stir-fry.

SERVES 4

PER SERVING   10.5g carbohydrate; 7.9g total fat (1.2g sat. fat);
843kJ (181 cal); 16.6g protein

CARB TIP   Serve with steamed jasmine rice.

sweet chilli and lime mixed vegetable salad

PREPARATION TIME: 20 minutes
COOKING TIME: 5 minutes

200g asparagus, trimmed, chopped coarsely
100g fresh baby corn, sliced lengthways
1 small red pepper (150g), sliced thinly
100g fresh shiitake mushrooms, sliced thinly
1 cucumber (130g), seeded, sliced thinly
12 spring onions, sliced thinly
100g bean sprouts
1 fresh small red Thai chilli, sliced thinly
2 tablespoons finely chopped fresh coriander
2 tablespoons lime juice
1 tablespoon sweet chilli sauce
2 teaspoons sesame oil
2 teaspoons fish sauce
1 clove garlic, crushed

1 Boil, steam or microwave asparagus and corn, separately, until just tender; drain. Cool 10 minutes.

2 Place asparagus and corn in large bowl with red pepper, mushrooms, cucumber, onion, sprouts, chilli and coriander.

3 Place remaining ingredients in screw-top jar; shake well. Drizzle salad with dressing; toss gently to combine.

SERVES 4

PER SERVING 13.3g carbohydrate; 3g total fat (0.4g sat. fat); 385kJ (92 cal); 5.2g protein
CARB TIP Serve with bean thread noodles.

MAIN MEAL RECIPES

barbecued balsamic and garlic octopus

PREPARATION TIME: 20 minutes (plus refrigeration time)
COOKING TIME: 5 minutes

1kg cleaned baby octopus
2 cloves garlic, crushed
1 tablespoon olive oil
2 tablespoons balsamic vinegar
2 teaspoons brown sugar
2 teaspoons finely chopped fresh thyme
150g curly endive

1 Cut each octopus in half crossways. Combine garlic, half of the oil, half of the vinegar, sugar and thyme in large bowl, add octopus; toss to coat octopus in marinade. Cover; refrigerate 3 hours or overnight.

2 Cook octopus, in batches, on heated oiled grill plate (or grill or barbecue) until browned all over and just cooked through.

3 Serve octopus with curly endive, drizzled with combined remaining oil and remaining vinegar.

SERVES 4

PER SERVING   4.1g carbohydrate; 8.9g total fat (1.6g sat. fat); 1413kJ (338 cal); 59.7g protein

CARB TIP   Serve with crusty Italian bread.

minted prawn salad

PREPARATION TIME: 30 minutes

32 cooked medium king prawns (1.5kg)
1 cucumber (130g)
1 tablespoon fish sauce
60ml lime juice
125ml coconut milk
2 tablespoons caster sugar
1 clove garlic, crushed
2cm piece fresh ginger (10g), grated
1 fresh small red Thai chilli, sliced thinly
80g curly endive
60g watercress
160g bean sprouts
60g thinly sliced fresh mint

1   Shell and devein prawns, leaving tails intact. Halve cucumber lengthways, slice thinly on the diagonal.

2   Whisk sauce, juice, coconut milk, sugar, garlic, ginger and chilli in large bowl. Add prawns, cucumber and remaining ingredients; toss mixture gently to combine.

SERVES 4

PER SERVING   10.5g carbohydrate; 7.9g total fat (5.9g sat fat); 1183kJ (283 cal); 41.9g protein

CARB TIP   Serve with rice stick noodles.

prawn, scallop and asparagus salad with ginger dressing

PREPARATION TIME: 25 minutes
COOKING TIME: 10 minutes

400g uncooked medium king prawns
400g sea scallops
250g asparagus, trimmed, halved
35g coarsely chopped fresh chives
120g baby spinach leaves
1 large red pepper (350g), chopped coarsely

ginger dressing
5cm piece fresh ginger
    (25g), grated
2 teaspoons olive oil
2 tablespoons lemon juice
1 teaspoon sugar

1   Shell and devein prawns, leaving tails intact.

2   Cook prawns, scallops and asparagus, in batches, on heated oiled grill plate (or grill or barbecue) until cooked as desired.

3   Meanwhile, make ginger dressing. Press grated ginger between two spoons over small bowl to extract juice; discard fibres. Whisk in oil, juice and sugar.

4   Place prawns, scallops, asparagus, chives, spinach, red pepper and dressing in large bowl; toss gently to combine.

SERVES 4

PER SERVING   6g carbohydrate; 3.8g total fat (0.6g sat. fat); 702kJ (168 cal); 25g protein

CARB TIP   Serve with warmed ciabatta loaf.

chilli lime seafood stir-fry

PREPARATION TIME: 25 minutes
COOKING TIME: 15 minutes

200g squid hoods
200g firm white fish fillets
8 uncooked medium king prawns (360g)
200g cleaned baby octopus
1 tablespoon peanut oil
1 clove garlic, crushed
2 fresh small red Thai chillies, sliced thinly
1 medium carrot (120g), halved, sliced thinly
1 medium red pepper (200g), sliced thinly
1 tablespoon fish sauce
1 teaspoon oyster sauce
1 tablespoon lime juice
4 spring onions, sliced thinly

1   Cut squid down centre to open; score in a diagonal pattern. Cut squid and fish
    into 3cm pieces; shell and devein prawns, leaving tails intact. Cut each octopus
    in half crossways.

2   Heat half of the oil in wok; stir-fry seafood, in batches, until prawns are changed
    in colour, fish is cooked as desired, and squid and octopus are tender. Cover to
    keep warm.

3   Heat remaining oil in same wok; stir-fry garlic, chilli and carrot until carrot is
    just tender. Add red pepper; stir-fry until pepper is just tender. Return seafood to
    wok with sauces and juice; stir-fry gently, until heated through.

4   Serve stir-fry topped with onion.

SERVES 4

PER SERVING   4.5g carbohydrate; 7.5g total fat (1.6g sat. fat);
                  1056kJ (252 cal); 41.1g protein

CARB TIP   Serve with steamed white long-grain rice.

fish and spinach with olive and basil sauce

PREPARATION TIME: 5 minutes
COOKING TIME: 10 minutes

750g spinach, trimmed, chopped coarsely
2 teaspoons olive oil
4 x 200g firm white fish fillets
1 tablespoon lemon juice
¼ teaspoon dried chilli flakes
1 clove garlic, crushed
50g seeded black olives
35g finely shredded fresh basil

1   Boil, steam or microwave spinach until just wilted; drain. Cover to keep warm.

2   Meanwhile, heat half of the oil in large frying pan; cook fish until browned both sides and cooked as desired. Remove from pan; cover to keep warm.

3   Place remaining oil in same cleaned pan with remaining ingredients; cook, stirring, until heated through. Divide spinach among serving plates; top with fish, drizzle with olive and basil sauce.

SERVES 4

PER SERVING   3.6g carbohydrate; 7.1g total fat (1.8g sat. fat); 1058kJ (253 cal); 43.3g protein

CARB TIP   Serve with mashed potatoes.

fish fillets with pancetta and caper herb butter

PREPARATION TIME: 15 minutes
COOKING TIME: 10 minutes

40g butter, softened
1 tablespoon finely chopped fresh flat-leaf parsley
1 tablespoon drained capers, rinsed, chopped finely
2 cloves garlic, crushed
2 spring onions, chopped finely
4 x 200g white fish fillets
4 slices pancetta (60g)
2 teaspoons olive oil
250g asparagus, trimmed

1 Combine butter, parsley, capers, garlic and onion in small bowl.

2 Spread quarter of the butter mixture over each fillet; top with a slice of pancetta.

3 Heat oil in large frying pan; cook fish, pancetta side down, until pancetta is crisp. Turn fish carefully; cook, uncovered, until fish is cooked as desired.

4 Meanwhile, boil, steam or microwave asparagus until tender; drain.

5 Serve fish and asparagus drizzled with any pan juices.

SERVES 4

PER SERVING 1.4g carbohydrate; 17g total fat (7.9g sat. fat); 1417kJ (339 cal); 45g protein

CARB TIP Serve with polenta made with chopped parsley and cream.

fish Provençale with herbed fresh tomato

PREPARATION TIME: 10 minutes
COOKING TIME: 20 minutes

2 medium yellow courgettes (240g), quartered lengthways
3 medium green courgettes (360g), quartered lengthways
2 teaspoons olive oil
4 x 200g white fish fillets
2 medium plum tomatoes (150g), seeded, chopped finely
2 tablespoons lemon juice
1 tablespoon coarsely chopped fresh dill
1 tablespoon coarsely chopped fresh flat-leaf parsley
1 tablespoon coarsely chopped fresh tarragon

1 Boil, steam or microwave both courgettes until just tender; drain.

2 Meanwhile, heat half of the oil in large frying pan; cook fish, uncovered, until cooked as desired. Remove from pan; cover to keep warm.

3 Heat remaining oil in same cleaned pan; cook tomato and juice, stirring, until just heated through. Remove from heat; stir in herbs. Serve vegetables with fish and herbed tomato.

SERVES 4

PER SERVING 3g carbohydrate; 7.1g total fat (1.7g sat. fat); 1041kJ (249 cal); 42.8g protein

CARB TIP Serve with fettuccine.

swordfish with Thai dressing

PREPARATION TIME: 5 minutes
COOKING TIME: 10 minutes

4 x 200g swordfish steaks
⅓ cup (80ml) sweet chilli sauce
1 tablespoon fish sauce
125ml lime juice
5cm stick (10g) finely chopped fresh lemon grass
2 tablespoons finely chopped fresh coriander
60g finely chopped fresh mint
1cm piece fresh ginger (5g), grated
150g mesclun

1   Cook fish on heated oiled grill plate (or grill or barbecue) until cooked as desired.

2   Place sauces, juice, lemon grass, herbs and ginger in screw-top jar; shake well.
    Divide mesclun among serving plates; top with fish, drizzle with dressing.

SERVES 4

PER SERVING   5.3g carbohydrate; 5.1g total fat (1.4g sat. fat);
                  1012kJ (242 cal); 42.2g protein

CARB TIP   Serve with fresh rice noodles.

tuna with peas and spring onion

PREPARATION TIME: 15 minutes
COOKING TIME: 15 minutes

1 tablespoon vegetable oil

4 x 200g tuna steaks

2 cloves garlic, crushed

2 medium brown onions (300g), sliced thinly

180ml fish stock

2 tablespoons lemon juice

185g frozen peas

8 spring onions, cut into 4cm lengths

1 tablespoon finely grated lemon rind

1 teaspoon sea salt flakes

1 Heat half of the oil in heated large frying pan; cook fish until browned lightly both sides. Remove from pan; cover to keep warm.

2 Heat remaining oil in same pan; cook garlic and brown onion, stirring, until onion softens. Add stock, juice, peas and green onion; bring to a boil. Reduce heat; simmer, uncovered, 2 minutes.

3 Return fish to pan; sprinkle with rind and salt. Cook, uncovered, until fish is cooked as desired.

SERVES 4

PER SERVING 8.1g carbohydrate; 16.4g total fat (5.2g sat. fat); 1664kJ (398 cal); 55g protein

CARB TIP Serve with mashed potatoes.

red snapper parcels with caper anchovy salsa

PREPARATION TIME: 30 minutes
COOKING TIME: 15 minutes

2 cloves garlic, crushed
1 baby fennel bulb (130g), sliced thinly
4 x 200g red snapper fillets
4 large fresh basil leaves
⅓ cup (80ml) dry white wine
35g coarsely chopped fresh chives
35g loosely packed fresh tarragon leaves
40g loosely packed fresh basil leaves
60g loosely packed fresh chervil leaves
35g watercress
1 tablespoon lemon juice
1 teaspoon olive oil

caper anchovy salsa

1 small red pepper (150g), chopped finely
2 tablespoons finely chopped seeded black olives
1 tablespoon drained baby capers, rinsed
8 drained anchovy fillets, chopped finely
35g chopped fresh basil
1 tablespoon balsamic vinegar

1 Preheat oven to hot. Combine garlic and fennel in small bowl.

2 Place fillets, skin-side down, on four separate squares of lightly oiled foil large enough to enclose fish. Top each fillet with equal amounts of the fennel mixture; top each with one basil leaf, drizzle each with 1 tablespoon of the wine. Gather corners of foil squares together above each fish; twist to enclose securely.

3 Place parcels on oven tray; bake in hot oven about 15 minutes or until fish is cooked as desired.

4 Meanwhile, make caper anchovy salsa. Combine ingredients in small bowl.

5 Place remaining ingredients in medium bowl; toss gently to combine salad.

6 Unwrap parcels just before serving; divide fish, fennel-side up, among serving plates. Top with salsa; accompany with salad.

SERVES 4

PER SERVING	3.6g carbohydrate; 5.3g total fat (1.5g sat. fat); 1068kJ (255 cal); 43.9 protein
CARB TIP	Serve with sliced steamed potatoes.

salmon steaks with fennel salad

PREPARATION TIME: 20 minutes
COOKING TIME: 5 minutes

2 tablespoons red wine vinegar

2 teaspoons olive oil

2 teaspoons sugar

2 teaspoons dijon mustard

1 tablespoon finely chopped fresh chives

1 tablespoon finely chopped fresh dill

4 x 200g salmon steaks

200g baby spinach leaves

2 medium apples (300g), sliced thinly

2 baby fennel bulbs (260g), sliced thinly

1 cucumber (130g), seeded, sliced thinly

60g coarsely chopped fresh chives

35g coarsely chopped fresh dill

1   Place vinegar, oil, sugar and mustard in screw-top jar; shake well.

2   Combine 1 tablespoon of the dressing with finely chopped chives and finely chopped dill in large bowl, add fish; turn to coat fish in mixture. Cook fish in heated oiled large frying pan about 5 minutes each side or until fish is cooked as desired.

3   Place spinach, apple, fennel, cucumber, coarsely chopped chives and coarsely chopped dill in large bowl with remaining dressing; toss gently to combine. Serve fish with salad.

SERVES 4	
PER SERVING	11.3g carbohydrate; 16.8g total fat (3.5g sat fat); 1508kJ (360 cal); 41g protein
CARB TIP	Serve with rice stick noodles.

poached chicken with ruby grapefruit salad

PREPARATION TIME: 40 minutes
COOKING TIME: 10 minutes

625ml water
625ml chicken stock
700g chicken breast fillets
4 ruby red grapefruit (2kg)
1 small red onion (100g), cut into thin wedges
4 spring onions, sliced thinly
2 fresh small red Thai chillies, sliced thinly
1 cup coarsely chopped fresh coriander
35g toasted unsalted peanuts
100g baby spinach leaves
2 cloves garlic, crushed
1 tablespoon grated palm sugar
1 tablespoon lime juice
1 tablespoon soy sauce

1 Combine the water and stock in large frying pan; bring to a boil. Add chicken; return to a boil. Reduce heat; simmer, covered, about 10 minutes or until cooked through. Cool chicken in poaching liquid 10 minutes. Remove chicken from pan; discard poaching liquid. Slice chicken thinly.

2 Segment grapefruit over large bowl to catch juice; add grapefruit segments to bowl with chicken, onions, chilli, coriander, nuts and spinach.

3 Place remaining ingredients in small jug; whisk until sugar dissolves. Pour dressing over salad; toss gently to combine.

SERVES 4

PER SERVING 7g carbohydrate; 8g total fat (1.5g sat. fat); 1066kJ (255 cal); 37.8g protein

CARB TIP Rice stick noodles can be used as a bed for this salad.

chicken and Thai basil stir-fry

PREPARATION TIME: 20 minutes
COOKING TIME: 15 minutes

2 teaspoons peanut oil

600g chicken breast fillets, sliced thinly

2 cloves garlic, crushed

1cm piece fresh ginger (5g), grated

2 fresh small red Thai chillies, sliced thinly

4 fresh kaffir lime leaves, shredded finely

1 medium brown onion (150g), sliced thinly

100g mushrooms, quartered

1 large carrot (180g), sliced thinly

60ml oyster sauce

1 tablespoon soy sauce

1 tablespoon fish sauce

80ml chicken stock

80g bean sprouts

90g loosely packed fresh Thai basil leaves

1 Heat half of the oil in wok; stir-fry chicken, in batches, until browned all over and cooked through.

2 Heat remaining oil in wok; stir-fry garlic, ginger, chilli, lime leaves and onion until onion softens and mixture is fragrant. Add mushrooms and carrot; stir-fry until carrot is just tender. Return chicken to wok with sauces and stock; stir-fry until sauce thickens slightly. Remove from heat; toss sprouts and basil through stir-fry.

SERVES 4

PER SERVING   8.4g carbohydrate; 6.2g total fat (1.4g sat. fat); 1012kJ (242 cal); 37.8g protein

CARB TIP   Serve with steamed jasmine rice.

tarragon chicken with carrot mash and leek

PREPARATION TIME: 20 minutes *(plus refrigeration time)*
COOKING TIME: 25 minutes

Soak 12 bamboo skewers in water for about 1 hour before using to prevent them from scorching.

4 single chicken breast fillets (700g), sliced thickly
1 tablespoon finely chopped fresh tarragon
1 tablespoon wholegrain mustard
30g butter
2 large leeks (500g), trimmed, chopped finely
4 medium carrots (480g), chopped coarsely
375ml chicken stock
pinch nutmeg

1   Thread equal amounts of chicken onto 12 skewers. Using fingers, press combined tarragon and mustard all over chicken, cover skewers; refrigerate for 30 minutes.

2   Meanwhile, melt butter in large frying pan; cook leek, stirring, until softened. Cover to keep warm.

3   Preheat oven to moderately hot.

4   Boil or microwave carrot in stock until just tender; drain in strainer over small bowl. Reserve 180ml of the stock; discard the remainder. Blend or process carrot with nutmeg until smooth. Cover to keep warm.

5   Meanwhile, place chicken and reserved stock in large shallow baking dish; cook, uncovered, in moderately hot oven about 15 minutes or until chicken is cooked through.

6   Divide carrot mash among serving plates; top with chicken and leek.

SERVES 4	
PER SERVING	8.8g carbohydrate; 10.9g total fat (5.3g sat. fat); 1254kJ (300 cal); 41.8g protein
CARB TIP	Serve with potato and carrot mash.

Portuguese-style chicken thighs

PREPARATION TIME: 15 minutes
COOKING TIME: 15 minutes

8 chicken thigh fillets (800g), halved
3 medium oranges (720g), segmented
300g baby spinach leaves
1 medium red onion (170g), sliced thinly

spicy dressing
2 teaspoons cracked black pepper
1 fresh small red Thai chilli, chopped finely
½ teaspoon hot paprika
1 clove garlic, crushed
1 teaspoon finely grated orange rind
60ml orange juice
2 tablespoons red wine vinegar
2 teaspoons olive oil

1   Make spicy dressing. Combine ingredients in medium bowl. Reserve about a quarter of the dressing in small jug; use hands to rub remaining dressing over chicken pieces.

2   Cook chicken, in batches, on heated oiled grill plate (or grill or barbecue) until cooked through.

3   Toss orange segments, spinach and onion in large bowl. Divide among serving plates; top with chicken. Drizzle with reserved dressing.

SERVES 4

PER SERVING   14g carbohydrate; 17.1g total fat (4.7g sat fat); 1572kJ (376 cal); 41.2g protein

CARB TIP   Serve with slices of crusty bread.

lemon pepper chicken with courgette salad

PREPARATION TIME: 20 minutes
COOKING TIME: 40 minutes

1 tablespoon finely grated lemon rind
2 teaspoons cracked black pepper
80ml lemon juice
2 teaspoons olive oil
4 single chicken breast fillets (700g)
4 medium green courgettes (480g)
4 medium yellow courgettes (480g)
1 clove garlic, crushed
4 spring onions, chopped finely
1 cup coarsely chopped fresh flat-leaf parsley
35g coarsely chopped fresh tarragon

1   Combine rind, pepper, 1 tablespoon of the juice and half of the oil in medium bowl, add chicken; toss to coat chicken in marinade. Cover; refrigerate until required.

2   Peel courgettes randomly; slice into thin strips diagonally. Cook courgettes slices, in batches, on heated oiled grill plate (or grill or barbecue) until browned lightly and tender.

3   Cook chicken on same grill plate until cooked through.

4   Meanwhile, whisk remaining juice and remaining oil with garlic in large bowl. Add courgettes, onion and herbs to bowl; toss gently to combine.

5   Serve chicken with courgette salad.

SERVES 4	
PER SERVING	4.1g carbohydrate; 7.6g total fat (1.5g sat. fat); 1221kJ (292 cal); 50g protein
CARB TIP	Serve with steamed tiny new potatoes.

chilli pork with oyster sauce

PREPARATION TIME: 15 minutes
COOKING TIME: 20 minutes

2 teaspoons peanut oil

600g pork fillets, sliced thinly

1 medium white onion (150g), sliced thinly

1 clove garlic, crushed

1 large red pepper (350g), sliced thinly

1 small green courgette (90g), sliced thinly

1 small yellow courgette (90g), sliced thinly

60ml oyster sauce

1 tablespoon sweet chilli sauce

35g coarsely chopped fresh flat-leaf parsley

1　Heat oil in wok; stir-fry pork, in batches, until browned.

2　Stir-fry onion and garlic in same wok until onion softens. Add peppers and both courgettes; stir-fry until vegetables are just tender.

3　Return pork to wok. Add sauces; stir-fry until heated thorugh. Serve sprinkled with parsley.

SERVES 4

PER SERVING　10.3g carbohydrate; 6.2g total fat (1.6g sat. fat); 1016kJ (243 cal); 35.8g protein

CARB TIP　Serve with thick fresh rice noodles.

pork and broccolini stir-fry

PREPARATION TIME: 15 minutes
COOKING TIME: 20 minutes

2 teaspoons peanut oil
600g pork steaks, sliced thinly
2 medium red onions (340g), sliced thinly
2 medium red peppers (400g), sliced thinly
1 clove garlic, crushed
1cm piece fresh ginger (5g), grated
300g broccolini, halved
2 tablespoons lemon juice
60ml water
60ml sweet chilli sauce
1 teaspoon fish sauce
1 tablespoon soy sauce
1 teaspoon sesame oil
35g coarsely chopped fresh coriander

1   Heat half of the peanut oil in wok; stir-fry pork, in batches, until browned.

2   Heat remaining peanut oil in wok; stir-fry onion, peppers, garlic and ginger until vegetables are just tender.

3   Return pork to wok with broccolini, juice, the water, sauces and sesame oil; stir-fry about 2 minutes or until mixture boils. Remove from heat; stir in coriander just before serving.

SERVES 4

PER SERVING   12.7g carbohydrate; 6g total fat (1.2g sat. fat); 1137kJ (272 cal); 40.8g protein

CARB TIP   Serve with steamed jasmine rice.

pork, lime and peanut salad

PREPARATION TIME: 25 minutes (plus refrigeration time)
COOKING TIME: 15 minutes

60ml lime juice
4cm piece fresh ginger (20g), grated
800g pork fillets, sliced thinly
500g choy sum, chopped coarsely
2 tablespoons water
2 medium carrots (240g), cut into matchsticks
35g firmly packed fresh basil leaves
1 cup firmly packed fresh coriander leaves
4 spring onions, sliced thinly
35g coarsely chopped toasted
   unsalted peanuts

sweet chilli dressing
1 tablespoon fish sauce
1 tablespoon sweet chilli sauce
2 tablespoons lime juice
1 fresh small red Thai chilli,
   chopped finely

1   Combine juice and ginger in large bowl, add pork; toss pork to coat in marinade.
    Cover; refrigerate 3 hours or overnight.

2   Make sweet chilli dressing. Place ingredients in screw-top jar; shake well.

3   Stir-fry pork, in batches, in heated oiled wok until cooked as desired. Cover to
    keep warm. Stir-fry choy sum with the water in same wok until just wilted.

4   Place pork, choy sum and dressing in large bowl with carrot, herbs and onion;
    toss gently to combine. Sprinkle with nuts.

SERVES 4

PER SERVING   6.8g carbohydrate; 10.4g total fat (2.2g sat fat);
                  1344kJ (321 cal); 48.8g protein
CARB TIP   Serve with rice vermicelli.

roasted pork fillets with orange salad

PREPARATION TIME: 10 minutes (plus standing time)
COOKING TIME: 35 minutes

800g pork fillets
2 cloves garlic, sliced thinly lengthways
8 small fresh sage leaves
1 teaspoon fennel seeds
1 tablespoon olive oil
1 small brown onion (80g), sliced thickly
125ml chicken stock
1 tablespoon orange juice
150g mesclun
2 medium oranges (480g)

orange vinaigrette
2 tablespoons orange juice
1 tablespoon lemon juice
1 clove garlic, crushed
2 teaspoons olive oil

1 Cut a few small slits along the top of pork; push in garlic and sage. Sprinkle pork with seeds; stand 30 minutes.

2 Preheat oven to hot.

3 Heat half of the oil in medium flameproof baking dish; cook pork until browned all over. Remove from dish.

4 Heat remaining oil in same dish; cook onion, stirring, until browned lightly. Return pork to dish; drizzle with stock and juice. Roast, uncovered, in hot oven about 10 minutes or until pork is cooked as desired. Cover pork; stand 5 minutes. Slice thickly.

5 Make orange vinaigrette. Place ingredients in screw-top jar; shake well.

6 Place mesclun in medium bowl. Segment oranges over mesclun to catch juice, add vinaigrette; toss gently to combine.

7 Serve sliced pork with pan juices and salad.

SERVES 4

PER SERVING 10.1g carbohydrate; 9.6g total fat (2.3g sat. fat);
1308kJ (313 cal); 46.1g protein

CARB TIP Serve with roasted kipfler potatoes.

---

stir-fried lamb in black bean sauce

PREPARATION TIME: 15 minutes
COOKING TIME: 15 minutes

1 teaspoon five-spice powder
2 teaspoons sesame oil
600g lamb strips
2 teaspoons peanut oil
2 cloves garlic, crushed
1cm piece fresh ginger (5g), grated
1 medium brown onion (150g), sliced thinly
1 small red pepper (150g), sliced thinly
1 small yellow pepper (150g), sliced thinly
6 spring onions, sliced thinly
125ml chicken stock
1 tablespoon soy sauce
2 tablespoons black bean sauce

1   Combine five-spice and sesame oil in medium bowl, add lamb; toss to coat lamb in mixture.

2   Heat half of the peanut oil in wok; stir-fry lamb, in batches, until lightly browned.

3   Heat remaining peanut oil in same wok; stir-fry garlic, ginger and brown onion until onion just softens. Add peppers and spring onion; stir-fry until peppers are just tender.

4   Add stock and sauces to wok; stir-fry until sauce boils and lamb is cooked as desired.

SERVES 4

PER SERVING   7g carbohydrate; 10.6g total fat (3.3g sat. fat); 1116kJ (267 cal); 35.7g protein

CARB TIP   Serve with steamed jasmine rice.

teriyaki lamb stir-fry

PREPARATION TIME: 15 minutes
COOKING TIME: 15 minutes

2 teaspoons olive oil
800g lean lamb strips
2 teaspoons sesame oil
2 cloves garlic, crushed
1 medium brown onion (150g), sliced thickly
1 fresh long red chilli, sliced thinly
80ml teriyaki sauce
60ml sweet chilli sauce
500g baby bok choy, quartered
175g broccolini, chopped coarsely

1 Heat olive oil in wok; stir-fry lamb, in batches, until cooked as desired.

2 Heat sesame oil in same wok; stir-fry garlic, onion and chilli until fragrant. Add sauces; bring to a boil. Add bok choy and broccolini; stir-fry until bok choy just wilts and broccolini is just tender. Return lamb to wok; stir-fry until heated through.

SERVES 4

PER SERVING 7.3g carbohydrate; 12.6g total fat (3.9g sat. fat); 1426kJ (341 cal); 48.4g protein

CARB TIP Serve with steamed white long-grain rice.

lamb steaks with walnut gremolata tomatoes

PREPARATION TIME: 15 minutes (plus refrigeration time)
COOKING TIME: 30 minutes

2 tablespoons finely chopped fresh oregano
2 tablespoons finely chopped fresh flat-leaf parsley
1 tablespoon finely chopped fresh rosemary
80ml dry red wine
1 tablespoon olive oil
4 x 200g lamb leg steaks
1 tablespoon coarsely chopped fresh flat-leaf parsley

walnut gremolata tomatoes
4 medium tomatoes (750g), halved
1 tablespoon balsamic vinegar
2 tablespoons finely chopped walnuts
1 tablespoon finely grated lemon rind
1 clove garlic, crushed
60g finely chopped fresh flat-leaf parsley

1   Combine oregano, finely chopped parsley, rosemary, wine and oil in shallow dish, add lamb; turn to coat lamb in marinade. Cover; refrigerate 3 hours or overnight.

2   Make walnut gremolata tomatoes. Cook tomatoes on heated oiled grill plate (or grill or barbecue) until soft. Combine remaining ingredients in small bowl. Sprinkle tomatoes with walnut mixture.

3   Cook lamb on grill plate until cooked as desired. Cover lamb; stand 5 minutes.

4   Sprinkle lamb with coarsely chopped parsley; serve lamb with tomatoes.

SERVES 4

PER SERVING   3.7g carbohydrate; 12g total fat (2.7g sat. fat); 1333kJ (319 cal); 44.9g protein

CARB TIP   Serve with polenta made with chopped parsley and cream.

islander kebab

PREPARATION TIME: 15 minutes
COOKING TIME: 15 minutes

Soak 8 bamboo skewers in water for about 1 hour before using to prevent them from scorching.

800g lamb rump, cut into 2cm cubes
280g yogurt 2 teaspoons olive oil
2 tablespoons lemon juice
2 cloves garlic, crushed
2 teaspoons finely chopped fresh thyme
40g mesclun

chilli tomato sauce
1 small brown onion (80g),
  chopped coarsely
1 clove garlic, crushed
1 long green chilli, chopped coarsely
2 medium tomatoes (380g),
  chopped coarsely
1 tablespoon tomato paste
80ml dry red wine

1   Thread lamb onto skewers. Combine yogurt, juice, garlic and thyme in small bowl. Reserve two thirds of the yogurt mixture in separate small bowl. Brush lamb with remaining yogurt mixture.

2   Cook lamb skewers, in batches, on heated oiled grill plate (or grill or barbecue) until cooked as desired.

3   Meanwhile, make chilli tomato sauce. Heat oil in small frying pan; cook onion and garlic, stirring, until onion softens. Add remaining ingredients; bring to a boil. Reduce heat; simmer, uncovered, about 5 minutes or until sauce thickens slightly. Blend or process sauce until smooth.

4   Serve kebabs with reserved yogurt mixture, sauce and mesclun.

SERVES 4

PER SERVING   6.8g carbohydrate; 12.1g total fat (5.1g sat. fat); 1471kJ (351 cal); 48.8g protein

CARB TIP   Serve with pitta bread.

lamb and artichoke kebabs

preparation time 5 minutes
cooking time 15 minutes

Soak 8 bamboo skewers in water for about 1 hour before using to prevent them from scorching.

800g diced lamb

2 x 400g cans artichoke hearts, drained, halved

1 large red pepper (350g), cut into chunks suitable for skewer

300g mushrooms, halved

garlic basil dressing

125ml red wine vinegar

2 teaspoons olive oil

2 tablespoons finely shredded fresh basil

1 clove garlic, crushed

1 teaspoon sugar

1 teaspoon dijon mustard

1   Thread lamb, artichoke, red pepper and mushrooms onto skewers. Cook kebabs, in batches, on heated oiled grill plate (or grill or barbecue) until cooked as desired.

2   Meanwhile, make garlic basil dressing. Place ingredients in screw-top jar; shake well.

3   Serve kebabs with dressing.

SERVES 4

PER SERVING   7.1g carbohydrate; 10.3g total fat (3.5g sat. fat); 1379kJ (330 cal); 50.5g protein

CARB TIP   Serve with lavash.

---

lamb shanks in five-spice, tamarind and ginger

PREPARATION TIME: 20 minutes
COOKING TIME: 2 hours 10 minutes

2 teaspoons five-spice powder

1 teaspoon dried chilli flakes

1 cinnamon stick

2 star anise

60ml soy sauce

125ml Chinese rice wine

2 tablespoons tamarind concentrate

2 tablespoons brown sugar

8cm piece fresh ginger (40g), grated

2 cloves garlic, chopped coarsely

310ml water

8 French-trimmed lamb shanks (1.6kg)

500g choy sum, chopped into 10cm lengths

350g gai larn (Chinese broccoli)

1 Preheat oven to moderate.

2 Dry-fry five-spice, chilli, cinnamon and star anise in small heated frying pan, stirring, until fragrant. Combine spices with sauce, wine, tamarind, sugar, ginger, garlic and the water in medium jug.

3 Place lamb, in single layer, in large shallow baking dish; drizzle with spice mixture. Cook, covered, in moderate oven, turning lamb occasionally, about 2 hours or until meat is almost falling off the bone. Remove lamb from sauce in dish; cover to keep warm. Skim and discard fat from surface of sauce; strain into small saucepan.

4 Boil, steam or microwave choy sum and gai larn, separately, until tender. Drain well.

5 Bring sauce to a boil; boil, uncovered, 2 minutes. Divide vegetables among serving plates; top with lamb, drizzle with sauce.

SERVES 4

PER SERVING   10.8g carbohydrate; 20.2g total fat (9g sat. fat);
1912kJ (456 cal); 50.5g protein

CARB TIP   Serve with steamed basmati rice.

warm lamb with
caramelised onions and cress salad

PREPARATION TIME: 15 minutes
COOKING TIME: 25 minutes

10g butter
2 medium red onions (340g), sliced thinly
80ml red wine vinegar
1 tablespoon brown sugar
60ml water
600g lamb loin fillet
500g asparagus, trimmed
350g watercress
1 tablespoon dijon mustard
2 cloves garlic, crushed
1 tablespoon lemon juice
2 teaspoons olive oil

1   Melt butter in large frying pan; cook onion, stirring, until soft. Add vinegar, sugar and the water; cook, stirring, until sugar dissolves, then bring to a boil. Reduce heat; simmer, uncovered, stirring occasionally, about 10 minutes or until onion caramelises.

2   Meanwhile, cook lamb, in batches, on heated oiled grill plate (or grill or barbecue) until cooked as desired. Cover lamb; stand 5 minutes. Slice thickly.

3   Boil, steam or microwave asparagus until just tender; drain. Place asparagus in large bowl with watercress and combined remaining ingredients; toss gently to combine. Serve salad topped with lamb and caramelised onions.

SERVES 4

PER SERVING   9g carbohydrate; 10.4g total fat (4.1g sat. fat); 1216kJ (291 cal); 39.1g protein

CARB TIP   Toss cooked risoni through salad.

grilled lamb steak with ratatouille

PREPARATION TIME: 20 minutes
COOKING TIME: 25 minutes

5 baby aubergines (300g), peeled,
  chopped coarsely
2 medium red peppers (400g),
  chopped coarsely
1 medium yellow pepper (200g),
  chopped coarsely
4 medium plum tomatoes (540g),
  chopped coarsely
1 medium brown onion (150g),
  chopped coarsely
2 cloves garlic, sliced thickly
cooking-oil spray
4 x 200g lamb steaks

balsamic dressing
2 teaspoons olive oil
1 tablespoon lemon juice
1 tablespoon balsamic vinegar
1 clove garlic, crushed
35g loosely packed fresh
  oregano leaves

1   Preheat oven to hot. Make balsamic dressing. Place ingredients in screw-top jar;
    shake well.

2   Combine vegetables and garlic, in single layer, in two large shallow baking
    dishes; coat vegetables lightly with cooking-oil spray. Cook, uncovered, in hot
    oven about 25 minutes or until ratatouille is just tender, stirring occasionally.

3   Meanwhile, cook lamb on heated oiled grill plate (or grill or barbecue) until
    cooked as desired.

4   Place ratatouille and half of the dressing in large bowl; toss gently to combine.
    Divide ratatouille and lamb among plates; drizzle with remaining dressing.

SERVES 4

PER SERVING   11g carbohydrate; 10.4g total fat (4g sat. fat);
                  1154kJ (276 cal); 33.7g protein

CARB TIP   Serve with a warm French bread stick.

veal steaks with lemon thyme sauce

PREPARATION TIME: 10 minutes *(plus refrigeration time)*
COOKING TIME: 20 minutes

30g butter
2 tablespoons sweet chilli sauce
2 teaspoons finely grated lemon rind
80ml lemon juice
1 tablespoon finely chopped fresh thyme
8 x 100g veal leg steaks
500g choy sum

1 Melt butter in small saucepan, add sauce, rind and juice; cook, stirring, without boiling, until sauce thickens slightly. Transfer to small bowl; stir in thyme. Cover; refrigerate until firm.

2 Spread half of the sauce over both sides of each steak; cook steaks on heated oiled grill plate (or grill or barbecue) until cooked as desired.

3 Meanwhile, boil, steam or microwave choy sum until just wilted; drain.

4 Just before serving, spread steaks with remaining sauce; serve with choy sum.

SERVES 4

PER SERVING 5.2g carbohydrate; 8.3g total fat (4.6g sat. fat); 828kJ (198 cal); 24.8g protein

CARB TIP Serve with buttered egg noodles.

veal with anchovy butter and mixed beans

PREPARATION TIME: 10 minutes
COOKING TIME: 15 minutes

30g butter, softened
4 drained anchovy fillets, chopped finely
2 teaspoons lemon juice
1 tablespoon coarsely chopped fresh dill
8 x 100g veal leg steaks
300g green beans, trimmed
300g yellow string beans, trimmed

1 Combine butter, anchovies, juice and dill in small bowl.

2 Cook veal, in batches, on heated oiled grill plate (or grill or barbecue) until cooked as desired.

3 Meanwhile, boil, steam or microwave beans until just tender; drain.

4 Serve veal with beans; top with anchovy butter.

SERVES 4

PER SERVING 3.7g carbohydrate; 9.7g total fat (5.2g sat. fat); 878kJ (210 cal); 26.6g protein

CARB TIP Serve with mashed potatoes.

veal and mushroom casserole

PREPARATION TIME: 15 minutes
COOKING TIME: 1 hour 10 minutes

800g diced veal
2 medium brown onions (300g), chopped coarsely
1 clove garlic, crushed
½ teaspoon hot paprika
4 medium tomatoes (760g), chopped coarsely
60g tomato paste
375ml beef stock
500ml water
200g mushrooms, halved
1 tablespoon fresh oregano leaves
300g baby carrots, trimmed
20g butter

1 Heat oiled large saucepan; cook veal, in batches, until browned all over. Cook onion and garlic in same pan, stirring, until onion softens. Add paprika; cook, stirring, until fragrant.

2 Return veal to pan with tomato, paste, stock and the water; bring to a boil. Reduce heat; simmer, uncovered, about 45 minutes or until veal is tender. Add mushrooms; bring to a boil. Reduce heat; simmer, uncovered, until mushrooms are tender. Stir in oregano.

3 Meanwhile, boil, steam or microwave carrots until tender; drain. Place carrots in medium bowl with butter; toss to coat carrots in butter.

4 Serve casserole with carrots.

SERVES 4

PER SERVING 13.3g carbohydrate; 11.8g total fat (4.8g sat. fat); 1534kJ (367 cal); 51g protein

CARB TIP Serve with boiled baby new potatoes.

beef and vegetable teppanyaki

PREPARATION TIME: 10 minutes *(plus refrigeration time)*
COOKING TIME: 15 minutes

¼ cup (60ml) japanese soy sauce
2 tablespoons mirin
2 tablespoons sake
1cm piece fresh ginger (5g), grated
2 teaspoons brown sugar
1 clove garlic, crushed
4 x 200g beef fillet steaks
200g sugar snaps (snow peas), trimmed
250g asparagus, trimmed

1 Combine soy, mirin, sake, ginger, sugar and garlic in large bowl, add beef; turn to coat beef in marinade. Cover; refrigerate 3 hours or overnight.

2 Boil, steam or microwave peas and asparagus, separately, until just tender; drain. Drain beef over medium bowl; combine vegetables in bowl with marinade.

3 Cook beef on heated oiled grill plate (or grill or barbecue) until cooked as desired. Cover beef; stand 5 minutes.

4 Meanwhile, drain vegetables; discard marinade. Cook vegetables on same grill plate, until browned all over.

5 Serve beef with vegetables.

SERVES 4

PER SERVING   10.4g carbohydrate; 8.6g total fat (3.6g sat. fat); 1398kJ (334 cal); 46.8g protein

CARB TIP   Serve with koshihikari rice.

Thai-style steak with pickled cucumber salad

PREPARATION TIME: 25 minutes *(plus refrigeration time)*
COOKING TIME: 10 minutes

2 tablespoons sweet chilli sauce

1 teaspoon fish sauce

1 clove garlic, crushed

2 tablespoons lime juice

1 tablespoon fresh coriander,
   coarsely chopped

4 x 200g beef rib-eye steaks

pickled cucumber salad

2 tablespoons caster sugar

125ml white vinegar

2 cucumbers (260g),
   seeded, sliced thinly

1 fresh small red Thai chilli, sliced
   thinly

35g coarsely chopped toasted
   unsalted peanuts

1 tablespoon fressh coriander,
   coarsely chopped

1   Make pickled cucumber salad. Combine sugar and vinegar in small saucepan;
    stir over heat, without boiling, until sugar dissolves. Reduce heat; simmer,
    uncovered, about 5 minutes or until reduced to half. Combine hot vinegar
    mixture with remaining ingredients in small bowl. Cover; refrigerate 3 hours
    or overnight.

2   Combine sauces, garlic, juice and coriander in large bowl, add beef; turn to coat
    beef in marinade. Cover; refrigerate 3 hours or overnight.

3   Drain beef; discard marinade. Cook beef on heated oiled grill plate (or grill
    or barbecue) until cooked as desired. Cover beef; stand 5 minutes.

4   Serve beef with drained cucumber salad.

SERVES 4

PER SERVING   14.6g carbohydrate; 15g total fat (5.1g sat. fat);
                  1471kJ (352 cal); 39.8g protein

CARB TIP   Serve with bean thread noodles.

Vietnamese beef, chicken and tofu soup

PREPARATION TIME: 20 minutes
COOKING TIME: 1 hour 5 minutes

3 litres water
500g gravy beef
1 star anise
2.5cm piece fresh galangal (45g), halved
60ml soy sauce
2 tablespoons fish sauce
350g chicken breast fillets
120g bean sprouts
1 cup loosely packed fresh coriander leaves
4 spring onions, sliced thinly
2 fresh small red Thai chillies, sliced thinly
80ml lime juice
300g firm tofu, diced into 2cm pieces

1   Combine the water, beef, star anise, galangal and sauces in large saucepan; bring to a boil. Reduce heat; simmer, covered, 30 minutes. Uncover; simmer, 20 minutes. Add chicken; simmer, uncovered, 10 minutes.

2   Combine sprouts, coriander, onion, chilli and juice in medium bowl.

3   Remove beef and chicken from pan; reserve stock. Discard fat and sinew from beef; slice thinly. Slice chicken thinly. Return beef and chicken to pan; reheat soup.

4   Divide tofu among serving bowls; ladle hot soup over tofu, sprinkle with sprout mixture. Serve with lime wedges, if desired.

SERVES 4	
PER SERVING	3.6g carbohydrate; 18.8g total fat (6.5g sat fat); 1410kJ (337 cal); 37.6g protein
CARB TIP	Serve with bean thread noodles.

Moroccan minted beef

PREPARATION TIME: 15 minutes
COOKING TIME: 20 minutes

2 teaspoons vegetable oil

1 large brown onion (200g), sliced thinly

2 teaspoons ground cumin

1 teaspoon finely grated lemon rind

425g can crushed tomatoes

200g green beans, trimmed

800g beef strips

2 tablespoons toasted slivered almonds

35g finely shredded fresh mint

1   Heat oil in medium frying pan; cook onion, stirring, until soft. Add cumin and rind; cook, stirring, until fragrant. Stir in undrained tomatoes; bring to a boil. Reduce heat; simmer, uncovered, stirring occasionally, about 5 minutes or until mixture thickens slightly.

2   Meanwhile, boil, steam or microwave beans until just tender; drain. Cover to keep warm.

3   Cook beef, in batches, in heated oiled large frying pan until cooked as desired. Return beef to pan; stir in tomato mixture, nuts and mint; serve beef mixture with beans.

SERVES 4

PER SERVING   7.5g carbohydrate; 17.5g total fat (5.5g sat. fat); 1530kJ (366 cal); 45.9g protein

CARB TIP   Serve with steamed couscous.

mustard T-bone
with chilli garlic mushrooms

PREPARATION TIME: 10 minutes
COOKING TIME: 20 minutes

2 teaspoons olive oil

10g butter

3 cloves garlic, crushed

1 fresh small red Thai chilli, chopped finely

500g mushrooms

4 x 250g beef T-bone steaks

2 tablespoons dijon mustard

1 tablespoon lemon juice

35g coarsely chopped fresh flat-leaf parsley

1 tablespoon coarsely chopped fresh rosemary

1   Heat oil and butter in large saucepan; cook garlic, chilli and mushrooms, stirring, about 5 minutes or until mushrooms are tender.

2   Meanwhile, brush beef all over with mustard; cook on heated oiled grill plate (or grill or barbecue) until cooked as desired. Cover beef; stand 5 minutes.

3   Serve beef and mushrooms sprinkled with juice and herbs.

SERVES 4

PER SERVING   2.7g carbohydrate; 13g total fat (5.2g sat. fat); 1179kJ (282 cal); 38.4g protein

CARB TIP   Serve with a potato salad.

beef steaks with green pepper salsa

PREPARATION TIME: 15 minutes
COOKING TIME: 10 minutes

4 x 200g beef eye fillet steaks
100g rocket leaves

green pepper salsa
2 small green peppers (300g), chopped finely
1 small red onion (100g), chopped finely
1 fresh small red Thai chilli, chopped finely
6 spring onions, sliced thinly
60ml lime juice
2 tablespoons finely chopped fresh mint

1   Make green pepper salsa. Combine ingredients in medium bowl.

2   Cook beef on heated oiled grill plate (or grill or barbecue) until cooked as desired.

3   Divide rocket among serving plates; top with beef and salsa.

SERVES 4

PER SERVING   3.9g carbohydrate; 8.1g total fat (3.3g sat. fat); 1087kJ (260 cal); 42g protein

CARB TIP   Serve with barbecued corn cobs.

stir-fried beef, bok choy and gai larn

PREPARATION TIME: 10 minutes
COOKING TIME: 25 minutes

2 teaspoons peanut oil

600g beef strips

2 cloves garlic, crushed

2cm piece fresh ginger (10g), grated

5cm stick (10g) finely chopped fresh lemon grass

1 fresh small red Thai chilli, sliced thinly

1kg baby bok choy, chopped coarsely

500g gai larn (Chinese broccoli), chopped coarsely

4 spring onions, sliced thinly

2 tablespoons kecap manis (sweet soy sauce)

1 tablespoon fish sauce

60ml sweet chilli sauce

60ml lime juice

35g coarsely chopped fresh mint

35g coarsely chopped fresh coriander

1   Heat half of the oil in wok; stir-fry beef, in batches, until browned all over.

2   Heat remaining oil in same wok; stir-fry garlic, ginger, lemon grass and chilli until fragrant. Add bok choy and gai larn; stir-fry until vegetables just wilt. Return beef to wok with onion, sauces and juice; stir-fry until heated through. Remove from heat; stir in herbs.

SERVES 4

PER SERVING   10.6g carbohydrate; 14.4g total fat (4.6g sat. fat); 1375kJ (329 cal); 39.2g protein

CARB TIP   Serve with steamed jasmine rice.

ginger beef stir-fry

PREPARATION TIME: 20 minutes
COOKING TIME: 10 minutes

6cm piece fresh ginger (30g)
2 teaspoons peanut oil
800g beef rump steak, sliced thinly
2 cloves garlic, crushed
120g snake beans, cut into 5cm lengths
8 spring onions, sliced thinly
2 teaspoons grated palm sugar
2 teaspoons oyster sauce
1 tablespoon fish sauce
1 tablespoon soy sauce
60g loosely packed fresh Thai basil leaves

1   Slice peeled ginger thinly; stack slices, then slice again into thin strips.

2   Heat half of the oil in wok; stir-fry beef, in batches, until browned all over.

3   Heat remaining oil in wok; stir-fry ginger and garlic until fragrant. Add beans; stir-fry until just tender.

4   Return beef to wok with onion, sugar and sauces; stir-fry until beef is cooked as desired. Remove from heat; toss basil through stir-fry.

SERVES 4

PER SERVING   4.4g carbohydrate; 15.9g total fat (6.4g sat. fat); 1463kJ (350 cal); 47.1g protein

CARB TIP   Serve with fresh rice noodles.

mixed vegetable and herb frittata

PREPARATION TIME: 25 minutes
COOKING TIME: 20 minutes

2 teaspoons olive oil
2 cloves garlic, crushed
2 medium courgettes (240g), sliced thinly
100g chestnut mushrooms, sliced thinly
180g baby spinach leaves
3 eggs
8 egg whites
35g coarsely chopped fresh basil
20g coarsely grated parmesan cheese

tomato salad
250g yellow teardrop tomatoes, halved
250g cherry tomatoes, halved
35g loosely packed fresh baby basil leaves
2 tablespoons balsamic vinegar

1   Make tomato salad. Combine tomatoes and basil in medium serving bowl. Stir in vinegar just before serving.

2   Heat oil in large frying pan; cook garlic and courgettes, stirring, until courgettes are just tender. Add mushrooms and spinach; cook, stirring, until spinach is just wilted.

3   Whisk eggs and egg whites in medium bowl until just combined; stir in basil.

4   Pour egg mixture into pan over vegetables; cook, uncovered, over medium heat about 10 minutes or until set. Sprinkle with cheese; place under preheated grill until frittata is browned lightly. Serve with salad.

SERVES 4

PER SERVING   4.6g carbohydrate; 8.5g total fat (2.6g sat. fat); 696kJ (166 cal); 17.2g protein

CARB TIP   Serve with toasted Italian bread.

vegetable curry with yogurt

PREPARATION TIME: 25 minutes
COOKING TIME: 15 minutes

2 teaspoons vegetable oil

4cm piece fresh ginger (20g), grated

3 spring onions, sliced thinly

2 cloves garlic, crushed

1 long green chilli, chopped finely

¼ teaspoon ground cardamom

1 teaspoon garam masala

1 tablespoon curry powder

1 teaspoon ground turmeric

2 medium granny smith apples (300g), coarsely grated

1 tablespoon lemon juice

500ml vegetable stock

½ small cauliflower (500g), cut into florets

4 yellow patty-pan squash (100g), halved

2 small green courgettes (180g), sliced thickly

150g baby spinach leaves

200g yogurt

1   Heat oil in large saucepan; cook ginger, onion, garlic, chilli, cardamom, garam masala, curry powder and turmeric until fragrant. Add apple, juice and stock; cook, uncovered, 5 minutes, stirring occasionally.

2   Add cauliflower, squash and courgettes; cook, uncovered, until vegetables are just tender. Remove from heat; stir spinach and yogurt into curry just before serving.

SERVES 4

PER SERVING   14.6g carbohydrate; 5.2g total fat (0.7g sat. fat); 599kJ (143 cal); 8.9g protein

CARB TIP   Serve with steamed basmati rice.

PANTRY LIST

PANTRY
anchovies
caperberries
capers
caster sugar
chinese rice wine
coconut milk
cornichons
cracked black pepper
dried chilli flakes
dried fruit of all types
fennel seeds
garlic
golden syrup
linseed, sunflower and
     almond blend
mirin
palm sugar

pepitas
preserved lemon
red wine
rolled oats
sake
sambal oelek
sea salt flakes
semi-dried tomatoes
sesame seeds
spices
sunflower seed kernels
tamarind concentrate
tomato paste
vanilla bean
vinegar
white wine

canned products
artichokes
beans
beetroot
chickpeas
salmon
tomatoes
tuna

mustards
dijon
wholegrain

oils
cooking-oil spray
olive
peanut
sesame
vegetable

pickles
butter cucumbers
pickled garlic
pickled ginger
pickled onions

sauces
black bean
bottled pasta
fish
kecap manis (sweet soy
     sauce)
oyster
soy
sweet chilli
teriyaki

REFRIGERATOR
bacon
butter
buttermilk
eggs
ham
herbs
milk
muesli

olives
orange juice
pancetta
seasonal fruit and
     vegetables of all types
smoked salmon
tofu
yogurt

cheeses
cheddar
cottage
gouda
low-fat ricotta
mozzarella
parmesan
pecorino
ricotta

FREEZER
chillies
galangal
ginger, peeled before
     freezing, grate frozen
homemade casseroles
homemade soups
kaffir lime leaves
lemon grass
meal-sized servings of
     meat, chicken and
     seafood of all types
nuts
peas

**CARB INGREDIENTS
FOR PANTRY**
cous cous
polenta
potatoes

RICE
basmati
jasmine
white long-grain

BREAD
ciabatta
French stick
fruit toast
lavash
pitta
sliced
sourdough
Turkish

PASTA & NOODLES
bean thread
chow mein
fettuccine
macaroni
rice stick
rice vermicelli
risoni
soba

**CARB INGREDIENTS
FOR REFRIGERATOR**
corn
noodles
     egg
     fresh rice

CARB, FAT &
KILOJOULE COUNTER

	Carb	Fat	Sat. Fat	kJ	Cal	Ptn
almonds, blanched, untoasted, 1 tablespoon	0.5	7.3	0.4	322	77	2.7
almond meal, 33g	1.3	16.6	1	736	176	6
almonds, with skin, untoasted, 1 tablespoon	0.6	7.1	0.5	314	75	2.5
anchovy fillet, canned in oil, drained, 1	0	0.3	0.1	25	6	0.8
apple sauce, 1 tablespoon	4.5	0	0	75	18	0
apple, canned, no added sugar, 100g	9	0	0	155	37	0.3
apple, canned, sweetened, 100g	20.9	0.1	0	343	82	0.2
apple, dried, 33g	13.9	0.1	0	230	55	0.3
apple, granny smith, fresh, unpeeled, small, 130g	13.1	0.1	0	222	53	0.3
apple, red, fresh, unpeeled, small, 130g	11	0.1	0	192	46	0.3
apricot, canned, in natural juice, drained, 100g	8.9	0	0	171	41	1
apricot, dried, 33g	15.2	0.1	0	280	67	1.5
apricot, fresh, medium, 50g	3.5	0.1	0	71	17	0.4
artichoke, canned, in brine, drained, 100g	1.2	0.3	0	67	16	1.9
artichoke, globe, boiled, 100g	1.4	0.2	0	88	21	3.1
artichoke, jerusalem, boiled, 100g	3.3	0.1	0	105	25	2.3
asparagus, canned in brine, drained, 100g	1.5	0.1	0	71	17	1.9
asparagus, cooked, 100g	1.6	0.1	0	79	19	2.8
aubergine, raw, small, 230g	6	0.7	0	167	40	2.5
avocado, fresh, small, 200g	0.6	31.6	6.9	1229	294	2.7
bacon, middle rasher, fried, rind removed, 40g	0.3	6.5	2.4	431	103	10.7
bacon, middle rasher, fried, with rind, 70g	0.6	21.3	8.1	1083	259	17.2
bacon, middle rasher, grilled, rind removed, 40g	0.3	5.4	2.1	405	97	11.9
bacon, middle rasher, grilled, with rind, 70g	0.6	15.7	5.9	936	224	20.7
bamboo shoots, canned, drained, 100g	1.2	0	0	33	8	0.8
banana chips, 33g	10.5	6	5.2	397	95	0.2
banana, fresh, small, 130g	17.3	0.1	0	309	74	1.5
basil, fresh, 1 tablespoon chopped	0	0	0	2	0.4	0
bean curd (see tofu)						
bean sprouts, raw, 100g	1.6	0.1	0	84	20	3.1
bean, broad, raw, boiled, 100g	2	0.5	0.1	171	41	6.9
bean, butter, raw, boiled, 100g	2.1	0.2	0.1	84	20	2.3
bean, cannellini, canned, drained, 100g	10.6	0.6	0	309	74	6.2

	Carb	Fat	Sat. Fat	kJ	Cal	Ptn
bean, green, raw, 100g	2.4	0.2	0	88	21	2.2
bean, lima, canned, drained, 100g	9.8	0.2	0	247	59	5.2
bean, lima, dried, boiled, 100g	10.2	0.3	0	297	71	6.4
bean, mixed, canned, drained, 100g	14.3	0.4	0.1	355	85	6.4
bean, red kidney, canned, drained, 100g	14.4	0.6	0.1	380	91	6.6
bean, red kidney, dried, boiled, 100g	14.2	0.4	0.1	481	115	12.8
bean, refried, canned, 100g	13.1	1.1	0.3	339	81	6.2
bean, snake, boiled, 100g	1.6	0.3	0	96	23	3.3
bean, soy, canned, drained, 100g	2.9	5.5	0.8	380	91	8.6
bean, soy, dried, boiled, 100g	1.4	7.7	1.1	539	129	13.5
beef stock, 60ml	0.4	0.1	0	21	5	0.7
beef, boneless, grilled, lean, 100g	0	6.3	2.8	765	183	31.3
beef, corned, deli, 100g	0	6.4	2.7	539	129	17.7
beef, eye fillet, grilled, 200g	0	19.2	8.6	1722	412	59.6
beef, eye fillet, grilled, lean, 200g	0	16.6	7.4	1639	392	60
beef, eye fillet, raw, 200g	0	12	5	1158	277	42
beef, eye fillet, raw, lean, 200g	0	8.4	3.6	1041	249	43
beef, mince, simmered, 100g	0	11.8	5.2	895	214	27
beef, mince, simmered, lean, 100g	0	8.4	3.7	782	187	26.7
beef, roast, deli, 100g	0	4.5	2.1	606	145	25.8
beef, rump steak, grilled, 250g	0	23.8	10.8	2232	534	79.5
beef, rump steak, grilled, lean, 250g	0	16.8	7.5	2006	480	82.8
beetroot, canned, drained, 100g	8.9	0.1	0	169	40.4	1.3
beetroot, fresh, small, 250g	18.5	0	0	380	91	4.2
berries, mixed, frozen, 100g	8.7	0.3	0	180	43	0.9
blackberry, fresh, 100g	7.5	0.3	0	159	38	1.4
blackcurrant, fresh, 100g	8	0.4	0	192	46	1.4
blueberry, fresh, 100g	11.3	0.1	0	205	49	0.6
bok choy, cooked, 100g	0.9	2.7	0.7	130	31	1
brazil nut, untoasted, 42g	1	27.4	5.9	1124	269	5.8
broccoli, boiled, 100g	0.4	0.3	0	100	24	4.7
broccoli, raw, 100g	0.6	0.3	0	105	25	4.7
brussels sprouts, boiled, 100g	1.9	0.3	0	103	24.6	3.5

	Carb	Fat	Sat. Fat	kJ	Cal	Ptn
butter, 1 teaspoon	0	4.1	2.7	150	36	0
butter, reduced-fat, 1 teaspoon	0	2	1.3	79	19	0.3
buttermilk, 60ml	3.4	1.3	0.8	150	36	2.6
cabbage, Chinese, cooked, shredded, 160g	1.3	4.6	1.1	221	53	1.8
cabbage, Chinese, raw, shredded, 80g	0.7	0	0	28	6.7	0.9
cabbage, green, cooked, shredded, 160g	3.8	0.2	0	104	25	2.1
cabbage, green, raw, shredded, 80g	2.1	0.1	0	59	14	1.2
cabbage, red, cooked, shredded, 160g	4.5	0.5	0	147	35	3.2
cabbage, red, raw, shredded, 80g	2.5	0.3	0	79	19	1.8
capers, drained, 1 teaspoon	0.3	0	0	8	2	0
carrot, baby, raw, 100g	5.5	0.1	0	109	26	0.7
carrot, raw, small, 70g	3.2	0.1	0	63	15	0.5
cashews, untoasted, 1 tablespoon	2	5.7	0.9	276	66	2
cauliflower, boiled, 100g	2	0.2	0	79	19	2.2
cauliflower, raw, 100g	2.1	0.2	0	79	19	2.2
celeriac, boiled, peeled, 100g	5.6	0.2	0	134	32	1.8
celery, raw, 1 trimmed stalk, 100g	2.2	0.1	0	50	12	0.6
champagne, 250ml	2.5	0	0	673	161	0.5
cheese, blue-vein, 30g	0	9.7	6.2	464	111	6.1
cheese, bocconcini, 30g	0	4.6	3	255	61	5.2
cheese, brie, 30g	0	8.7	5.6	422	101	5.8
cheese, camembert, 30g	0	7.9	5.1	385	92	5.6
cheese, cheddar, 30g	0	10.1	6.5	506	121	7.6
cheese, colby, 30g	0	9.7	6.2	481	115	7.2
cheese, cottage, 30g	0.7	1.7	1.1	155	37	4.6
cheese, cottage, low-fat, 100g	0.6	0.4	0.2	113	27	5.3
cheese, cream, 30g	0.8	9.9	6.4	422	101	2.6
cheese, cream, reduced-fat, 30g	0.9	5	3.3	242	58	2.5
cheese, edam, 30g	0	8.2	5.2	443	106	8.4
cheese, feta, 30g	0.1	7	4.6	351	84	5.3
cheese, goats, 30g	0.3	4.7	3.1	247	59	3.9
cheese, gouda, 30g	0	9.2	5.9	477	114	7.8
cheese, haloumi, 30g	0.5	5.1	3.3	305	73	6.4

	Carb	Fat	Sat. Fat	kJ	Cal	Ptn
cheese, mascarpone, 30g	0.5	17.2	11.3	652	156	0.4
cheese, mozzarella, 30g	0	6.6	4.2	376	90	7.8
cheese, parmesan, 30g	0	9.7	6.2	556	133	11.4
cheese, pecorino, 30g	0.1	8.2	5.2	447	107	8.4
cheese, pizza, 30g	0	6.6	4.2	389	93	8.6
cheese, ricotta, 30g	0.4	3.4	2.2	184	44	3.2
cheese, ricotta, low-fat, 30g	0.6	2.6	1.7	159	38	3.1
cheese, smoked, 30g	0.1	8.2	5.2	418	100	6.4
cheese, Swiss, 30g	0.1	9	5.7	481	115	8.5
cherries, canned in syrup, drained, 100g	17	0.1	0	297	71	0.9
cherries, fresh, 100g	11.9	0.2	0	226	54	1
chicken stock, 60ml	0.4	0.2	0.1	27	6.4	0.7
chicken, breast, fillet, grilled, 170g	0	13.6	3.9	1313	314	47.8
chicken, drumstick, with skin, grilled, 150g	0	15.9	4.8	1032	247	24.8
chicken, livers, fried, 100g	1.4	11.4	2.3	836	200	23.1
chicken, maryland, grilled, 350g	0	47.1	14.4	2771	663	61
chicken, mince, fried, 100g	0	10.6	3	849	203	26.9
chicken, sausage, grilled, 100g	5.3	16.2	5.3	999	239	18.3
chicken, smoked, 100g	0	7	2	677	162	24.6
chicken, tenderloin, grilled, 75g	0	6.1	1.7	585	140	21.2
chicken, thigh, fillet, grilled, 110g	0	14.1	4.2	995	238	27.9
chicken, wing, grilled, 85g	0	12.4	3.5	669	160	12.6
chickpea, canned, drained, 100g	13.7	2.1	0.3	405	97	6.3
chilli, green, 1 teaspoon chopped	0.1	0	0	4	1	0.1
chilli, red, 1 teaspoon chopped	0.2	0	0	4	1	0.1
chives, fresh, 1 tablespoon chopped	0.1	0	0	4	1	0.1
coconut milk, canned, 60 ml	2.3	12.4	10.9	514	123	1.2
coconut, desiccated, 1 tablespoon	0.4	4	3.5	163	39	0.4
coconut, fresh, 100g	3.6	27.4	24.2	1120	268	3
coffee, instant powder, 1 teaspoon	0.4	0	0	17	4	0.5
corn, kernel, canned, drained, 100g	18.6	1	0.1	401	96	3
corn, raw, 100g	16.4	1.2	0.1	393	94	4.2
courgette, raw, small, 90g	1.4	0.3	0	46	11	0.7

	Carb	Fat	Sat. Fat	kJ	Cal	Ptn
cream, single, 60ml	2.6	12.9	8.2	548	131	1.8
cream, double, 60ml	1.7	25.7	17.3	995	238	1.1
cream, sour, 60ml	1.7	23.8	15.7	978	234	1.4
cream, sour, reduced-fat, 60ml	2.7	11.8	7.8	527	126	2.2
cream, thickened, 60ml	1.9	22.1	14.5	869	208	1.3
cucumber, dill, pickled, 50g	0	0	0	15	3.6	0.2
cucumber, raw, 1, 130g	2.3	0.1	0	54	13	0.6
curly endive, raw, 100g	0.4	0.2	0	42	10	1.5
curry paste, 1 tablespoon	1.8	7.2	0.7	318	76	1.2
date, dried, 55g	31.6	0.1	0	531	127	0.9
date, fresh, 55g	17.6	0.1	0	297	71	0.6
devon, 100g	5.9	18.2	6.9	978	234	12.3
duck, baked, lean, 100g	0	9.5	2.8	765	183	24.3
duck, baked, with skin, 100g	0	26	7.8	1296	310	19.7
egg, fried, 1, 60g	0.2	9	2.7	477	114	8.3
egg, hard-boiled, 1, 60g	0.2	6.5	2	380	91	7.9
egg, poached, 1, 60g	0.2	6.7	2	376	90	7.4
fennel, raw, small, 200g	3.6	0.1	0	88	21	1.1
fig, dried, 55g	28.6	0.4	0.1	506	121	1.9
fig, fresh, medium, 60g	4.9	0.2	0	100	24	0.8
fish (see seafood)						
fish stock, 60ml	0.4	0.1	0	21	5	0.7
flour, potato, 35g	28	0.2	0.1	481	115	0
flour, soy, 30g	7.2	2	0.3	431	103	14
gai larn, cooked, 100g	1.1	0.1	0	63	15	2.4
garlic, raw, 1 clove	0.3	0.1	0	13	3	0.2
ginger, raw, 1cm piece, 5g	0.2	0	0	4	1	0
golden syrup, 1 tablespoon	21.7	0	0	347	83	0.1
grapefruit, fresh, small, 350g	10.9	0.5	0	251	60	2.1
grapes, white/green, fresh, 100g	15	0.1	0	255	61	0.6
ham, shaved, deli, 100g	0	3.6	1.3	451	108	18.8
hazelnuts, untoasted, 1 tablespoon	0.5	6	0.3	255	61	1.4
honey, 1 tablespoon	23.5	0	0	376	90	0.1

	Carb	Fat	Sat. Fat	kJ	Cal	Ptn
honeydew, fresh, 100g	6.5	0.3	0	134	32	0.7
ice-cream, vanilla, low-fat, 1 scoop, 125g	24	3.9	2.5	619	148	5.6
juice, orange, 1 cup	19.2	0.3	0	355	85	1.3
kecap manis, 1 tablespoon	13.1	0	0	230	55	0.4
kiwi fruit, fresh, medium, 85g	7.1	0.1	0	146	35	1
leek, raw, small, 200g	4.7	0.5	0	134	32	2.4
lemon juice, 1 tablespoon	0.5	0	0	21	5	0.1
lemon rind, grated, 1 teaspoon	0.1	0	0	3	0.8	0
lemon, fresh, medium, 140g	2.5	0.3	0	134	32	0.8
lemonade, soft drink, diet, 60ml	0	0	0	13	3	0
lettuce, iceberg, 100g	0.4	0.1	0	25	6	0.9
lime juice, 1 tablespoon	0.3	0	0	17	4	0.2
lime, fresh, 1, 80g	0.8	0.1	0	63	15	0.6
lychee, fresh, 1, 25g	16.2	0.1	0	284	68	1.1
mango, fresh, small, 300g	25.5	0.4	0	477	114	2
milk, 60ml	2.9	2.4	1.6	167	40	2
milk, no-fat, 60ml	3.4	0.1	0	109	26	2.7
mint, fresh, 1 tablespoon chopped	0.2	0	0	8	2	0.1
mushroom, button, raw, 100g	1.5	0.3	0	96	23	3.6
mushroom, shiitake, cooked, 100g	12.2	0.2	0	230	55	1.6
mustard, all types, 1 teaspoon	0.2	0.1	0	8	2	0.2
oil, olive, 1 tablespoon	0	18.2	2.6	673	161	0
oil, peanut, 1 tablespoon	0	18.2	3.3	673	161	0
oil, sesame, 1 tablespoon	0	18.4	2.6	681	163	0
oil, vegetable, 1 tablespoon	0	18.4	2.3	681	163	0
olives, black, pickled in brine, 38g	9	0.4	0.1	171	41	0.3
olives, green, pickled in brine, drained, 38g	9	0.4	0.1	171	41	0.3
onion, raw, small, 80g	2.8	0.1	0	67	16	1
onion, green, raw, 1, 10g	0.5	0	0	13	3	0.2
onion, pickled, 50g	7.1	0.1	0	134	32	0.3
orange rind, grated, 1 teaspoon	0.3	0	0	8	2	0
orange, fresh, small, 180g	10.1	0.1	0	201	48	1.3
pancetta, 15g slice	0.1	2.1	0.8	125	30	2.9

	Carb	Fat	Sat. Fat	kJ	Cal	Ptn
parsley, flat-leaf, fresh, 1 tablespoon chopped	0	0	0	4	1	0.1
passionfruit, fresh, 1, 1 tablespoon pulp	1.1	0.1	0	38	9	0.6
pawpaw, fresh, 100g	6.9	0.1	0	121	29	0.4
peanuts, unsalted, untoasted, 1 tablespoon	1.6	5.8	0.7	288	69	2.8
pepper, green, raw, small, 150g	2.3	0.1	0	67	16	1.5
pepper, red, raw, small, 150g	4.2	0.2	0	109	26	1.7
pine nuts, untoasted, 1 tablespoon	0.7	10.1	0.6	418	100	2
pineapple, fresh, 100g	8	0.1	0	159	38	1
plum, fresh, medium, 110g	6.4	0.1	0	134	32	0.5
potato, peeled, boiled, small, 120g	15.4	0.1	0	314	75	3
potato, peeled, roasted, small, 120g	18.1	2.9	0.4	468	112	3.2
prosciutto, 1 slice, 15g	0.1	0.9	0.3	79	19	2.7
radish, red, 1, 35g	0.7	0.1	0	17	4	0.3
rocket, 100g	2.2	0.7	0	105	25	2.6
rockmelon, fresh, 100g	4.7	0.1	0	92	22	0.5
salt, 1 teaspoon	0	0	0	0	0	0
sauce, black bean, 1 tablespoon	4.3	0.6	0.1	109	26	0.9
sauce, fish, 1 tablespoon	0.9	0.1	0	42	10	1.4
sauce, hoisin, 1 tablespoon	8.1	1.2	0.2	184	44	0.4
sauce, oyster, 1 tablespoon	4.6	0.2	0	105	25	0.6
sauce, pasta, bottled, 125ml	8.2	0.1	0	184	44	2.1
sauce, soy, 1 tablespoon	0.6	0	0	33	8	1.1
sauce, sweet chilli, 1 tablespoon	8.5	0.2	0	155	37	0.1
seafood, clams, cooked, 100g	0.2	0.1	0	67	16	3.5
seafood, ocean trout, raw, 200g	0	7.6	1.8	945	226	38.8
seafood, octopus, cooked, 100g	0.9	1.7	0.4	477	114	23.6
seafood, salmon, raw, 220g	0	15.6	3.5	1304	312	42.9
seafood, salmon, smoked, 1 slice, 30g	0	1.4	0.3	167	40	6.9
seafood, tuna, canned in springwater, drained, 100g	0	2.6	1	518	124	24.8
seafood, tuna, raw, 100g	0	5.7	2.3	635	152	25.1
seaweed, 1 sheet	0	0.1	0	10	2.5	0.5
sesame seeds, 1 teaspoon	0	1.6	0.2	67	16	0.6

	Carb	Fat	Sat. Fat	kJ	Cal	Ptn
shallot, raw, 1, 25g	0.7	0	0	17	4	0.3
snow pea sprouts, raw, 100g	23.6	0.7	0.2	573	137	8.8
snow peas (sugar snaps), raw, 100g	4.7	0.2	0	134	32	3
spinach, raw, 100g	0.6	0.3	0	63	15.1	2.4
squash, raw, 100g	3.3	0.2	0	109	26	2.6
sugar, brown, 1 tablespoon	12.6	0	0	201	48	0
sugar, caster, 1 tablespoon	18	0	0	288	69	0
sultanas, 1 tablespoon	10.2	0.1	0	171	41	0.4
sunflower seed kernels, 1 tablespoon	0.4	9.2	0.6	414	99	4.1
sweetener, 1 teaspoon	0.5	0	0	8	2	0
tahihi, 1 tablespoon	0.2	14	1.7	598	143	4.7
tofu, 100g	1.3	6.8	1	472	113	11.9
tomato paste, 1 tablespoon	2.3	0.1	0	54	13	0.7
tomato, cherry, fresh, 100g	2.2	0.1	0	50	12	0.5
tomato, crushed, canned, 100g	3.2	0.2	0	75	18	0.8
tomato, egg, fresh, small, 60g	1.4	0.1	0	38	9	0.6
tomato, fresh, small, 90g	1.7	0.1	0	50	12	0.9
tomato, sun-dried, drained, 50g	17.1	3.9	0.5	535	128	5.4
Vegemite, 1 teaspoon	0.4	0.1	0	29	7	1.2
vegetable stock, 60ml	1.8	1	0.1	117	28	2.8
vinegar, all types, 1 tablespoon	0	0	0	12	2.8	0
walnuts, untoasted, 1 tablespoon	0.3	6.2	0.4	255	61	1.3
watercress, raw, 100g	0.8	0.4	0	79	19	2.9
wine, dry red, 60ml	0	0	0	351	84	0.3
wine, dry white, 60ml	0.4	0	0	355	85	0.3
yogurt, frozen, soft serve, fruit, low-fat, 125g	27.3	2.1	1.4	627	150	6.5
yogurt, plain, 140g	6.6	4.8	3.1	426	102	6.6
yogurt, plain, low-fat, 140g	10.6	2.4	1.5	410	98	7

	Carb	Fat	Sat. Fat	kJ	Cal	Ptn
Grain-based foods *						
bread roll, sourdough, 1, 65g	34.2	2.6	0.4	773	185	6.1
bread, French stick, white, 50g	26.5	1.9	0.3	594	142	4.5
bread, fruit, 1 slice, 30g	16.4	1.1	0.2	355	85	2.3
bread, white, 1 slice, 30g	13.4	0.8	0.1	301	72	2.5
ciabatta, 100g	44.8	2.6	0.4	999	239	8.4
couscous, cooked, 100g	9.5	0.1	0	196	47	1.6
lavash, white, 1, 65g	36.2	1.3	0.2	765	183	6.1
linseed, sunflower and almond blend, 70g	19	27.9	7.8	1618	387	16.7
muesli, 55g	32.2	4.9	1.4	803	192	5.1
noodle, bean thread, cooked, 100g	25.3	0	0	431	103	0
noodle, egg, dry, cooked, 100g	25.6	0.6	0.1	548	131	5.3
noodle, rice, dry, cooked, 100g	21.4	0.4	0	414	99	2
noodle, rice, fresh, cooked, 100g	21.4	0.4	0	414	99	2
oats, rolled, cooked, 100g	8.5	1.1	0.2	213	51	1.6
pasta, regular, cooked, 100g	24.6	0.3	0	497	119	4
pitta, lebanese bread, white, 100g	51.9	2.3	0.3	1120	268	9.3
polenta, cooked, 100g	9.9	2.3	1.3	301	72	3.1

* used in recipes or carb tips

GLOSSARY

ALMONDS flat, nuts with pointed ends; a pitted brown shell enclosing a creamy-white kernel covered by a brown skin.

slivered small pieces cut lengthways.

ARTICHOKE HEARTS tender centre of the globe artichoke, itself the large flower-bud of a member of the thistle family; having tough petal like leaves, edible in part when cooked. Artichoke hearts can be harvested fresh from the plant or purchased in brine canned or in glass jars.

AUBERGINE also known as eggplant; belongs to the same family as tomatoes, chillies and potatoes. Ranging in size from tiny to very large and in colour from pale green to deep purple, eggplant has a variety of flavours.

BACON RASHERS also known as slices of bacon, made from pork side, cured and smoked. Middle rashers are the familiar bacon shape, ie, a thin strip of belly pork having a lean, rather round piece of loin at one end; streaky bacon is the same cut minus the round loin section.

BEAN SPROUTS also known as bean shoots; tender new growths of beans and seeds germinated for consumption as sprouts.

BEANS

cannellini small white dried beans similar in appearance and flavour to other *Phaseolus vulgaris* varieties – great northern and navy or haricot beans. Sometimes sold as butter beans.

green sometimes called French or string beans (although the tough string they once had has generally been bred out of them), these long fresh beans are consumed pod and all.

snake long (about 40cm), thin, round, fresh green beans, Asian in origin, with a taste similar to green or french beans. Used most frequently in stir-fries, they are also called yard-long beans because of their length.

yellow string also known as wax, french, runner and (incorrectly) butter beans; a yellow-coloured fresh green bean.

BOK CHOY also known as bak choy, pak choi, Chinese white cabbage or Chinese chard, has a fresh, mild mustard taste; use stems and leaves, stir-fry or braise. Baby bok choy, also known as pak kat farang or Shanghai bok choy, is small and more tender than bok choy. Its mildly acrid, distinctively appealing taste has brought baby bok choy to the forefront of commonly used Asian greens.

BROCCOLINI a cross between broccoli and chinese kale, it is milder and sweeter than broccoli. Each long stem is topped by a loose floret that closely resembles broccoli; from floret to stem, broccolini is completely edible.

BUTTER use salted or unsalted (sweet) butter; 125g is equal to one stick of butter.

BUTTERMILK found in the refrigerated dairy compartments of supermarkets. Originally just the liquid left after cream was separated from milk, today it is commercially made in a similar way to yogurt.

CANTELOUPE also known as rockmelon.

CAPERS the grey-green buds of a warm climate (usually Mediterranean) shrub, sold either dried and salted or pickled in a vinegar brine; tiny young baby capers, are also available.

CARDAMOM native to India and used extensively in its cuisine; can be purchased in pod, seed or ground form. Has a distinctive aromatic, sweetly rich flavour and is one of the world's most expensive spices.

CHEESE

cheddar the most common cow milk 'tasty' cheese; should be aged, hard and have a pronounced bite.

mozzarella soft, spun-curd cheese; it originated in southern Italy where it is traditionally made from water buffalo milk.

parmesan also known as parmigiano, parmesan is a hard, grainy cow milk cheese which originated in the Parma region of Italy. The curd is salted in brine for a month before being aged for up to two years in humid conditions.

pecorino is the generic Italian name for cheese made from sheep milk. It's a hard, white to pale yellow cheese, usually matured for eight to 12 months and known for the region in which it's produced – Romano from Rome, Sardo from Sardinia, Siciliano from Sicily and Toscano from Tuscany.

ricotta soft white cow milk cheese; roughly translates as 'cooked again'. It's made from whey, a by-product of other cheese making, to which fresh milk and acid are added. Ricotta is a sweet, moist cheese with a fat content of around 8.5% and a slightly grainy texture.

CHILLI available in many different types and sizes. Use rubber gloves when seeding and chopping fresh chillies as they can burn your skin. Removing seeds and membranes lessens the heat level.

flakes deep-red dehydrated extremely fine slices and whole seeds; good for cooking or for sprinkling over cooked food in the same way as salt and pepper.

green generally unripened thai chillies but sometimes different varieties that are ripe when green, such as habanero, poblano or serrano chillies.

thai, red small, medium hot, and bright red in colour.

CHOY SUM also known as pakaukeo or flowering cabbage, a member of the bok choy family; easy to identify with its long stems, light green leaves and yellow flowers. It is eaten, stems and all, steamed or stir-fried.

CIABATTA in Italian, the word means slipper, the traditional shape of this crisp-crusted white bread.

CINNAMON STICK dried inner bark of the shoots of the cinnamon tree. Also available in ground form.

CLOVE dried flower bud of a tropical tree; can be used whole or in ground form. Has a strong scent and taste so should be used sparingly.

COCONUT MILK not the juice found inside the fruit, which is known as coconut water, but the diluted liquid from the second pressing of the white meat of a mature coconut (the first pressing produces coconut cream). Available in cans and cartons from supermarkets.

COOKING-OIL SPRAY we used a cholesterol-free cooking spray made from canola oil.

COURGETTE the French name for zucchini, which is a small variety of marrow.

COUSCOUS a fine, grain-like cereal product, originally from North Africa; made from semolina.

CUMIN also known as zeera, available in ground or seed form; purchased from supermarkets.

CURLY ENDIVE also known as frisée, this is a curly-leafed green vegetable, mainly used in salads.

CURRY POWDER a blend of ground spices used when making Indian food. Can consist of some of the following spices in varying proportions: dried chilli, cinnamon, coriander, cumin, fennel, fenugreek, mace, cardamom and turmeric. Available in mild or hot varieties.

EGGS some recipes in this book call for raw or barely cooked eggs; exercise caution if there is a salmonella problem in your area.

FENNEL also known as finocchio or anise; eaten raw in salads or braised or fried as an accompaniment. Also the name given to dried seeds which have a licorice flavour.

FIVE-SPICE POWDER a fragrant mixture of ground cinnamon, cloves, star anise, sichuan pepper and fennel seeds.

GAI LARN also known as kanah, gai lum, chinese broccoli and chinese kale; appreciated more for its stems than its coarse leaves. Can be served steamed or stir-fried, in soups or noodle dishes.

GALANGAL also known as ka, a rhizome with a hot ginger-citrusy flavour; used similarly to ginger and garlic as a seasoning and as an ingredient. Sometimes known as thai, siamese or laos ginger, it also comes in a dried powdered form called laos. Fresh ginger can be substituted for fresh galangal but the flavour of the dish will not be the same.

GARAM MASALA a blend of spices, originating in North India; based on varying proportions of cardamom, cinnamon, cloves, coriander, fennel and cumin, roasted and ground together. Black pepper and chilli added give a hotter version.

GINGER also known as green or root ginger; the thick gnarled root of a tropical plant. Can be kept, peeled, covered with dry sherry, in a jar and refrigerated, or frozen in an airtight container.

GRANNY SMITH APPLES crisp, juicy apples with a rich green skin, which are not only good to eat, but are ideal for cooking, too. Granny smith apples originated in Sydney, first grown by Maria Anne Smith in 1867.

GRAVY BEEF boneless stewing beef which, when slow cooked, imbues stocks, soups and casseroles with a mild yet redolent flavour.

HERBS when specified, we used dried (not ground) herbs in the proportion of one to four for fresh herbs, eg, 1 teaspoon dried herbs equals 4 teaspoons (1 tablespoon) chopped fresh herbs.

basil used extensively in Italian dishes, it is one of the main ingredients in pesto.

chervil also known as cicily; mildly fennel-flavoured herb with curly dark-green leaves.

chives related to onions and leeks, with a subtle onion flavour. Garlic chives, also known as chinese chives, are strongly flavoured, have flat leaves and are eaten as a vegetable, usually in stir-fry dishes.

coriander also known as pak chee, cilantro or chinese parsley; green-leafed herb with a pungent flavour. Often stirred into, or sprinkled over, a dish just before serving for maximum impact. Both the stems and roots of coriander are also used in Thai cooking; wash well before chopping.

dill has soft, feathery sprigs; add to dishes at the end of cooking time as it will lose its flavour if overcooked.

oregano often used in Mediterranean cooking, it adds a sweet flavour to tomato sauces, meats and pizzas.

parsley, flat-leaf also known as continental or italian parsley.

sage pungent herb with narrow, grey-green leaves; slightly bitter with a musty mint aroma.

tarragon has a strong anise-like flavour, use sparingly.

Thai basil with purplish stems and smaller leaves than sweet basil, it has a slight licorice or aniseed taste and is one of the flavours that typify Thai cuisine.

thyme a basic herb of French cuisine, widely used in Mediterranean countries to flavour meats and sauces. Has tiny grey-green leaves that give off a pungent, mint, lemon aroma.

KAFFIR LIME LEAVES look like two glossy dark green leaves joined end to end, forming a rounded hourglass shape. Found fresh or dried in many Asian dishes, it is used like bay leaves or curry leaves, especially in Thai cooking. Sold fresh, dried or frozen, the dried leaves are less potent, so double the number called for in a recipe if you are using them instead of fresh leaves.

KECAP MANIS a dark, thick, sweet soy sauce used in South-East Asian cuisines. Depending on the brand, the soy's sweetness is derived from the addition of either molasses or palm sugar when brewed.

KIPFLER POTATO small and finger-shaped, with a nutty flavour; used baked and in salads.

KIWI FRUIT also known as chinese gooseberry.

LAVASH flat, unleavened bread of Mediterranean origin.

LEBANESE CUCUMBER short, slender and thin-skinned; also known as the european or burpless cucumber.

LEEK a member of the onion family; resembles the green onion but is much larger.

LEMON GRASS a tall, clumping, sharp-edged grass, smelling and tasting of lemon; the white lower part of the stem is used, finely chopped, in cooking.

MESCLUN is a salad mix of assorted young lettuce and other leaves, including baby spinach leaves, mizuna and curly endive.

MINCE MEAT also known as ground beef.

MIRIN is a Japanese champagne-coloured wine made of glutinous rice and alcohol expressly for cooking; seasoned sweet mirin is called manjo mirin and made of water, rice, corn syrup and alcohol.

MIXED SPICE a blend of ground spices usually consisting of cinnamon, allspice and nutmeg.

MUSHROOMS
button small, cultivated white mushrooms with a mild flavour.

shiitake when fresh are also known as chinese black, forest or golden oak mushrooms; although cultivated, have the earthiness and taste of wild mushrooms. Large and meaty; often used as a substitute for meat in Asian vegetarian dishes. When dried, are known as donko or dried chinese mushrooms; rehydrate before use.

swiss brown light to dark brown mushrooms with full-bodied flavour also known as roman or cremini. Button or cap mushrooms can be substituted.

MUSTARD
dijon a pale brown, distinctively flavoured mild French mustard.

wholegrain also known as seeded. A French-style coarse-grain mustard made from crushed mustard seeds and dijon-style French mustard.

NOODLES
bean thread made from extruded mung bean paste; also known as cellophane or glass noodles because they are transparent when cooked. White in colour (not off-white like rice vermicelli), very delicate and fine; available dried in various-sized bundles. Must be soaked to soften before use, but deep-frying requires no pre-soaking.

egg also known as ba mee or yellow noodles; made from wheat flour and eggs, and sold fresh or dried. Range in size from fine strands to wide, spaghetti-like pieces as thick as a shoelace.

fresh rice also known as ho fun, khao pun, sen yau, pho or kway tiau, depending on the country of manufacture. The most common form of noodles used in Thailand; can be purchased in various widths or large sheets weighing about 500g which are cut into the width of noodle desired. Chewy and pure white, they do not need pre-cooking before use.

rice stick popular South-East Asian dried rice noodles. Come in different widths – thin used in soups, wide in stir-fries – but all should be soaked in hot water until soft.

NUTMEG the dried nut of an evergreen tree native to Indonesia; it is available in ground form or you can grate it with a fine grater.

OIL

olive made from ripened olives. Extra virgin and virgin are the first and second presses, respectively, and are considered the best, while extra light and light are diluted and refer to taste, not fat levels.

peanut pressed from ground peanuts; most commonly used oil in Asian cooking because of its high smoke point (capacity to handle high heat without burning).

sesame made from roasted, crushed, white sesame seeds; a flavouring rather than a cooking medium.

vegetable any of a number of oils sourced from plants rather than animal fats.

ONION

green also known as scallion or (incorrectly) shallot; an immature onion, picked before the bulb has formed, with a long, bright-green edible stalk.

red also known as Spanish, red Spanish or Bermuda onion; a sweet-flavoured, large, purple-red onion.

PANCETTA an Italian bacon cured in spices and salt. Can be purchased from delicatessens.

PAPAYA also known as pawpaw, it's a large, pear-shaped, reddish orange tropical fruit; sometimes used unripe (green) in cooking.

PAPRIKA ground dried red capsicum; available sweet or hot.

PATTY-PAN SQUASH also known as crookneck or custard marrow pumpkin; a round, slightly flat summer squash that is yellow to pale green in colour with a scalloped edge. Harvested young, it has firm, white flesh and a distinctive flavour.

PEPPER also known as bell pepper or capsicum. Native to Central and South America, it can be red, green, yellow, orange or purplish black. Seeds and membranes should be discarded before use.

PINE NUT also known as pignoli; not in fact a nut but a small, cream-coloured kernel from pine cones.

PITTA also known as lebanese bread. This wheat-flour pocket bread is sold in large flat pieces that separate into two thin rounds. Also available in small thick pieces called pocket pitta.

POLENTA also known as cornmeal, this is a flour-like cereal made of dried corn (maize) sold ground in several different textures; also the name of the dish made from it.

PRAWNS also known as shrimp.

RICE

basmati a white, fragrant, long-grain rice. It should be washed several times before cooking.

jasmine fragrant long-grain rice; white rice can be substituted but it will not taste the same.

koshihikari small, round-grain white rice. Substitute white short-grain rice and cook by the absorption method.

long-grain elongated grain, remains separate when cooked; popular steaming rice in Asia.

risoni rice-shaped small pasta; very similar to orzo pasta.

ROCKET also known as arugula, rugula and rucola; a peppery green leaf which can be used similarly to baby spinach leaves, eaten raw in salad or used in cooking. Baby rocket leaves are both smaller and less peppery.

SAFFRON stigma of a member of the crocus family, available in strands or ground form; imparts a yellowish orange colour to food once infused. Quality varies greatly; the best is the most expensive spice in the world. Should be stored in the freezer.

SAKE Japan's favourite rice wine, is used in cooking, marinating and as part of dipping sauces. If unavailable, dry sherry, vermouth or brandy can be used as a substitute. When consumed as a drink, it is served warm; stand the container in hot water for about 20 minutes before serving.

SAUCES

black bean a Chinese sauce made from fermented soy beans, spices, water and wheat flour

fish called naam pla on the label if it is made in Thailand; the Vietnamese version, nuoc naam, is almost identical. Made from pulverised salted fermented fish (most often anchovies); it has a pungent smell and strong taste

oyster Asian in origin, this rich, brown sauce is made from oysters and their brine, cooked with salt and soy sauce, and thickened with starches.

soy also known as sieu, is made from fermented soy beans. Several variations are available.

sweet chilli a thin, mild Thai sauce made from red chillies, sugar, garlic and vinegar; used more as a a condiment.

teriyaki a homemade or commercially bottled sauce usually made from soy sauce, mirin, sugar, ginger and other spices; it imparts a distinctive glaze when brushed on grilled meat.

SESAME SEEDS black and white are the most common forms of this small oval seed, however, there are red and brown varieties also. A good source of calcium; used as an ingredient in cooking and as a condiment. To toast: spread seeds evenly on oven tray, toast in moderate oven briefly.

SHALLOTS also called French shallots, golden shallots or eschalots; small, elongated, brown-skinned members of the onion family. They grow in tight clusters in a similar way to garlic.

SOBA pale brown, thin, spaghetti-like noodle from Japan made from buckwheat and varying proportions of wheat flour.

SPINACH also known as English spinach and, incorrectly, silverbeet. Tender green leaves are good uncooked in salads or added to soups, stir-fries and stews just before serving.

STAR ANISE a dried star-shaped pod whose seeds have an astringent aniseed flavour; used to flavour stocks and marinades.

SUGAR use coarse, granulated table sugar, also known as crystal sugar, unless otherwise specified.

brown a soft, fine granulated sugar retaining molasses which give its colour and flavour.

caster also known as superfine or finely granulated table sugar.

palm also known as nam tan pip, jaggery, jawa or gula melaka; made from the sap of sugar cane and palm trees. Light brown to black in colour and usually sold in rock-hard cakes; substitute it with brown sugar if unavailable.

SUGAR SNAP PEA fresh small pea which can be eaten, whole, pod and all, similarly to snow peas and mange tout ('eat all').

TAMARIND CONCENTRATE (OR PASTE) the commercial result of the distillation of tamarind juice into a condensed, compacted paste. Thick and purplish black, it is ready-to-use, with no soaking or straining required; can be diluted with water according to taste. Use tamarind concentrate to add zing to sauces, chutneys, curries and marinades.

TOFU also known as bean curd, an off-white, custard-like product made from the 'milk' of crushed soy beans; comes fresh as soft or firm, and processed as fried or pressed dried sheets. Leftover fresh tofu can be refrigerated in water (which is changed daily) for up to four days.

firm tofu made by compressing bean curd to remove most of the water. Good in stir-fries because it can be tossed and not fall apart.

silken tofu refers to the manufacturing method of straining the soy bean liquid through silk.

TOMATOES

cherry also known as tiny tim or tom thumb tomatoes, these are small and round.

egg also called plum or roma, these are small, oval-shaped tomatoes used in Italian cooking or salads.

paste tomato puree that is triple concentrated and used to flavour soups, stews, sauces and casseroles.

semi-dried partially dried tomato pieces in olive oil; softer and juicier than sun-dried, these are not a preserve and do not keep as long as sun-dried.

teardrop small, yellow pear-shaped tomatoes.

TURKISH BREAD comes in long (about 45cm) flat loaves as well as individual rounds; made from wheat flour and sprinkled with sesame or black onion seeds.

TURMERIC also known as kamin, is a rhizome related to galangal and ginger, and must be grated or pounded to release its somewhat acrid aroma and pungent flavour. Known for the golden colour it imparts to the dishes of which it's a part, fresh turmeric can be substituted with the more common dried powder (use 2 teaspoons of ground turmeric plus a teaspoon of sugar for every 20g of fresh turmeric called for in a recipe).

VANILLA BEAN dried, long, thin pod from a tropical golden orchid grown in Central and South America and Tahiti; the minuscule black seeds inside the bean are used to impart a luscious vanilla flavour in baking and desserts.

VINEGAR

balsamic originally from Modena, Italy; there are now many balsamic vinegars on the market ranging in pungency and quality depending on how, and how long, they have been aged. Quality can be determined up to a point by price; use the most expensive sparingly.

red wine this vinegar is based on fermented red wine.

rice a colourless vinegar made from fermented rice and flavoured with sugar and salt. Also known as seasoned rice vinegar. Sherry can be substituted.

white vinegar made from spirit of cane sugar.

white wine vinegar made from white wine.

WATERCRESS a member of the cress family, a large group of peppery greens used raw in salads, dips and sandwiches, or cooked in soups. It is perishable, so use as soon as possible.

WINE the adage is that you should never cook with wine you wouldn't drink; in our recipes, we use good-quality dry white and red wines.

Chinese rice wine made from rice, wheat, sugar and salt, with 13.5% alcohol; available from Asian food stores. Mirin or sherry can be substituted.

FACTS & FIGURES

Wherever you live, you'll be able to use our recipes with the help of our easy-to-follow conversions. While these conversions are approximate only, the difference between an exact and the approximate conversion of various liquid and dry measures is minimal and will not affect your cooking results.

measuring equipment

The most accurate way of measuring dry ingredients is to weigh them. When measuring liquids, use a clear glass or plastic jug with the metric markings.

how to measure

When using graduated metric measuring cups, shake dry ingredients loosely into the appropriate cup. Do not tap the cup on a bench or tightly pack the ingredients unless directed to do so. Level top of measuring cups and measuring spoons with a knife. When measuring liquids, place a clear glass or plastic jug with metric markings on a flat surface to check the accuracy at eye level.

Note: Tablespoons are 15ml. All cup and spoon measurements are level. Use large eggs with an average weight of 60g.

DRY MEASURES

metric	imperial
15g	½oz
30g	1oz
60g	2oz
90g	3oz
125g	4oz (¼lb)
155g	5oz
185g	6oz
220g	7oz
250g	8oz (½lb)
280g	9oz
315g	10oz
345g	11oz
375g	12oz (¾lb)
410g	13oz
440g	14oz
470g	15oz
500g	16oz (1lb)
750g	24oz (1½lb)
1kg	32oz (2lb)

LIQUID MEASURES

metric	imperial
30ml	1 fluid oz
60ml	2 fluid oz
100ml	3 fluid oz
125ml	4 fluid oz
150ml	5 fluid oz (¼ pint/1 gill)
190ml	6 fluid oz
250ml	8 fluid oz
300ml	10 fluid oz (½ pint)
500ml	16 fluid oz
600ml	20 fluid oz (1 pint)
1000ml (1 litre)	1¾ pints

HELPFUL MEASURES

metric	imperial
3mm	⅛in
6mm	¼in
1cm	½in
2cm	¾in
2.5cm	1in
5cm	2in
6cm	2½in
8cm	3in
10cm	4in
13cm	5in
15cm	6in
18cm	7in
20cm	8in
23cm	9in
25cm	10in
28cm	11in
30cm	12in (1ft)

OVEN TEMPERATURES

These oven temperatures are only a guide. Always check the manufacturer's manual.

	°C (Celsius)	°F (Fahrenheit)	Gas mark
Very slow	120	250	½
Slow	140 – 150	275 – 300	1 – 2
Moderately slow	170	325	3
Moderate	180 – 190	350 – 375	4 – 5
Moderately hot	200	400	6
Hot	220 – 230	425 – 450	7 – 8
Very hot	240	475	9

GENERAL INDEX

RECIPE INDEX